IMMUNOGLOBULIN D:
STRUCTURE AND FUNCTION

Z - 861

FLUR 8ч3

ANNALS OF THE NEW YORK ACADEMY OF SCIENCES
Volume 399

IMMUNOGLOBULIN D: STRUCTURE AND FUNCTION

Edited by G. Jeanette Thorbecke and Gerrie A. Leslie

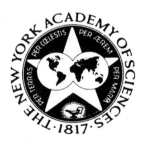

The New York Academy of Sciences
New York, New York
1982

Library of Congress Cataloging in Publication Data

Main entry under title:

Immunoglobulin D.

(Annals of the New York Academy of Sciences; v. 399)
"This series of papers is the result of a conference . . . held 13–15 January 1982, by the New York Academy of Sciences"—
    Bibliography: p.
    Includes index.
    1. Immunoglobulin D—Congresses. I. Thorbecke, G. Jeanette. II. Leslie, Gerrie A. III. New York Academy of Sciences. IV. Series. [DNLM: 1. IGD—Congresses. W1 AN626YL v. 399 / QW 601 I324 1982]
Q11.N5 vol. 399 [QR186.8.D2]   500s   82-18984
ISBN 0-89766-188-5   [599'.0293]
ISBN 0-89766-189-3 (pbk.)

SP
Printed in the United States of America
ISBN-0-89766-188-5 (cloth)
ISBN-0-89766-189-3 (paper)

ANNALS OF THE NEW YORK ACADEMY OF SCIENCES
VOLUME 399
December 6, 1982

IMMUNOGLOBULIN D: STRUCTURE AND FUNCTION*

Editors and Conference Chairs
G. JEANETTE THORBECKE and GERRIE A. LESLIE

———————◆———————

CONTENTS

*This series of papers is the result of a conference entitled Immunoglobulin D: Structure and Function, held 13–15 January, 1982, by The New York Academy of Sciences.

Financial assistance was received from:
- E.I. DU PONT DE NEMOURS & COMPANY
- MERCK SHARP & DOHME RESEARCH LABORATORIES
- NATIONAL CANCER INSTITUTE, NATIONAL INSTITUTES OF HEALTH
- NATIONAL INSTITUTE OF ALLERGY AND INFECTIOUS DISEASES, NATIONAL INSTITUTES OF HEALTH
- NATIONAL SCIENCE FOUNDATION
- OFFICE OF NAVAL RESEARCH
- WYETH LABORATORIES

INTRODUCTORY REMARKS

Gerrie A. Leslie

Department of Microbiology and Immunology
Oregon Health Sciences University
Portland, Oregon 97201

Firstly I'd like, on behalf of Dr. Jeanette Thorbecke and myself, to welcome you to this meeting, the first ever dedicated strictly to trying to understand what IgD does. We all like to think that it does something important and I'm sure we're going to get some new insights. We hope to get some "sparks flying" and generate some new ideas and by the end of the conference know more than we did before we got here.

I'd like to thank The New York Academy of Sciences for their willingness to sponsor this meeting and for the outstanding cooperation that we have had from the staff of The New York Academy. The weather is a little bit different than when Dr. Thorbecke and I sat down to think about whether we really could get a conference together on IgD—that happened to be in Paris—but neither she nor I are responsible for the weather. It is significant to me that this first meeting strictly devoted to IgD is being held in New York City, because when I became actively interested in IgD I happened to get six years of support from the John A. Hartford Foundation, from New York, and I wish they were still in the business of supporting individual researchers.

Those of you who have been working with IgD for quite some time know that it's only recently that many people paid any attention to IgD. When I first got interested in IgD, I tried to get my clinical colleagues to send interesting sera to me. I wanted to show that serum IgD was a legitimate antibody. The old story would be, well, you tell me what it does and I'll get you the samples. My response was, "Well, if you don't get me the samples, how are we ever going to find out what it does?"

It's nice to see Dr. David Rowe in the audience. David is, in many ways, the one responsible for discovering this creature, IgD. It was a cold January 1st, 1964, that, in collaboration with Dr. John Fahey at National Institutes of Health, he put together the information that said, "Hey, we've got a new immunoglobulin here." I didn't ask him why he called it IgD, probably because I often get asked, due to work that I have done on lower vertebrates, why do I call IgG, IgY? It sort of escapes me now why that particular nomenclature was used but I assure you it made great sense at the time.

The original studies on IgD focused their attention on its presence in the serum of humans. Many scientists tried to show antibody activity associated with IgD. In the first paper that I published on IgD with Drs. Rowe and Clem, we suggested, based on physical chemical properties of the delta chain, that there would be an extra homology region associated with this chain and we predicted unusual biological characteristics of IgD. It appears that we were wrong in terms of the extra homology region (an extended hinge would account for our error), but I still think that we are going to find some interesting biological characteristics associated with IgD. David and John's first two papers on IgD were published in the *Journal of Experimental Medicine* in 1965. As a graduate student I must say that they were in fact the first two immunology papers that I ever received as a result of my "exposure" to *Current Contents*.

It was also David and his collaborators who gave IgD that extra "boost in the arm," which made it respectable in the sense of showing its possible importance as a B-lymphocyte receptor. It is now clear that IgD is a predominant isotype on the surface of most B-cells. Many of the papers presented at this meeting will focus on this point. A major question is, however, does surface IgM and IgD interaction with ligand deliver different "signals" to the B-cell? In 1977 a graduate student in my laboratory, John Ruddick, suggested that the valence of membrane IgM may be different from membrane IgD and that the interactions of these isotypes with identical antigens may deliver different signals to the B-cells. This is an important concept that will be discussed further, I'm sure.

The studies that have been published from my laboratory, as well as those from others, strongly suggest that IgD can be a humoral antibody, especially in autoimmune diseases and situations of chronic antigen exposure. I suggest that animal models of autoimmunity and carcinogenesis be carefully evaluated for IgD antibodies. Furthermore, IgD as a secretory immunoglobulin should be further investigated.

I hope that during this meeting we are going to hear many new ideas and variations on themes that we thought about or heard before. Let's keep an open mind on such questions as: Is IgD a legitimate serum antibody? What is its role as an antigen receptor on the surface of the B-cell? Does IgD play an important immunoregulatory role? Is it a blocking antibody? I think we are going to see that in most animal systems there is very little serum IgD. Why? I personally hope that someone will give us information that says IgD is a respectable humoral antibody as well as a B-cell antigen receptor.

GENETIC ASPECTS OF IgD EXPRESSION:
I. ANALYSIS OF THE Cμ-Cδ COMPLEX IN COMMITTED AND UNCOMMITTED DNA

F. R. Blattner,* J. E. Richards,* A. Shen,* M. Knapp,† S. Strober,†
A. C. Gilliam,‡ S. Jones,‡ H.-L. Cheng,‡ J. F. Mushinski,§
and P. W. Tucker‡

*Department of Genetics
University of Wisconsin
Madison, Wisconsin 53706

†Department of Medicine
University of Stanford Medical School
Stanford, California 94305

‡Department of Microbiology
University of Texas Southwestern Medical School
Dallas, Texas 75235

§Department of Cell Biology
National Cancer Institute
Bethesda, Maryland 20205

INTRODUCTION

Most of the available knowledge concerning the organization and structure of immunoglobulin genes has come from the use of recombinant DNA techniques to compare DNA from cells either committed (e.g., B-lymphocytes and plasma cells) or noncommitted (e.g., liver, embryo and sperm tissue) to Ig expression. In germline DNA, these approaches have shown that the heavy (H) chain locus is comprised of variable segment (V) genes,[1,2] short D segments,[3] four J_H segments,[4,5] and eight tandemly arranged constant region (C_H) genes corresponding to Ig class.[6] By the time the B-cell has reached the terminally differentiated state of the plasmacytoma, two types of DNA rearrangements can occur.[5,7,8] The first involves the translocation of one V_H segment and one D segment from their respective pools of several hundred to the immediate 5′ side of one of the J_H genes to produce an intact gene for the variable region. This joining event is mediated by homologous recombination and site-specific deletion in a manner analogous to integration and excision of virus and transposons.[9] VDJ joining occurs very early in B-cell development, presumedly at the pre-B cell level. This event commits that clone to expression of a given variable region by initially forming a functional transcriptional unit including the most 5′ C_H gene, Cμ. The actual joining of the VDJ complex to Cμ is accomplished at the RNA level by removal of the approximately 8 kilobase pairs (Kbp) of intervening RNA sequence from the precursor transcript.

The second DNA rearrangement concerns the mechanism of the switch recombination whereby the same VDJ can be expressed with C_H genes other than Cμ. The rearrangement in plasmacytomas is associated with deletion of all C_H genes 5′ to the expressed C_H gene on the allelic chromosome.[2,6,10–12] Switching appears to be mediated by homologous recombination between short, repeated

1

0077-8923/82/0399-0001$01.75/0 © 1982, NYAS

DNA sequences located a few Kbp 5' to the C_H genes. It is unclear at what stage in B-cell development the class switch gene rearrangement occurs.

Dual and continued expression of more than one C_H gene presents a significant contradiction to the deletion model. The majority of virgin B-cells bear both IgM and IgD on their cell surface. Moreover, the expression of Igs by memory B-cells is complex in that the majority of cells bear two Ig classes on their surface including combinations other than IgM and IgD.[13,14] Although B-cells express surface IgM and IgD about equally,[15] the level of secretory IgD in plasma is some 1000-fold lower than IgM.[16] Rare populations of normal plasma cells[17] and plasmacytomas[18] secrete IgD in the absence of detectable IgM expression. This suggests that different mechanisms might be involved when IgD is expressed alone than when expressed simultaneously with IgM.

We have studied the molecular genetics of IgD expression in mouse DNA derived from the three appropriate tissue types discussed above. We have shown[19] that in uncommitted DNA, the $C\mu$ and $C\delta$ genes are separated by a short intervening sequence of only about 2.3 kbp. Since this is much closer together than any of the other C_H genes, their proximity may be a key factor in their dual expression. We have recently extended this analysis[20,21] to a cell line (BCL$_1$) which shows many of the characteristics of a mature virgin B-cell[22] and which is committed to simultaneous expression of both IgM and IgD on its surface.[23] These studies show that the germ line arrangement of the $C\mu$ and $C\delta$ genes are preserved in the dual expressing cell with no concomitant DNA rearrangement other than VDJ joining. And finally, we have analyzed the DNA from two plasmacytomas, TEPC 1017 and 1033[18] that are committed to IgD secretion without expression of IgM. In these highly differentiated cells the germline arrangement of the $C\delta$ gene has been rearranged with concomitant deletion of $C\mu$ alleles in the majority of their aneuploid chromosomes in a manner akin to the Honjo deletion model.[6]

In this communication, we will review these studies carried out at the DNA level and will present recent nucleotide sequence determined between and flanking the $C\mu$ and $C\delta$ genes that might be involved in regulatory events. In the second paper, we present our progress to date toward understanding the complex transcription of the $C\delta$ gene. In the final paper, we deal with the functional implications of the δ chain protein as indicated from the nucleotide sequence and gene organization.

Organization of $C\mu$-$C\delta$ Locus in Germline DNA

A first step toward understanding the molecular mechanism of δ and μ chain expression has been determination of the organization of the $C\delta$ gene and its relationship to the $C\mu$ gene and J_H gene cluster in germline DNA. A summary of our results obtained from the molecular cloning of these DNA segments is given in FIGURE 1. The J_H cluster which encodes the carboxyl end of the V_H chains is located approximately 8 Kbp 5' to the four constant region exons of the $C\mu$ gene.[4,5] Exons shown by Rogers et al.[24] and Early et al.[25] to encode the membrane (m) terminus of μ chains are located about 1.8 Kbp 3' to $C\mu4$ of which the 3' end encodes the altenative secreted (s) carboxyl terminus. To our surprise we found[19] that the three exons constituting the constant region of the $C\delta$ gene were located only about two Kbp downstream (3') (e.g., the distance between $\mu M2$ and $C\delta1$). Later Moore et al.[26] and Maki et al.[27] confirmed these results using restriction mapping and electron micrographic approaches. More recently we have estab-

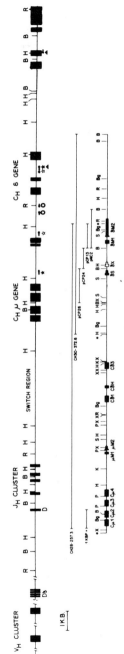

FIGURE 1. Physical map of the C_μ-$C\delta$ germline locus. The upper portion shows the J cluster, C_μ and $C\delta$ genes and their respective membrane exons drawn to scale. The V_H cluster. The V_H cluster and D segments are separated from J_H by an unknown distance except for the most rightward D. Sets of repeating DNA sequences are indicated under the map by arrows (denoting their location and 5' → 3' orientation) and their content: the identical symbols representing identical sequences (cf. text for details). The lower portion of the figure presents a more detailed map of the C_μ and $C\delta$ region. Exons are always denoted by boxes, with the lowered portion representing 3' untranslated regions. Recombinant DNA clones used to derive the map are shown above as arrows, where CH refers to the Charon 28 bacteriophage cloning vector, and PCP to subclones in pBR322. Restriction sites are abbreviated as follows: R, Eco RI; B, Bam HI; H, Hind III; X, Xba I; Bg, Bgl II; P, Pst I; S, Sph I; *, Mbo I.

lished the exact spacing by determining the complete nucleotide sequence between Cμ and Cδ (discussed below). This short distance suggested to us[19,28] and others[26,27] a model for dual expression of Cμ and Cδ. A manageable transcript containing one V_H region (VDJ) and both Cμ and Cδ regions could be spliced in several ways to yield mRNA for μ or δ chains in M, S, and possible other forms.

Electron micrographic data of Maki et al.[27] and our recent nucleotide sequence and mapping results[28-30] have established the topology of the exons encoding the alternative S and M carboxyl termini of the δ chain. Unlike the case in μ, the δs terminus is encoded some 4.7 Kbp distal to the terminal constant region domain (Cδ3). The δm terminus is coded by two exons, δM1 and δM2, located approximately 1.5 Kbp further downstream. We have also detected a region of DNA between the δS and δM exons that we term δX since its function and expression remain at this time a mystery. A detailed discussion of the alternative expression of secreted and membrane forms of δ chain is presented in the subsequent papers.

Unusual Repeating Sequences in the Cμ-Cδ Region of Germline DNA

We have identified several clusters of unusual DNA sequences within and flanking the Cμ-Cδ region that might influence expression of these genes. Two such sets were first revealed on examination in the electron microscope of a Cμ-Cδ bacteriophage clone which was denatured then allowed to reanneal slowly on the EM grids. The pair of secondary structures formed (FIGURE 2) are due to inverted repeat sequences whose location relative to the genomic map are indicated in FIGURE 1. The small, inner stem is produced by pairing of two sequences within the intervening DNA between Cμ and Cδ. The outer stem, which loops out a considerable portion of Cδ, is provided by a sequence some 200 bp 3' to the μM2 exon pairing with its inverse complement located in the large intron between the CδH and Cδ3 exons.

To analyze these structures in detail we determined the complete nucleotide sequence of the Cμ-Cδ intron (2275 bp) and the intron between CδH and Cδ3 (990 bp). The relationship between the two repeat structures and the palindromes observed in the EM are shown in FIGURE 3. The most 5' arm of the outer stem structure (indicated in FIGURE 1 by *). It has two distinct components: A tandem duplication of the type $(GGGAGA)_{12}$, which constitutes a series of Mn1 I restriction endonuclease sites and a second tandem repeat of the type $(AG)_{28}$. The stem results from annealing of the $(AG)_{28}$ portion to its exact inverted complement (CT_{30}) located between CδH and Cδ3. The inner secondary structure (denoted in FIGURE 1 by *) results from a small stem (85 bp)-loop (287 bp) structure with nearly perfect pairing. The sequence of this inner structure is complex and contains no repetitive regions.

DNA sequencing has revealed two additional sets of sequence, whose locations are indicated in FIGURES 1 and 3. Both of these are related to the stem of the outer loop. The most 5', in the intron between Cμ4 and μM1, is a tandem repeat of the type $(CA)_{33}$ which is directly duplicated in the CδH-Cδ3 intron as $(CA)_{30}$. Far 3', within the CδX exonic region (FIGURE 1), there is a tandem repeat $(GA)_{16}$ followed shortly by $(AT)_5(GT)_6$. Two longer forms of the GA repeat have been discussed above and occur in both direct and inverse-complementary orientation relative to this sequence. Although the appropriate clone has not been tested, one would predict that a secondary structure of the "outer" type above

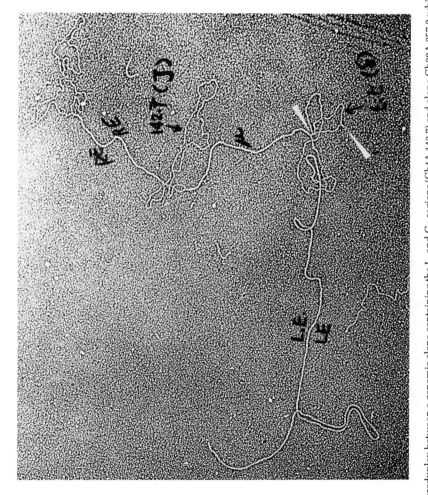

FIGURE 2. Heteroduplex between a genomic clone containing the J_H and $C\mu$ regions (Ch4A 142.7) and clone Ch28A 257.3 which contains the $C\mu$ and $C\delta$ locus. The regions common to both clones ($C\mu$ and $C\mu$–$C\delta$ intron up to the Eco RI site noted in FIGURE 1) form a contiguous duplex structure. Regions corresponding to the J_H cluster and $C\delta$ form the single-stranded segments. The inverted repeats around the $C\delta$ gene are denoted by the white arrows, and left and right vector arms are denoted by LA and RA, respectively.

could also be formed between the CδX exon and Cδ hinge intron repeats. The cartoon of FIGURE 3 illustrates how both outer structures could be formed simultaneously. The function of these outer stem-loops may be the establishment of secondary structure in δ mRNA. For example, the resulting configuration of the CδX-hinge intron stem, which places the CδS terminal exon in a loop, may influence the splicing efficiency of secreted δ chain mRNA in normal B-cells since expression of the secreted protein is exceedingly low.

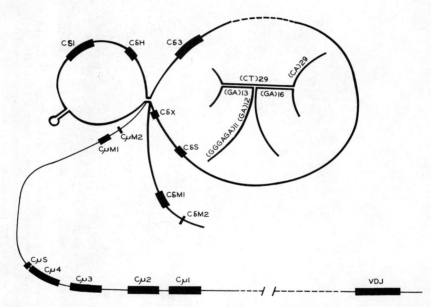

FIGURE 3. Possible secondary structures present in a Cμ-Cδ transcript. A schematic representation of pairing of both GA sequence repeats with the inverse complement present in the intron between CδH and Cδ3. DNA sequence has been determined for the entire 30 kbp region (the VDJ region corresponding to that of BCL₁) except for the portion denoted by broken lines. The drawing is approximately to scale except where indicated by double slashes. DNA sequences (*) that participate in the hypothetical pairing are emphasized by the inset in the large loop.

Tumor Cells as Models of B-Cell Expression

The use of tumors arising from the B-cell lineage for studies at the nucleic acid level has made it possible to analyze gene arrangements and rearrangements at different stages of B-cell development. This approach is based on the assumption that such tumors can serve as models of the normal situation. In our studies we have used the B lymphoma BCL₁ to represent a virgin B-cell committed to dual expression of IgM and IgD on the cell surface. To model a plasma cell secreting IgD, we have used the plasmacytomas (myelomas) TEPC 1017 and TEPC 1033.

Analysis of BCL₁ DNA as a Model for Mature Virgin B-Cell DNA

The BCL_1 tumor arose spontaneously in a BALB/c mouse and grows predominantly in the spleen with subsequent spread to the blood.[22] This lymphoma maintains many of the characteristics of splenic small lymphocytes including dual expression of IgM and IgD on virtually all cells as measured by the cell sorter.[22,23] The cells also retain the ability to secrete IgM after stimulation with lipopolysaccharide.[23] In studies in which surface proteins were labeled with ^{125}I, immunoprecipitated with anti-λ, anti-μ, and anti-δ antisera, and separated on polyacrylamide gels, both μ and δ chains were found to be present.[20] The amount of δ was much lower than the amount of μ however. Incubation of the labeled proteins with an anti-idiotypic reagent derived from rats showed that both μ and δ chains from the cloned line share idiotypic determinants, and suggests that the chains have a common variable region. BCL_1 cells are diploid and have only one copy of the H chain bearing chromosome 12.[20]

All C_H Genes in BCL₁ DNA Are in the Germline Arrangement and Share a Single V_H Gene

A detailed examination of genes expressed in BCL_1 was carried out in three ways. First, the variable region being expressed by the tumor was thoroughly characterized, cloned, and sequenced both at the DNA level (FIGURE 4) and partially from an RNA clone. This DNA sequence was further confirmed by comparison with the amino acid sequence of the first 22 residues of the purified μ chain secreted from a hybridoma BCL.F2/8 made from BCL_1 (D. Capra, unpublished results). The protein sequence predicted is clearly that of a variable region of V_H subgroup II (31) and uses $J_H 2$. As indicated in FIGURE 4, the sequence is very similar to that of the MOPC 104E μ chain (~75% match), although different J_H and D segments are used. Like other V_H and V_L sequences reported,[32,33] the $BCL_1 V_H$ has a 20 amino acid leader peptide segment interrupted by an 82 bp intron.

Determination of the genomic location of this V_H gene in BCL_1 DNA through Southern blot analysis was facilitated by the existence of *Pst* I and *Xba* I restriction sites (FIGURE 4) within the V_H gene. We thus compared DNA digests with these enzymes of genomic DNA and genomic DNA clones by subsequent hybridization to $J_H 2$, Cμ, and Cδ probes. The patterns observed established that the VDJ complex in the cloned DNA occupies the same position in the BCL_1 genome and that there is only one copy of VDJ complex in the BCL_1 genome.

The relationship of the VDJ complex to Cμ in BCL_1 and germline DNA was also determined using *Kpn* I digestion, which is known to produce a single fragment in the germline that contains both Cμ and the entire J_H cluster. Each DNA when probed for Cμ and $J_H 2$ sequences contained a single band to which both probes hybridized. This band measured 15.7 kbp in BCL_1 DNA and 14.7 kbp in the germline. These analyses thus showed that there is a single copy of the Cμ gene in BCL_1 DNA and that it is located on the 3′ side of the VDJ complex we have sequenced.

The next question was whether the C_H gene also uses this copy of the VDJ complex or whether a second copy of VDJ might be present between Cμ and Cδ. We thus compared the organization of the Cμ, Cδ, and other C_H genes in BCL_1 DNA and germline DNA by Southern blotting and hybridization with the C_H probes (FIGURE 5). Using the established germline map (FIGURE 1) as a guide, we

```
CCCTGTCTCATGAATATGCAAATCAGGTGAGTCTATGGTGGTAAATATAGGGATATCTACACACCTCAAAAACTTAAGATCACAGTAGTCTCTACAGTCA
---------+---------+---------:+---------+---------+---------+---------+---------+---------+---------+

CAGGAGTACACAGGGCATTGCCATGGGTTGGAGCTGTATCATCTTCTTTCTGGTAGCAACAGCTACAGGTAAGGGGCTCACAGTAGTTTGTTTGAGGTCT
---------+---------+---------+---------+---------+---------+---------+---------+---------+---------+
PEPTIDE LEADER:      M  G  W  S  C  I  I  F  F  L  V  A  T  A  T  G
```

```
                                                                    PST1
GGCAATACACTTAGGTGACAATGATATCCACTCTGTCCTTCCCTTCACAGGTGTGCACTCCCAGGTTCAGCTGCAGCAGTCTGGGCCTGAGGTGGTGAGG
---------+---------+---------+---------+---------+---------+---------+---------+---------+---------+
            V REGION OF BCL1:              V  H  S  Q  V  Q  L  Q  Q  S  G  P  E  V  V  R
            V REGION OF M104E:                E                                L        K
                                              1                             10
```

```
                                                                              XBA1
CCTGGGGTCTCAGTGAAGATTTCCTGCAAGGGGTTCCGGCTACACATTCACTGATTATGCTATGCACTGGGTGAAGCAGAGTCATGCAAAGAGTCTAGAGT
---------+---------+---------+---------+---------+---------+---------+---------+---------+---------+
P  G  V  S  V  K  I  S  C  K  G  S  G  Y  T  F  T  D  Y  A  M  H  W  V  K  Q  S  H  A  K  S  L  E  W
   A           M           A                 Y     K                       G
   20                      30                            40
```

```
GGATTGGAGTTATTAGTACTTACAATGGTAATACGAGCTACAACCAGAAGTTTAAGGGCAAGGCCACAATGACTGTAGACAAATCCTCCAGCACAGTCCA
---------+---------+---------+---------+---------+---------+---------+---------+---------+---------+
 I  G  V  I  S  T  Y  N  G  N  T  S  Y  N  Q  K  F  K  G  K  A  T  M  T  V  D  K  S  S  S  T  V  H
    D        N  P  N        G                             L                                  A  Y
    50                      60                            70                                 80
```

```
TATGGAACTTGCCAGATTGACATCTGAGGATTCTGCCAATCTATACTGTGCAAGATACTATGGTAACTACTTTGACTACTGGGGCCAAGGCACCACTCTC
---------+---------+---------+---------+---------+---------+---------+---------+---------+---------+
M  E  L  A  R  L  T  S  E  D  S  A  N  L  Y  C  A  R  Y  Y  G  N  Y  F  D  Y  W  G  Q  G  T  T  L
Q     N  S              V  Y              D     D  W           V        A        V
            90                      100                          110
```

```
ACAGTCTCCTCAGGTGAGTCCTTACAACCTCTCTCTTCTATTCAGCTTAAATAGATTTTACTGCATTTGTTGGGGGGGAAATGTGTGTATCTGAATTTCA
---------+---------+---------+---------+---------+---------+---------+---------+---------+---------+
T  V  S  S  R
         118
```

FIGURE 4. Nucleotide sequence of the BCL$_1$ VDJ$_2$ complex and flanking DNA from clone CH28-289.1. The predicted amino acid sequence is shown below. Below these are substitutions found in the variable region of the μ chain of MOPC 104E. The positions of two useful enzyme sites are indicated above the DNA sequence.

selected enzymes which should sensitively reveal rearrangements in sequences flanking C$_H$ genes. In the case of Cμ and Cδ, we also compared restriction maps in the regions of interest between BCL$_1$ and liver recombinant phage clones (FIGURE 6). In all cases, the fragments generated were identical in both BCL$_1$ and germline DNA. Thus, the context of Cμ, Cδ and the other C$_H$ genes examined (Cγ_3, Cγ_1, Cγ_{2b}, and Cα) are identical in BCL$_1$ and germline, proving that these genes are not

A

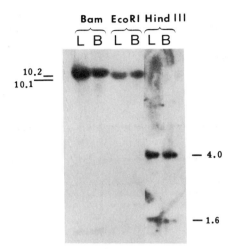

Probe: pδ54 (δcDNA)

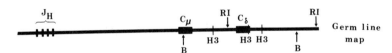

B

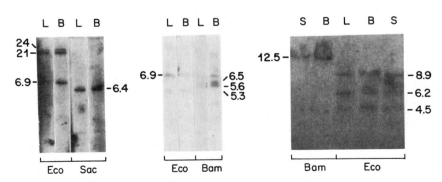

FIGURES 5A & 5B. Comparisons of the genomic contexts of the Cδ and other C_H genes in BCL₁ (B) and BALB/c liver (L) DNA by Southern blot analysis. DNA was digested with the indicated enzymes and probed with appropriate cDNA plasmids. **(A)** Cδ context, **(B)** Cγ3, Cγ2b, and Cα context. In all cases, identity of germline and BCL₁ bands are observed.

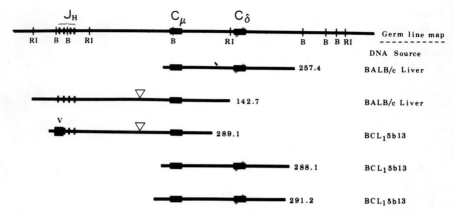

FIGURE 6. Schematic representations of VDJ, Cμ and Cδ genomic clones isolated from BCL$_1$ DNA. Restriction maps were constructed by comparison to germline Cμ and Cμ-Cδ.[19] The maps are identical to the right of the VDJ$_2$ complex.

rearranged in the tumor and that no copy of the BCL$_1$ VDJ complex has been inserted upstream of the Cδ gene. Recent studies of Maki et al.[27] using a mouse-guinea pig hybrid cell GCL2.8 and electron microscopic approaches have arrived at essentially identical conclusions regarding the germline configuration of the J$_H$-Cμ-Cδ locus in virgin B-cells.

Analysis of DNA of TEPC 1017 and TEPC 1033 as a Model for Secretory IgD

The TEPC tumors were obtained by Potter after induction of BALB/c mice with 2-pristane and for some years they existed in his collection of myelomas classified as secreting no known class of Ig. With the availability of anti-δ serum they were characterized as IgD secreters by Finkelman et al.[18] These tumors bear small amounts of IgD on the cell surface in addition to secreting enormous quantities of it as K$_2\delta_2$. TEPC 1017 mRNA clones provided the starting point for the nucleic acid level analysis of murine IgD, but the gene arrangement in these cells has not been extensively characterized at the DNA level.

To study the gene arrangement in this secretory cell we have used Southern hybridization analysis (FIGURE 7) to compare the arrangements of the Cδ gene in DNA from liver and from TEPC 1017 and TEPC 1033. The results indeed show that a deletion involving the Cμ gene is present in the tumors. As shown in FIGURE 7, TEPC 1017 contains most of its Cδ sequences on a 3.3 Kbp Hind III fragment and TEPC 1033 contains Cδ on a larger 4.6 Kbp fragment. Both are different from the germline size of 4.0 Kbp. Densitometric scanning of autoradiographs showed that both tumors in addition, have about 25% of their δ hybridizing DNA in the 4.0 Kbp form seen in the liver. The fact that both tumors are pseudotetraploid (G. Klein and S. Ohno, personal communication) suggests that one of the four chromosomes remains unrearranged while the other three have undergone a rearrangement resulting in removal of the Hind III site located 2 Kbp to the left of Cδ1 (see germline map). On the other hand, Cδ genes in liver and both tumors are contained on a single *Eco* RI fragment of 9.8 Kbp. This data is consistent with a relocation of different VDJ complexes 5' to the Cδ1 domain, between the *Hind* III site 2.0 Kbp 5' to Cδ1 and the *Eco* RI site 0.5 kbp 5' to Cδ1. When the Southern transfer was reprobed for Cμ, only a very faint germline signal was detected (data not shown). No IgM has been detected on the surface of or within these plasmacytoma cells (F. D. Finkelman, personal communication), and no μ chain mRNA has been identified in these cells (data not shown). These observations collectively suggest that the majority of Cμ alleles in these tumors have been deleted and the remaining, unrearranged Cμ allele is not expressed. Interpretations of Southern blots are clearly limited since some rearrangements observed might be abortive in nature. Molecular cloning of the TEPC genomes will be required to determine if more complex DNA translocations occur.

Dual Expression of IgM and IgD Probably Requires Alternative Processing of μδ Transcript

The maintenance of a surface IgM and IgD phenotype on all cells of the cloned BCL_1 cell line for many generations argues that both IgM and IgD must be actively expressed from the single copy of chromosome 12 that is present in the cells. Since only one copy of the VDJ_H, Cμ, and Cδ genes is present in the BCL_1 genome and there is no translocation of a copy of the VDJ complex to a position

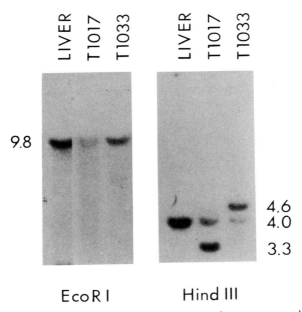

FIGURE 7. Southern blot analysis of the Cδ context in IgD plasmacytoma and BALB/c liver DNA. Liver, TEPC 1017, and TEPC 1033 DNAs were digested with the enzymes indicated and hybridized to a Cδ cDNA probe. The nonidentity in the Hind III bands indicates that tumor DNA has rearranged its Cδ locus.

between the $C\mu$ and $C\delta$ genes, we have concluded that δ chains are translated from mRNA which is derived by processing of a primary transcript which originally included sequences from both $C\mu$ and $C\delta$ genes.

A molecular model for alternative RNA processing of this sort, first proposed for the expression of the late genes of adenovirus,[34] has also been suggested[24,25,35] as applicable in the case of membrane vs secreted expression of IgM. It is now clear from our DNA sequencing data[19,29] that the proposed primary transcript, which would contain approximately 30 Kbp of RNA, has six polyadenylation recognition sites. These are located in the expected positions in the 3' untranslated regions of $C\mu4$ ($\equiv\mu S$), $\mu m2$, δS, and δ_x. Two poly (A) sites are located in the $\delta M2$ 3' untranslated region. Cleavage of the transcript at any one of the sites followed by poly(A) addition would result in production of six mRNA precursors that are subsequently spliced to yield mature μ and δ mRNAs. The control of this event must be developmentally linked since expression of membrane forms gives way to expression of secreted forms on B-cell triggering. Further, there is clearly a preference for certain sites since expression of the large δm transcript is highly favored over the smaller δm RNA (cf. following paper and refs. 29 and 30).

A major problem confronting this model is its requirement for skipping perfectly legitimate RNA splicing sites. For example, if δ mRNA is to be expressed, the splice from VDJ to $C\delta1$ must skip all acceptor sites in $C\mu$ that occur 5' to $C\delta1$. Here the influence of secondary structures of the type we discussed above may be crucial in establishing where to splice. Different donor and acceptor pairs may have varying strengths of association, but this alone cannot explain the switch that occurs on triggering. Selection of splice sites is precise in the $\mu\delta$ transcript so that exons of $C\mu$ are never reassorted with exons of $C\delta$, yet the alternative carboxyl terminal structures of either chain can be simultaneously expressed or shifted in response to cellular signals. An intriguing observation related to this fact is the phasing of RNA splicing in relation to translation. In both μ and δ, the splice from the M1 to M2 exon occurs in exact codon register. This is in contrast to all other splicings known in Ig mRNAs where the splice occurs after the first base of the codon register. The use of a different phasing relationship for the cytoplasmic side of the membrane may create a "barrier" for reassortment of interior with exterior domains, since this splicing would create problems of translational reading frame.

Secretion of IgD by Myelomas Involves DNA Rearrangement

Evidence reported here for TEPC 1017 and 1033 agrees with that of Moore et al.[26] and Maki et al.[27] and suggests that expression of IgD is the plasmacytomas is mediated by a DNA rearrangement 5' to the $C\delta$ locus with concomitant deletion of $C\mu$. This rearrangement is generally consistent, at the resolution so far analyzed, to the switch recombination observed for γ and α chain expression (reviewed in ref. 2). However, a major difference appears to be the nature of the switch sequences (S) used for the proposed $S\mu:S\delta$ recombination. Blocks of short DNA sequences GAGCT and GGGGT are a large portion of the $S\mu$ repetitive region and are thought to facilitate switch recombination.[36] The switch recombination sites of rearranged $C\gamma$ and $C\alpha$ genes also show a high degree of preference for the sequence AGGTTG 5' to either the $S\mu$ donor or the appropriate C_H S acceptor site.[37] Analysis of the $C\mu$-$C\delta$ intronic DNA sequence reveals no sequences homologous to either of these repeats. Furthermore, a cloned probe constructed from a Hind III-Hind III fragment that spans the $S\mu$ region does not hybridize to any region between $C\mu$ and $C\delta$ but does hybridize with variable strength to the appropriate S region fragments of $C\alpha$ and $C\gamma3$. The most likely candidate for a $S\delta$ site would appear to be the region of the GGGAGA repeat. We are currently analyzing genomic clones of TEPC 1017 and 1033 DNA in hopes of unraveling this mystery.

It is tempting to extrapolate that these results obtained from IgD myelomas are relevant to biological secretion of IgD. However, the evidence for normal IgD secreting plasma cells, other than in extremely old animals,[17] is not convincing. In fact, the unusual distal locations of the exon that codes for the δ secreted terminus (FIGURE 1) has suggested to us[29] that IgD may be secreted from B-cells whose $C\delta$ locus has not been rearranged. This proposal is justified in the third paper of this series.

A Combination of Both DNA Deletion and Alternative RNA Processing to Explain Other Double Producers

The simultaneous expression of at least two Ig classes on the surface of B-lymphocytes, including combinations other than IgM and IgD, has been reported by several investigators.[13,14] The BCL_1 model shows that IgM and IgD expression can occur by having two proximate C_H genes share a single V_H gene. It is not clear whether this is a special mechanism which is used by B-lymphocytes to express only the IgM and IgD combination, or whether this is a general mechanism by which nonsecreting lymphocytes can express other combinations of Ig classes simultaneously on the cell surface. It is conceivable that other C_H genes might be translocated to a position near the $C\mu$ gene by a deletional switch recombination mechanism while preserving the $C\delta$ gene context or, more probably, might replace the $C\delta$ gene. This later event might require the same "$S\delta$" sequence used for deletion of $C\mu$ in IgD secretion, or alternatively a different recognition site may be employed. For example, a B-cell expressing surface IgM and IgG may have a context similar to that of BCL_1 but with a $C\gamma$ gene holding the position of the $C\delta$ gene by virtue of a deletion of all C_H genes between $C\mu$ and the $C\gamma$ gene expressed. Thus, the Ig gene context during B-cell development may involve at least three gene rearrangements: 1) V_HJ_H translocation at the level of the pre-B-cell with commitment to a single idiotype; 2) a translocation at the level of the mature B-cell bringing C_H genes 3' to $C\delta$ close to the $C\mu$ gene for dual surface Ig expression; and 3) a translocation at the level of the mature Ig secreting plasma cell which brings the expressed C_H gene immediately proximate to the V_HJ_H gene complex, deleting all the intervening genes and restricting Ig synthesis to a single class.

REFERENCES

1. KEMP, D. J., S. CORY & J. M. ADAMS. 1979. Proc. Natl. Acad. Sci. U.S.A. **76**: 4627.
2. CORY, S. & J. M. ADAMS. 1980. Cell **19**: 37.
3. SCHILLING, J., B. CLEVINGER, J. M. DAVIE & L. HOOD. 1980. Nature **283**: 35.
4. NEWELL, N., J. E. RICHARD, P. W. TUCKER & F. R. BLATTNER. 1980. Science **209**: 1128.
5. SAKANO, H., R. MAKI, Y. KUROSAWA, W. ROEDER & S. TONEGAWA. 1980. Nature **286**: 676.
6. HONJO, T. & T. KATAOKA. 1978. Proc. Natl. Acad. Sci. U.S.A **75**: 2140.
7. DAVIS, M. M., K. CALAME, P. W. EARLY, D. L. LIVANT, R. JOHO, I. L. WEISSMAN & L. HOOD. 1980. Nature **283**: 733.

8. KATAOKA, T., T. KAWAKAMI, N. TAKAHASHI & T. HONJO. 1980. Proc. Natl. Acad. Sci. U.S.A. **77:** 919.
9. SIMON, M., ZIEG, J., M. SILVERMAN, G. MANDEL & R. DOOLITTLE. 1980. Science **209:** 1370.
10. RABBITTS, T. H., A. FORSTER, W. DUNNICK & D. L. BENTLEY. 1980. Nature **283:** 351.
11. DAVIS, M., S. K. KIM & L. HOOD. 1980. Science **209:** 1360.
12. DAVIS, M., S. K. KIM & L. HOOD. 1980. Cell **22:** 1.
13. PERNIS, B., L. FORNI & A. L. LUZZATI. 1976. Cold Spring Harbor Symp. Quant. Biol. **41:** 175.
14. COOPER, M. D., J. F. KEARNEY, P. M. LYDYARD, C. E. GROSSI & A. R. LAWTON. 1976. Cold Spring Harbor Symp. Quant. Biol. **41:** 139.
15. VITETTA, E. S. & J. W. UHR. 1977. Immunol. Rev. **37:** 50.
16. FINKELMAN, F. D., V. L. WOODS, A. BERNING & I. SCHER. 1979. J. Immunol. **123:** 1253.
17. BARGELLESI, A., G. CORTE, E. E. COSULICH & M. FERRARINI. 1979. Eur. J. Immunol. **9:** 490.
18. FINKELMAN, F. D., S. W. KESSLER, J. F. MUSHINSKI & M. POTTER. 1980. J. Immunol. **126:** 680.
19. LIU, C. P., P. W. TUCKER, J. F. MUSHINSKI & F. R. BLATTNER. 1980. Science **209:** 1348.
20. KNAPP, M., C.-P. LIU, N. NEWELL, P. W. TUCKER, S. STROBER & F. R. BLATTNER. 1982. Proc. Natl. Acad. Sci. U.S.A. In press.
21. KNAPP, M., C.-P. LIU, N. NEWELL, P. W. TUCKER, S. STROBER & F. R. BLATTNER. 1981. *In* B-Lymphocytes in the Immune Response. N. Klinman, D. E. Mosier, I. Scher & E. S. Vitetta, Eds. **15:** 43. Elsevier/North Holland.
22. KNAPP, M. R., P. P. JONES, S. J. BLACK, S. SLAVIN, E. S. VITETTA & S. STROBER. 1979. J. Immunol **123:** 992.
23. KNAPP, M. R., E. SEVERINSON-GRONOWICZ, J. SCHRODER & S. STROBER. 1979. J. Immunol. **123:** 1000.
24. ROGERS, J., P. EARLY, C. CARTER, K. CALAME, M. BOND, L. HOOD & R. WALL. 1980. Cell **20:** 303.
25. EARLY, P., J. ROGERS, M. DAVIS, K. CALAME, M. BOND, R. WALL & L. HOOD. 1980. Cell **20:** 313.
26. MOORE, K. W., J. ROGERS, T. HUNKAPILLER, P. EARLY, C. NOTTENBURG, R. WALL, I. WEISSMAN, H. BAZIN & L. HOOD. 1981. Proc. Natl. Acad. Sci. USA **78:** 1800.
27. MAKI, R., W. ROEDER, A. TRAUNECKER, C. SIDMAN, M. WABL, W. RASCHKE & S. TONEGAWA. 1981. Cell **24:** 353.
28. TUCKER. P. W., H-L. CHENG, J. F. MUSHINSKI, L. FITZMAURICE, C-P. LIU & F. R. BLATTNER. 1981. *In* B Lymphocytes in the Immune Response. M. Klenman, D. E. Mosier, I. Scher & E. S. Vitetta, Eds. **15:** 43. Elsevier/North Holland.
29. CHENG, H-L., F. R. BLATTNER, L. FITZMAURICE, J. F. MUSHINSKI & P. W. TUCKER. 1982. Nature. **296:** 410.
30. FITZMAURICE, L., J. OWENS, F. R. BLATTNER, H-L. CHENG, P. W. TUCKER & J. F. MUSHINSKI. 1982. Nature. In press.
31. KABAT, E. A., T. T. WU & H. BILOFSKY. 1979. NIH Publication No. 80-2008.
32. TONEGAWA, S., C. BRACK, N. HOZUMI, G. MATTHYSSENS & R. SCHULLER. 1977. Immunol. Rev. **36:** 73.
33. SEIDMAN, J. G. & P. LEDER. 1978. Nature **276:** 790.
34. ZIFF, E. B. 1980. Nature **287:** 491.
35. ALT, F. W., A. L. M. BOTHWELL, M. KNAPP, E. SIDEN, E. MATHER, M. KOSHLAND & D. BALTIMORE. 1980. Cell **20:** 293.
36. NIKAIDO, T., NAKAI, S. & T. HONJO. 1981. Nature **292:** 845.
37. LANG, R. B., L. W. STANTON & K. B. MARCU. 1982. Nucleic Acids Res. **10:** 611.

DISCUSSION OF THIS PAPER BEGINS ON PAGE 38.

GENETIC ASPECTS OF IgD EXPRESSION: II. MULTIPLE FORMS OF δ CHAIN mRNA IN NORMAL MOUSE SPLEEN, MOUSE B-CELL LYMPHOMAS AND MOUSE AND HUMAN MYELOMAS*

J. Frederic Mushinski,† Carol J. Thiele,† James D. Owens,†
Frederick R. Blattner,‡ A. L. Shen,‡ P. W. Tucker,§ and L. Fitzmaurice¶

†Laboratory of Cell Biology
National Cancer Institute
Bethesda, Maryland 20205

‡Department of Genetics
University of Wisconsin
Madison, Wisconsin 53706

§Department of Microbiology
University of Texas Southwestern Medical School
Dallas, Texas 75235

¶Laboratory of Immunology
National Institute of Allergy and Infectious Disease
Bethesda, Maryland 20205

Immunoglobulin D (IgD) was first described as a myeloma protein,[1] a secreted immunoglobulin (Ig) produced by malignant plasma cells. However, IgD-secreting myelomas are uncommon in man and mouse, and IgD-secreting plasma cells are rare in normal animals[2] so that IgD is a minor component of circulating antibodies.[3] The real importance of this Ig isotype seems to lie in its presence as a molecule found on the surface of B-lymphocytes. In fact it has been estimated that 80% of mature B-lymphocytes have IgD embedded in their membranes,[2] usually in conjunction with membrane-bound IgM. Although IgD is frequently found on B-cell membranes, the amount of this protein that can be isolated for analysis is very small. Thus, most of the structural information currently available for IgD has been derived from myeloma proteins, the secreted form of this Ig.[4,5] Although substantial protein sequence,[6] mRNA,[7] and DNA sequence[8] data have been determined for both the secreted and the membrane forms of IgM, very little has been published on the detailed structure of membrane IgD.[9]

Our studies on the expression of the IgD gene complex in mice have also had their origins in mRNA obtained from two IgD-secreting mouse plasmacytomas identified two years ago by Fred Finkelman[10] from a group of uncharacterized plasmacytomas induced by Michael Potter by intraperitoneal injections of pristane (tetramethylpentadecane) in BALB/c mice.[11] These plasmacytomas, TEPC1017 and TEPC1033, produce membrane IgD as well as secrete myeloma proteins,[12] but the cDNA clone, pδ54J, that we synthesized from TEPC1017

*C. J. Thiele is a recipient of a fellowship from the Cancer Research Institute, Inc; F. R. Blattner is a grantee of the National Institute of General Medical Sciences (GM21812), and P. W. Tucker is a grantee of the National Institute of Allergy and Infectious Diseases (AL16547).

15

mRNA[13] coded for the secreted form of IgD heavy chain (δ chain), designated δ_s.[5,14]

This δ cDNA was used to identify and isolate δ genomic clones from a bacteriophage library of DNA from BALB/c liver.[15] This DNA contains the germline or unrearranged form of the δ gene complex and consists of three constant region segments, Cδ1, CδH, and Cδ3, separated by small introns. Delta gene segments that encode alternate 3' termini for the secreted and membrane

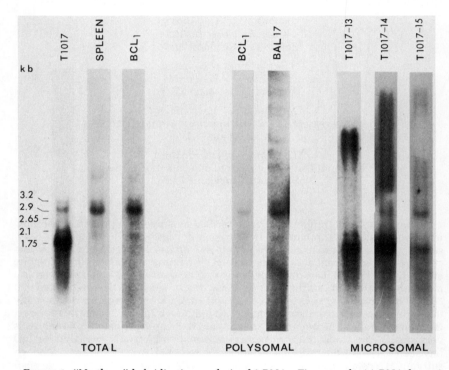

FIGURE 1. "Northern" hybridization analysis of δ RNAs. Five μg poly A$^+$ RNA from 1) Guanidinium thiocyanate (G-SCN) extracted RNA[26] from TEPC1017 tumors, 2) Lithium chloride-urea (Li-U) extracted RNA[27] from BALB/c spleens, 3) Li-U RNA from BCL$_1$ containing spleens,[28] 4) Phenol-chloroform extracted polyribosomes prepared from BCL$_1$-containing spleens, and 5) Phenol-chloroform extracted polyribosomes prepared from BAL17 cells,[29] as well as 0.5 μg of RNA from sucrose gradient fractions 13, 14 and 15 of poly (A)$^+$ RNA prepared from TEPC1017 microsomes[13] were denatured in 10 mM methyl mercury hydroxide[16] and electrophoresed in 1.0% agarose gel containing 5 mM methyl mercury hydroxide. The gel was stained with ethidium bromide and processed for transfer to diazotized paper.[17] The paper was hybridized[18] to a Cδ cDNA probe prepared from pδ54J[13] by digestion with Pvu II and Hind III and electrophoretic separation on polyacrylamide gel electrophoresis.[30] This probe was ^{32}P labeled by nick translation.[31] The approximate sizes of the hybridizing RNA bands (in kilobases) are shown to the left of the figure. The sizes were determined by reference to ethidium-bromide stained mouse 18S and 28S rRNAs which were assumed to be 2.0 and 4.7 kb, respectively, and by reference to TMV (6.34kb) and BMV (0.87, 2.3, 3.1, and 3.4 kb) RNAs fractionated in adjacent lanes.

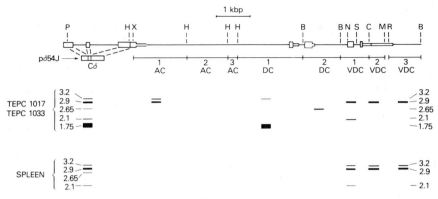

FIGURE 2. Physical map of the δ gene[15] showing restriction sites used to generate the probes used in RNA hybridization studies. B = BamHI, C = Cla I, H = Hind III, M = Mbo I (converted to BamHI when inserted into λ phage clone), N = Hinc II, P = Pvu II, R = EcoRI, S = RsaI, and X = XbaI. Fragments from phage λ clones of liver DNA indicated here were subcloned into plasmid vectors. Beneath each probe is drawn a summary of the hybridization results (FIGURE 1 and references 19 and 32) obtained with this probe on electrophoresed RNAs as shown. The widths of the lines is an approximation of the relative degrees of hybridization with each probe.

forms of δ chains are separated from the 3' end of Cδ3 and from each other by much larger introns.

We have used that portion of pδ54J cDNA which contains Cδ1, CδH, and Cδ3 as a probe for the constant regions of δ in order to study the RNAs produced by the expression of the δ gene. We have also used portions of the genomic clone as probes to determine the nature of the different forms of δ RNA found in plasmacytomas, spleens and B-cell lymphomas. The basic technique used was electrophoresis of poly(A)-containing RNA in methyl mercury hydroxide agarose gels[16] followed by blotting onto diazotized paper[17] and hybridization[18] with ^{32}P-labeled DNA probes.

It was expected that there might be two forms of δ mRNA in TEPC1017 and TEPC1033 cells which would correspond to secreted (δ_s) and membrane-bound (δ_m) forms of δ chain mRNA. Instead we found that five hybridizing bands of δ RNA could be identified in these cells[13,19] (FIGURE 1).

The size of these RNAs was determined by comparison with the distance migrated by standards, plant viral RNAs and mouse ribosomal RNAs. In the two plasmacytomas, the smallest δ mRNA, which contains 1,750 nucleotides or 1.75 kilobases (1.75 kb) of RNA, was by far the most abundant species. We believe that this RNA is the messenger for secreted δ chain, since these plasmacytomas secrete large amounts of IgD. The intense hybridization signal from such abundant RNAs frequently obscures minor bands. Therefore a roughly quantitative schematic summary of the results of hybridization studies of plasmacytoma and spleen RNAs, such as those presented in FIGURE 1 and reference 32, is depicted in FIGURE 2 beneath the part of the δ gene from which the probe was derived.

As expected, the 1.75 kb δ_s RNA is not seen in spleen RNA[19] or in RNA from B-lymphomas that appear to synthesize membrane IgD but no secretory IgD

(FIGURE 1). All these tissues contain much less δ RNA than the plasmacytomas. Prolonged exposure of autoradiograms revealed 2.1, 2.9 and 3.2 kb δ RNAs at least one of which is likely to encode the membrane form of δ chain. The 2.9 kb δ RNA is the most abundant of these RNAs in spleen and B-lymphomas and second in abundance only to the 1.75 kb species in the plasmacytomas. This suggests that it is the major functional δ_m mRNA.

In order to characterize further the unexpectedly large number of δ RNAs, probes derived from DNA located at some distance 3' to the constant domains were used to probe the RNA blots. These probes were derived from the bacteriophage clones of the germline δ gene by digestion with restriction endonucleases, as depicted in FIGURE 2. The only 3' DNA fragment that hybridized with the 1.75 kb RNA was the DC1 probe. A 250 base pair (0.25 kbp) stretch of DNA from this region was found by DNA sequence studies[14] to contain the 3' terminus of pδ54J as well as a 3' untranslated region ending with a AATAAA signal for poly(A) addition. The DNA sequence from the liver clone DC1 translates into a nonhydrophobic amino acid sequence identical with the amino acid sequence of a secreted mouse IgD protein.[5] This, indeed, must be the δ_s gene segment which, although separated from the δ constant region domains in genomic DNA, is joined to Cδ3 to form the 1.75 kb δ_s mRNA by one or more RNA splicing steps during processing of RNA from primary transcript to the mature mRNA. The DC1 probe also hybridizes with the 3.2 kb RNA of the plasmacytomas. This 3.2 kb δ RNA is not seen in RNA prepared from TEPC1017 microsomal RNA (FIGURE 1), which is expected to contain only those RNAs that are mature mRNAs available on polyribosomes for translation into protein. Thus the 3.2 kb δ RNA in plasmacytomas is unlikely to be an alternate form of δ_s mRNA. Since the 3.2 kb δ RNA also hybridizes with a probe from AC1 DNA it is more likely that the 3.2 kb δ RNA is a precursor of the 1.75 kb δ_s mRNA. The 1.75 kb δ_s RNA would then be derived from the 3.2 kb RNA by splicing out the AC1 sequences in one or more steps during processing of the primary RNA transcripts.

Neither AC1 nor DC1 hybridize to discrete bands of RNA from normal spleens; the absence of detectable δ_s mRNA is consistent with the fact that spleen cells synthesize little or no detectable δ_s protein. The 2.1, 2.9 and 3.2 kb δ RNAs in spleen and in the B-cell lymphomas are likely to be mRNAs for membrane-bound IgD δ chains (δ_m mRNAs). All three δ_m RNAs hybridize with DNA from the VDC1 region which contains a sequence encoding a hydrophobic polypeptide similar to that of membrane bound μ chain.[20] The two larger forms of δ_m RNA hybridize with VDC2 and VDC3 probes as well and could be precursors of the 2.1 kb δ_m RNA. However, the 2.9 kb form of δ_m RNA is the most abundant of the δ_m RNAs, making it unlikely to be a short-lived precursor of the less abundant 2.1 kb form. Furthermore, in contrast with the δ_s findings, all three δ_m RNAs are found in polysomal RNA preparations (FIGURE 1) strongly suggesting that all three forms are translationally active δ_m mRNAs. Thus it is possible that these three RNAs are alternative forms of δ_m RNA which differ only in the length of their 3' untranslated region but code for the same δ_m polypeptide. Since the δ_m mRNAs have not yet been isolated and sequenced, one cannot exclude the possibility that differential RNA splicing could generate RNAs that have differences in the coding region as well as RNAs that differ only in the untranslated region.

It may be significant that there are multiple forms of δ_m mRNA and only one form of δ_s mRNA. There are two reasons that make it unlikely that the multiple species are incomplete or aberrant RNAs resulting from some tumor-specific processing error or owing to the aneuploid nature of the tumor genome. Firstly, these multiple species exist in normal spleen cells, and secondly, all 3 δ_m mRNA species are found in polysomal RNA.

One possible interpretation is that a single δ_m chain is encoded by three or more mRNAs differing only in their 3' untranslated regions. Such a 3' heterogeneity has been demonstrated for mRNAs encoding the single polypeptide of dihydrofolate reductase.[21] The existence of multiple splicing and polyadenylation signals in the portion of the genome encoding δ chain membrane terminal sequences in consistent with this possibility.[20] Further, it is possible that such a redundancy of RNA processing patterns for the production of translatable δ_m mRNA would lessen the likelihood of loss of δ chain production due to mutational accidents and thus be advantageous to spleen B-cells.

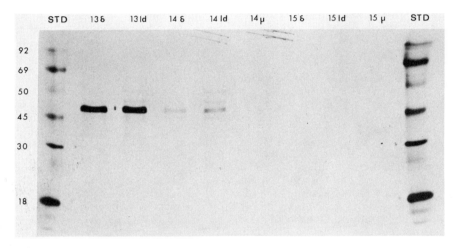

FIGURE 3. Fluorogram of a 15% polyacrylamide slab gel electrophoresis. Poly(A)$^+$ RNA from TEPC1017 microsomes was fractionated on a 5–40% sucrose gradient and the L-[^{35}S] methionine cell-free translation products of RNA from fractions 13–15 were analyzed after immune precipitation with affinity-purified rabbit anti-δ, (13δ, 14δ, and 15δ), rabbit anti-TEPC1017 idiotype (13Id, 14Id, and 15Id) and rabbit anti-μ (14μ and 15μ). Details of the cell-free translation and immune precipitation were published previously,[13] as were the preparation and characterization of the antibodies.[10] [^{14}C]-labeled molecular weight standards (New England Nuclear) were electrophoresed in lanes marked STD and their molecular weights $\times 10^{-3}$ are indicated to the left of the figure.

Another possibility is that the three δ_m mRNAs produce three different forms of δ_m polypeptide. Certainly more than three different functions have variously been attributed to membrane IgD. If there were slightly different forms of the δ_m chain, they might make different IgD molecules specially adapted for different functions. For example, slightly longer C-terminal ends might reach deeper into the cytoplasm to contact different subcellular organelles to which a surface signal might be transduced. We have some preliminary evidence that suggests that the multiple δ_m RNAs may be translated into multiple δ proteins (FIGURE 3). In this figure we see at least three faint bands of immunoprecipitable proteins (44,000,

52,000 and 57,000 daltons) present in the products synthesized by reticulocyte lysates stimulated by RNA from three sucrose gradient fractions of RNA from TEPC1017 (cf. FIGURE 1), in addition to the very abundant band of myeloma protein (46,000 daltons). The faint bands are most apparent when precipitated by an antiserum which is idiotypic for TEPC1017.[10] It is possible that the idiotypic antiserum, which is specific for the less glycosylated variable part of the heavy chain, is better able to precipitate the nonglycosylated products of cell-free synthesis than is the class specific anti-δ reagent, specific for determinants on the heavily glycosylated Fc region. We are attempting to confirm and extend these findings by translation of δ_m mRNAs purified from spleen and plasmacytoma RNA by hybridization to DNA from the membrane binding region of the δ gene, the VDC region.

Analysis of the DNA sequence in the VDC or membrane-binding region of δ DNA[20] cannot rule out either of the mechanisms for multiple δ_m mRNA production discussed above. RNA splicing signals are not understood clearly enough to predict the final mRNA products from examination of the sequence of genomic DNA alone. It is thought that there are specific signals consisting of DNA sequences that indicate where polyadenylation can take place. Addition of a stretch of adenosines is felt to define the 3′ end of a primary RNA transcript. AATAAA or ATTAAA have been identified as these signals, and we have found one such signal for δ_s and two for δ_m.[20] After polyadenylation, splicing out of intron RNA appears to take place at certain sites. The DNA sequence of introns characteristically begins with GT and ends with AG. These dinucleotide combinations occur very frequently in DNA, so additional flanking sequences must be involved in recognition of suitable splicing sites. It is also likely that a hierarchy of such signals exists, which makes splicings at some sites more likely than at others. Thus, many possibilities exist for generating three or more mature δ_m mRNAs from a single RNA transcript of the δ gene by different splicings within the VDC region. Until the δ_m mRNAs are cloned and sequenced we will not know whether δ_m mRNA multiplicity results in several different δ_m polypeptides or a single δ_m polypeptide.

There is one more δ RNA that has been detected using the Cδ cDNA probe. It has a size of 2.65 kb but is very difficult to detect because of the much greater hybridization of the Cδ probe to other δRNA bands. When RNA is hybridized with DC2, only this band hybridizes but this hybridization is apparent only after a very long exposure time. This unique hybridization suggests that this 2.65 kb RNA may be another form of δRNA, perhaps another secretory form. The possibility of it being a mutant or incomplete RNA has not been ruled out, but its lack of DC1 or VDC sequences is not consistent with such a possibility. This RNA needs further characterization before we can conclude much about its function.

We have recently begun a parallel study of the expression of human IgD to see if there is a similar multiplicity of δ mRNAs in the human Ig system. This study has been aided by the acquisition of a human myeloma cell line called ODA, which was adapted to culture in Japan by Dr. N. Ishihara[22] and kindly provided to us. Our studies are still in the initial stages but we do have evidence already for at least two different sized δ mRNAs. FIGURE 4 shows the immunoprecipitated products of cell-free translation of different sucrose gradient fractions of ODA poly(A)-containing RNA. Fraction 16 RNA directs the synthesis of a δ chain of about 58,000 daltons, and fraction 19 contains RNA specifying one of about 62,000 daltons as well as a remnant of the RNA coding for the smaller δ. We do not know if each sucrose gradient fraction contains more than one species of δ RNA since we do not yet have a human cDNA δ probe. We have tried to hybridize these human RNA fractions with our mouse cDNA δ probe, but we have not succeeded in obtaining specific hybridization.

It is possible that the two δ chains (58,000 and 62,000 daltons) synthesized by ODA mRNA could be $δ_s$ and $δ_m$ polypeptides. This is not necessarily the case, however, since ODA cells labeled in culture appear to secrete two δ proteins into the culture fluid. These proteins are poorly separated by SDS-PAGE (FIGURE 5, lane B), but they are separated well by nonequilibrium pH gradient gel electrophoresis. This analysis (data not shown) reveals two bands of protein, in roughly

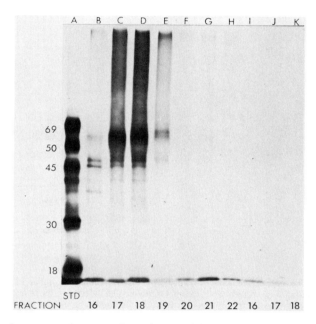

FIGURE 4. Fluorogram of a 15% polyacrylamide slab gel electrophoresis. Poly(A)$^+$ RNA from ODA cells was fractionated on a 5–40% sucrose gradient and the L-[^{35}S] methionine cell-free translation products of RNA from fractions 16–22 were analyzed after immune precipitation with an affinity purified rabbit anti-human δ reagent (lanes B–H) or normal rabbit serum (lanes I–K). [^{14}C]-labeled molecular weight standards (New England Nuclear) (lane A) with molecular weight $\times 10^{-3}$ indicated at left were utilized.

equal amounts. These secreted, glycosylated δ chains (68,000 daltons-pI 4.5–5.5 and 71,000 daltons-pI 5.5–5.6) also differ in size by about 3000 daltons. It is unlikely that equal amounts of secreted and membrane IgD are synthesized and secreted or shed into the culture fluid. These two proteins are more likely to be different forms of secreted IgD. Whether one represents a breakdown product of the other or an aberrant form of δ peculiar to the ODA line of plasma cell remains to be determined.

It is important to note that these human δ translation products are about 10,000 daltons larger than the mouse δ translation products.[13,23] This large difference in size between human and mouse δ myeloma proteins is also seen when the products secreted by myeloma cells in culture were labeled by radioactive amino acid precursors (FIGURE 5) with or without the presence of an inhibitor of glycosylation, tunicamycin. This evidence is consistent with the presence of at least one more constant region domain in the human myeloma protein δ chain than in those of mouse[15] or rat.[24] The studies of the δ gene in the mouse[14,15,23] (FIGURE 2) revealed no trace of a second Cδ domain in the bacteriophage genomic clone. The amino acid sequence studies on human myeloma protein WAH[25] suggested that the human δ gene differs significantly from the mouse and rat in

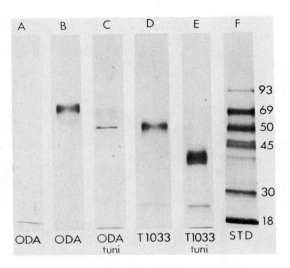

FIGURE 5. Fluorogram of a 15% polyacrylamide slab gel electrophoresis. L-[35S]-Methionine in vitro labeled secreted products of ODA and TEPC1033 cells were analyzed after immune precipitation with affinity purified heterologous antisera and formalin-fixed Staphylococcus aureus.[33] ODA cell supernatants were precipitated with normal rabbit serum (lane A), and rabbit anti-human δ reagent (lane B), while a tunicamycin-treated ODA cell supernatant was precipitated by the rabbit anti-human δ reagent (lane C). TEPC1033 cells (lane D) and tunicamycin-treated TEPC1033 cell supernatants (lane E) were precipitated with a rabbit anti mouse δ reagent.[10] [14C]-labeled molecular weight standards (New England Nuclear) (lane F) with molecular weights ×10^{-3} indicated at right were utilized.

that it contains a typical Cδ2 gene segment. It is also possible that DNA studies will reveal differences in the hinge region as well.

Clearly there are likely to be many more interesting similarities and differences between the genetic organization and expression of IgD in human and mouse cells which have yet to be revealed. We have shown here that both mouse and human cells contain two or more δ mRNAs and produce at least two δ proteins. Multiplicity or redundancies of δ proteins and mRNAs may be one feature that both species have in common, perhaps because of the essential nature of the expression of this Ig isotype.

SUMMARY

We have found at least five forms of δ chain mRNA and characterized them by electrophoresis and hybridization to a cloned Cδ cDNA probe and other δ probes. TEPC1017 and TEPC1033, plasmacytomas that synthesize secreted and membrane IgD, produce two RNAs (1.75 kb and 3.2 kb) encoding δ chain for secreted IgD (δ_s) and two RNAs (2.1 and 2.9 kb) encoding δ chain for membrane IgD (δ_m). The function of the fifth and least abundant δ chain mRNA (2.65 kb) is unknown. Normal mouse spleens, spleens containing the B-cell lymphoma BCL_1, and cultured B-cell lymphoma cells from BCL_1 and BAL17 do not contain the 1.75 kb δ_s mRNA but do contain 2.1, 2.9 and 3.2 kb δ chain mRNAs which appear to be different forms of δ_m mRNA. These δ_m mRNAs differ in their 3′ termini; they may encode the same structural protein and differ only in their untranslated regions, or the three δ_m mRNAs may encode different forms of membrane IgD.

The human myeloma cell line ODA contains at least two different-sized δ mRNAs encoding δ chain proteins of 58,000 and 62,000 daltons. These human δ chains are much larger than the δ_s protein encoded by mouse plasmacytoma mRNA (44,000–46,000 daltons) and may contain at least one constant region domain more than that of the mouse.

ACKNOWLEDGMENTS

We thank Dr. Fred Finkelman for the gifts of antiserum, Dr. Barbara Osborne for assistance in 2D gel electrophoresis, and Ms. Victoria Armstrong for her expert preparation of this manuscript.

REFERENCES

1. ROWE D. S. & J. L. FAHEY. 1965. A new class of human immunoglobulins. I. A unique myeloma protein. J. Exp. Med. **121:** 171–184.
2. BARGELLESI, A., G. CORTE, E. COSULICH & M. FERRARINI. 1979. Presence of IgD and IgD-containing plasma cells in the mouse. Eur. J. Immunol. **9:** 490–492.
3. FINKELMAN, F. D., V. L. WOODS, A. BERNING & I. SCHER. 1979. Demonstration of mouse serum IgD. J. Immunol. **123:** 1253–1259.
4. LIN, L.-C., F. W. PUTNAM. 1981. Primary structure of the Fc region of human immunoglobulin D: implications for the evolutionary origin and biological function. Proc. Nat. Acad. Sci. USA **78:** 504–508.
5. DILDROP, R. & K. BEYREUTHER. 1981. C-terminal sequence of the secreted form of mouse IgD heavy chain. Nature **292:** 61–63.
6. KEHRY, M., S. EWALT, R. DOUGLAS, C. SIBLEY, W. RASCHKE, D. FAMBROUGH & L. HOOD. 1980. The immunoglobulin μ chains of membrane-bound and secreted IgM molecules differ in their C-terminal segments. Cell **21:** 393–406.
7. ROGERS, J., P. EARLY, C. CARTER, K. CALAME, M. BOND, L. HOOD & R. WALL. 1980. Two mRNAs with different 3′ ends encode membrane-bound and secreted forms of immunoglobulin μ chain. Cell **20:** 293–301.
8. EARLY, P., J. ROGERS, M. DAVIS, K. CALAME, M. BOND, R. WALL & L. HOOD. 1980. Two mRNAs can be produced from a single immunoglobulin μ gene by alternative RNA processing pathways. Cell **20:** 313–319.
9. GODING, J. W. & L. A. HERZENBERG. 1980. Biosynthesis of lymphocyte surface IgD in the mouse. J. Immunol. **124:** 2540–2547.
10. FINKELMAN, F. D., S. W. KESSLER, J. F. MUSHINSKI & M. POTTER. 1981. IgD-secreting

murine plasmacytomas: identification and partial characterization of two IgD myeloma proteins. J. Immunol. **126**: 680-687.

11. POTTER, M. 1972. Immunoglobulin-producing tumors and myeloma proteins of mice.
Physiol. Rev. **52**: 631-719.

12. KESSLER, S. W., J. F. MUSHINSKI, M. POTTER & F. D. FINKELMAN. 1980. Dual processing of
δ chains for secretion and for membrane deposition in IgD-synthesizing plasmacytomas. Fed. Proc. **39**: 1055.

13. MUSHINSKI, J. F., F. R. BLATTNER, J. D. OWENS, F. D. FINKELMAN, S. W. KESSLER, L.
FITZMAURICE, M. POTTER & P. W. TUCKER. 1980. Mouse immunoglobulin D: construc-
tion and characterization of a cloned δ chain cDNA. Proc. Nat. Acad. Sci. USA **77**:
7405-7409.

14. TUCKER, P. W., C.-P. LIU, J. F. MUSHINSKI & F. R. BLATTNER. 1980. Mouse immunoglobulin D: messenger RNA and genomic DNA sequences. Science **209**: 1353-1360.

15. LIU, C.-P., P. W. TUCKER, J. F. MUSHINSKI & F. R. BLATTNER. 1980. Mapping of heavy
chain genes for mouse immunoglobulins M and D. Science **209**: 1348-1353.

16. BAILEY. J. M. & N. DAVIDSON. 1976. Methylmercury as a reversible denaturing agent for
agarose gel electrophoresis. Anal. Biochem. **70**: 75-85.

17. ALWINE, J. C., D. J. KEMP & G. R. STARK. 1977. Method for detection of specific RNAs in
agarose gels by transfer to diazobenzyloxymethyl-paper and hybridization with DNA
probes. Proc. Nat. Acad. Sci. USA **74**: 5350-5354.

18. WAHL, G. M., M. STERN & G. R. STARK. 1979. Efficient transfer of large DNA fragments
from agarose gels to diazobenzyloxymethyl paper and rapid hybridization by using
dextran sulfate. Proc. Nat. Acad. Sci. USA **76**: 3683-3687.

19. FITZMAURICE, L., J. OWENS, H.-L. CHENG, P. W. TUCKER, C.-P. LIU, A. L. SHEN, F. R.
BLATTNER & J. F. MUSHINSKI. 1981. Transcription of δ chain genes in mouse myeloma
cells and normal spleen. *In* Immunoglobulin Idiotypes and Their Expression. C.
Janeway, E. E. Sercarz, H. Wigzell & C. F. Fox, Eds. 263-269. Academic Press. New
York, N.Y.

20. TUCKER, P. W. Genetic aspects of IgD expression. III. Functional aspects of δ chain
sequences. Ann. N.Y. Acad. Sci. This volume.

21. SETZER, D. R., M. McGROGAN, J. H. NUNBERG & R. T. SCHIMKE. 1980. Size heterogeneity
in the 3' end of dihydrofolate reductase messenger RNAs in mouse cells. Cell **22**:
361-370.

22. ISHIHARA, N., T. SEIDO & S. OHBOSHI. 1977. Establishment and characterization of a
human IgD myeloma cell line. Proceed. Japan Cancer Assn. **36**: 120. (Abstract, in
Japanese).

23. MAKI, R., W. ROEDER, A. TRAUNECKER, C. SIDMAN, M. WABL, W. RASCHKE & S.
TONEGAWA. 1981. The role of DNA rearrangement and alternative RNA processing in
the expression of immunoglobulin delta genes. Cell **24**: 353-365.

24. ALCARAZ, G., A. BOURGOIS, A. MOULIN, H. BAZIN & M. FOUGEREAU. 1980. Partial
structure of a rat IgD molecule with a deletion in the heavy chain. Ann. Immunol.
(Inst. Pasteur) **131C**: 363-388.

25. PUTNAM, F. W., N. TAKAHASHI, D. TETAERT, B. DEBUIRE & L.-C. LIN. 1981. Amino acid
sequence of the first constant region domain and the hinge region of the δ heavy
chain of human IgD. Proc. Nat. Acad. Sci. USA **78**: 6168-6172.

26. CHIRGWIN, M. J., A. E. PRZYBYLA, R. J. MACDONALD & W. J. RUTTER. 1979. Isolation of
biologically active ribonucleic acid from sources enriched in ribonuclease. Biochemistry **18**: 5294-5298.

27. AUFFRAY, C. & F. ROUGEON. 1980. Purification of mouse immunoglobulin heavy chain
messenger RNA from total myeloma tumor RNA. Eur. J. Biochem. **107**: 303-314.

28. KNAPP, M. R., P. P. JONES, S. J. BLACK, S. SLAVIN, E. S. VITETTA & S. STROBER. 1979.
Characterization of a spontaneous murine B-cell leukemia (BCL$_1$). I. Cell surface
expression of IgM, IgD, Ia and FcR. J. Immunol. **123**: 992-999.

29. KIM, K. J., C. KANELLOPOULOS-LANGEVIN, R. M. MERWIN, D. H. SACHS & R. ASOFSKY.
1979. Establishment and characterization of BALB/c lymphoma lines with B-cell
properties. J. Immunol. **122**: 549-554.

30. MAXAM, A. M. & W. GILBERT. 1980. Sequencing end-labeled DNA with base-specific chemical cleavages. Methods Enzymol. **65:** 499–560.
31. RIGBY, P. J. W., M. DIECKMANN, C. RHODES, & P. BERG. 1977. Labeling of deoxyribonucleic acid to high specific activity *in vitro* by nick translation with DNA polymerase I. J. Mol. Biol. **113:** 237–251.
32. FITZMAURICE, L., J. OWENS, F. R. BLATTNER, H.-L. CHENG, P. W. TUCKER, & J. F. MUSHINSKI. 1982. Nature. **296:** 459–462.
33. KESSLER, S. W. 1975. Rapid isolation of antigens from cells with a staphylococcal protein A antibody absorbent: parameters of the interaction of antibody-antigen complexes with protein A. J. Immunol **115:** 1617–1624.

———————————◆———————————

DISCUSSION OF THIS PAPER BEGINS ON PAGE 38.

GENETIC ASPECTS OF IgD EXPRESSION:
III. FUNCTIONAL IMPLICATIONS OF THE SEQUENCE
AND ORGANIZATION OF THE Cδ GENE

P. W. Tucker,* H.-L. Cheng,* J. E. Richards,† L. Fitzmaurice,‡
J. F. Mushinski,‡ and F. R. Blattner†

*Department of Microbiology
University of Texas
Southwestern Medical School
Dallas, Texas 75235

†Department of Genetics
University of Wisconsin
Madison, Wisconsin 53706

‡Department of Cell Biology
National Institutes of Health
Bethesda, Maryland 20205

INTRODUCTION

The majority of mature B-lymphocytes strongly express both IgM and IgD on the cell surface with the same idiotype and ligand specificity, and hence, the same variable region.[1] When the B-cell differentiates into a plasma cell upon receipt of an antigen-dependent triggering, this same variable region is used for secreted antibody.[2,3] Although B-cells express surface IgM and IgD about equally,[4] the level of secretory IgD in plasma is about 1000-fold lower than IgM.[5,6] This may be due in part to the lower stability of IgD but it also must reflect the fact that cells committed to secretion of IgD must either be quite rare or they must secrete δ in small amounts.

The simultaneous expression of two receptors on the B-cell surface has led to several theories regarding their differential function (see reference 7 for a review). However, the intense interest in the function of mouse IgD had been hindered until recently by scarcity of data on its structure. The timely discovery of two murine plasmacytomas, TEPC 1017 and TEPC 1033,[8] finally made possible the isolation of sufficient amounts of δ chain mRNA. This has allowed us to construct[9] and sequence[10] a cDNA clone and use it as a probe for extensive sequence and organizational analysis[10-14] of the germline BALB/c Cδ gene. The structure we deduced for the tumor protein was unprecedented and provocative in that only two C_H domains (Cδ1 and Cδ3) separated by a hinge were found. This was particularly unexpected since a human myeloma δ chain had earlier been shown from peptide mapping data[15,16] to have a "normal" three constant region structure. A number of indirect lines of evidence suggested to us that this unusual two constant domain structure is characteristic of normal mouse membrane and secreted δ chains. The characterization of a two Cδ domain rat myeloma protein[17] was consistent with this interpretation, and indicated that deletion of a Cδ2 domain might be a common feature of the murine species.

Although our data answered some structural questions, they raise many more regarding function. Putnam and coworkers[18,19] have recently reported the entire

26

0077–8923/82/0399–0026$01.75/0 © 1982 NYAS

amino acid sequence of a human secreted δ chain, and we have completed the DNA sequence of the exons encoding the carboxyl terminal portions of mouse secreted and membrane δ chains.[20] In light of this new information, it seems appropriate to readdress the possible structure-function relationships of IgD and its differential role relative to IgM on B-cell membranes.

Organization of the Cδ Gene

The arrangement of the mouse Cδ gene (given in FIGURE 1) is topographically, and for that matter functionally, divided into two regions: the 5' most cluster of exons (Cδ1, CδH, and Cδ3) encodes the body of the δ chain constant region; the exons located some 5 killobase pairs (Kbp) 3' to the body of the gene code for alternative secreted (δs) or membrane (δM1 and δM2) carboxyl termini. The region designated δx is transcribed into mature δ chain mRNA (*cf* previous paper and references 20, 21), but there is no evidence that it is translated into protein and will not be considered further here.

Before discussing the functional significance of the sequences, we will comment briefly on the carboxyl terminal arrangement of secreted (s) and membrane (m) exons. The arrangement of Cδ is very similar to that of Cμ in that the membrane termini (M1 and M2) are coded distally for both genes. However, the organization of Cδ differs dramatically from Cμ and all other C$_H$ genes in that the δS terminus is also encoded distally to the body of the Cδ gene. The secreted tail of μ is encoded as a 21 amino acid extension of the last Cμ domain (Cμ4). The topographically analogous DNA sequence for Cδ (CδAC in FIGURE 1) is apparently never translated into protein.

Structure of the Constant Region Domains

FIGURE 2 gives the amino acid translation obtained for each exonic segment of the Cδ gene[10,20] with N terminal ends aligned to facilitate comparisons with the complete human[18,19] sequence. A discussion of the homology relationships and evolutionary features have been presented elsewhere[10,18,19] and will also be discussed at length in this volume by Putnam *et al.* We say here that for Cδ1, introduction of three gaps in the mouse sequence and one in the human allows a match of 26 of the 93 comparable residues for only a 28% homology. This is extremely low compared to matches of other pairs of human and mouse C$_H$1 domains which are from 40%-60% homologous.[22] Clearly the mouse Cδ1 has generic properties unique to C$_H$1 domains,[11,22] and the lack of homology to the human Cδ1 is a bonafide difference, not an error in interpretation of the DNA sequence data. Another difference of significance between human and mouse Cδ1 is the presence of two carbohydrate addition sites in the mouse that are not conserved in the human protein.

The Cδ3 domains of human and mouse match in 52 percent of the comparable positions up to the end of the Cδ3 exon in genomic DNA. Beyond this point the human secreted chain extends for seven amino acids, only one of which matches δS. A notable absence in the mouse Cδ3 is the two clusters of proline residues near both ends of the human domain. Putman *et al.*[19] point out that these residues are unique to the IgD class and may have functional significance in the human.

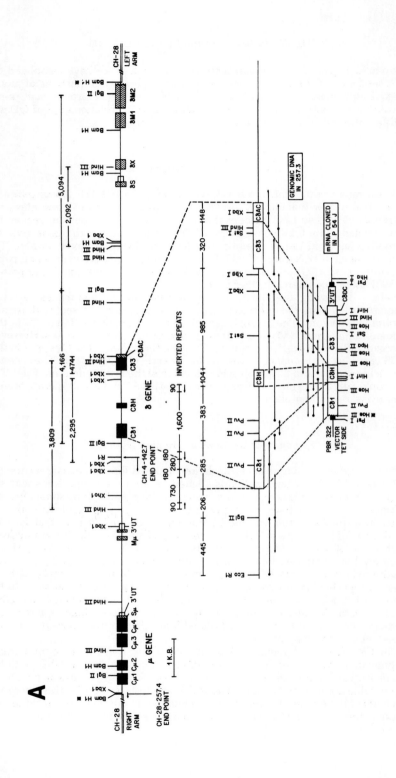

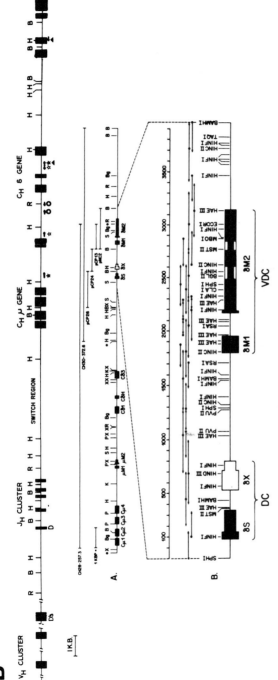

B

FIGURE 1 (A and B): DNA sequencing of the Cδ gene. **A.** Relationship of the body of the Cδ gene and TEPC 1017 δ chain mRNA. The region of the BALB/c genome cloned in Ch. 28-257.3 is shown in the upper portion with exons denoted as boxes. The lower panel shows the detailed restriction maps and DNA sequencing strategy for Cδ and the cDNA insert of clone pδ54]. Fragments were cleaved and labeled at the dots, and the direction and length of the sequence obtained from these sites using the chemical degration method are indicated by arrows. **B.** Relation of the membrane and secreted exons of Cδ. Restriction sites are abbreviated as follows: X, Xba. I, Bg, Bgl II; B, Bam HI; P, Pst I; H, Hind III; K, Kpn I; S, Sph I; R, Eco RI. A map of the area sequenced spanning the δ secreted (δS) and membrane (δM1 and δM2) regions is shown in the lower panel with the lowered portion of the exon boxes corresponding to 3' noncoding regions. Sequencing strategy is the same as in **A.** For more details on the localization of exons, see text and references 10, 11, 20, 21.

```
M Cδ1   GDKKEPDMF LLSECKAPENEXINLGCLVIGSQP  LKISNEPKKSSSVEVFPSENRNGNYTH   VLQVTVLASELNLNHTCTINKPKRKEKPKFP
         KPDF S C P N  L C L G P   N  S   FP R Y N    T L    C     K K F
H Cδ1   APTKAPDVFPIISSCRHPKDNSPVVLACLITGYHPSVTVTNYMGTQSQPQRTFPEIGRRDSYNTSSQLSTPLQQNRQGEYKCVVQHTASKSKKEIF


M HINGE  ESNDSQSSKRVTPTLQAKNHSTEAT KAITTKDIEG
          ES Q S T QA   AT TT  G
H HINGE  RNPESPKAQASSVPTAQPQAEGSLAKATTAPATTRNTGRGGEEKKKEKEEQEERETKTPECP


H Cδ2   SHTQPLGVYLLTPAVQDLLRLRDKIATFCFVVGSDLKDAHLTNEVAGKVPTGVVEGLLERHSNGSQSQHSRLTLPRSLNNAGTSVTCTLNH


M Cδ3            AAAPSNLTVNLLTTSTHPENSSHLLCEYSGFFPENIHLMLGVHSKMKSTNFVTANPTAQPGGT FQTNSVLRLPVALSSSLDTYTCVVEHEASKTKLNSKSLAIS
                 AAP  L N L S  PE  SHLLCEYSGF P NI LNNL      F A P QPG T F  NSVLR P  S    TYTCVV HE S T LNNS SL S
H Cδ3   PSLPPQRLNALREPAAQAPVKLSLNLLASSDPPEAASHLLCEYSGFSSPNILLNVLEDVQREYNTSGFAPARPPOPGSTTFNANSVLRVPAPPSPQPATYTCVVSHEDSRTLLNASRSLEVSY


M CδS   CTHLLPESDGPSRRPDGPALA
H CδS       D
        VTDNGPN


M CδX   DFLFKIYSKYKISARTSHKA


M CδM1  ITVNTQHSCINDEQSDSYNDLEEENGLNPTNCTVALFLTLLYSGFVTFIKVK
```

FIGURE 2. Comparison of the δ chain amino acid sequence between mouse and man. The mouse (M) sequence is that predicted from the DNA determination of the Cδ gene[10,20] and the human (H) sequence was determined directly at the protein level.[18,19] Residues appearing in the middle are conserved between the species when gaps are introduced to facilitate alignment. There is no proof that the mouse CδX sequence is expressed in δ-chain protein, although it is transcribed as mRNA. No equivalent has yet been determined for it or the membrane terminus (CδM1) in the human.

The Unusual δ Hinge

The mouse hinge region (CδH) in unusual is two respects. Its length (35 amino acids) is greater than any other sequenced mouse hinge, yet in contrast with other hinges, no cysteine residues are formed. Thus no covalent linkages between heavy chains are possible for this region of the sequence. The functional significance of this finding is discussed below. Its relatively high charge distribution (six basic and five acidic residues out of 35) and presence of a potential N-linked carbohydrate addition sequence as well as numerous O-linkage sites are also unique features among mouse hinge regions.

The human hinge is equally unusual in its extraordinary length (64 amino acids), presence of carbohydrate, and charge distribution.[19] All charged glutamic acid and lysine residues reside in the carboxyl terminal portion of the human hinge, whereas the charges are more or less randomly distributed in the mouse sequence. With a reasonable degree of gapping, the two sequences can be aligned in their N-terminal portions (FIGURE 3 and reference 19) with surprising homology (17 of the comparable 35 residues). Putnam *et al.* suggests[19] that the human sequence may have arisen as a duplication of the mouse hinge with subsequent mutation of the carboxyl terminal portion.

The Case of the Missing Cδ2 Domain

Although we feel confident that a two domain structure can account for the size of mouse δ, the absence of a Cδ2-like exon from the BALB/c genome would

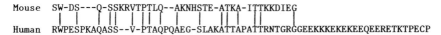

FIGURE 3. Comparison of the hinge regions of mouse and human IgD. Gaps required for best alignment are indicated by dashes and identities are shown by vertical lines.

constitute the greatest structural difference yet observed between the immune systems of murine and man. To shed light on this question, we determined the complete DNA sequence between the CδH and Cδ3 exons (data now shown). No domain-like features or homology with the human Cδ2 amino acid sequence were revealed. Instead this intron contains a striking tandem repeat of the type $CT_{29}AC_{29}$. We anticipated, based on our experience with the $C\gamma_{2b}$ gene,[23] that the δ intron might contain a pseudogene or evolutionary domain relic as a consequence of splice site mutation and hinge detachment (see also discussion in reference 24). Computer searches have not supported this hypothesis. One interesting rationalization for this is that the repeat sequence resulted from a primordial transposition (integration/excision) event or from insertion of a dispersed repetitive sequence such as the ribosomal nontranscribed spacer.[25] This would be responsible for even further evolutionary drift from the postulated Cδ2 relic. Regardless of the evolutionary mechanism, the absence of this region in murine DNA suggests that a Cδ2 is not important for the function of IgD. The alternative possibility, that different forms of murine IgD exist that possess the Cδ2, seems highly improbable in view of the now extensive characterization of this locus at the molecular level.

The Carboxyl Terminus of Tumor Secreted δ

The carboxyl terminal 23 amino acids of the δ chain produced by myeloma and hybridoma tumors are encoded on an exon located 4.7 kbp downstream of the terminal structural domain, Cδ3. As detailed in the legend to FIGURE 2, the genomic DNA sequence[20] differs slightly from the TEPC 1017 cDNA sequence that we published previously[11] due probably to a reverse transcription artifact. The actual B1-8.δ1 protein sequence[26] is identical to that which would be coded from our genomic sequence. As shown in FIGURE 4, δS is not homologous to the secreted terminal of either mouse μ,[27] α,[24] or human δ.[18]

An AATAAA poly(A) site, which presumably signals the 3' end of δs mRNA, is located 163 bp downstream of the end of the protein. Assuming the actual end of the message is about 20 bp beyond the poly(A) addition site, that 200 A residues

```
CYS                                                          /SPLICE
TGCATGGTGGGCCACGAGGCCTTGCCCATGAACTTCACCCAGAAGACCATCGACCGTCTGTCGGGTAAACCCACCA   ALPHA
TGTGTTGTAGGCCACGAGGCCCTGCCACACCTGGTGACCGAGAGGACCGTGGACAAGTCCACTGGTAAACCCACAC   MU
TGTGTGGTGGAACATGAGGCCTCAAAGACAAAGCTTAATGCCAGCAAGAGCCTAGCAATTAGTGGTAAGTCACAAC   DELTA
TGCTCTGTGTTACATGAGGGCCTGCACAACCACCATACTGAGAAGAGCCTCTCCCACTCTCCTGGTAAATGATCCC   GAMMA 1
TGCAACGTGAGACACGAGGGTCTGAAAAATTACTACCTGAAGAAGACCATCTCCCGGTCTCCGGGTAAATGAGCTC   GAMMA 2B


    CMVGHEALPMNFTQKTIDRLSGKPTNVNVSVIMSEGDGICY.    ALPHA
    CVVGHEALPHLVTERTVDKSTGKPTLYNVSLIMSDTGGTCY.    MU
    CVVEHEASKTKLNASKSLAISGCYHLLPESDGPSRRPDGPALA.  DELTA (DC)
    CSVLHEGLHNHHTEKSLSHSPGK.                      GAMMA1
    CNVRHEGLKNYYLKKTISRSPGK.                      GAMMA 2B
```

FIGURE 4. Carboxyl termini comparisons among various classes of H chains. The upper panel compares the DNA sequences of five immunoglobulin H chains aligned at the right hand invariant cysteine of the carboxyl terminal domain. A donor splice site appears in the same position in each chain. In the lower panel the amino acid sequences of the carboxyl termini for these chains are correspondingly aligned with positions of the invariant Cys and RNA splice site, indicated by lines. The δ (DC) sequence given is translated from genomic DNA and differs from the previously published cDNA sequence in two positions due to cloning artifacts (an extra T and A → G as indicated, TGC TAC CAC CTC CTG CCT GAG TCA GAC GGT CCT TCT AGG AGA CCT GAT GGT CCT GCC CTT GCC, resulting in a phase shift 12 codons from the beginning of the exon.

are added as a 3' tail and that a typical V region plus leader with 50 nucleotides of 5' untranslated region is present, the calculated length of the full δs mRNA would be about 1650 bases. This agrees with estimates of 1700 to 1800 bases by gel measurement,[9,21] (and *cf.* preceding paper). Likewise, the molecular weight for the secreted, nonglycosylated polypeptide chain calculated from the predicted amino acid sequence coded by the mRNA is 42.1 kilodaltons (kD). This is within 5%[28] and 12%[9] of reported size measurements of cell-free translation products of δ chain mRNA. The considerable higher estimates of δ chain length made *in vivo* are subject to the uncertain contribution of carbohydrate. However, one estimate[29] of the length following enzymatic removal of carbohydrate was 50,000 kd. This size value is consistent with our two-domain model for normal mouse δ chains.

The Membrane Terminus of Cell Surface δ

Since IgD is synthesized almost exclusively as a cell surface receptor, intense interest has been focused toward understanding its interaction with the membrane relative to IgM. In the case of IgM, studies by Rogers et al.,[30] Early et al.,[31] and Alt et al.,[32] showed that μm RNA differed from μs mRNA only in its 3′ base sequence, which encodes a 40 amino acid carboxyl terminus.[30] This peptide contained a 26 amino acid central core that was extremely hydrophobic and could easily span the lymphocyte membrane bilayer.

Examination of the Cδ DNA sequence near the beginning of the strongly expressed portion (referred to as VDC in FIGURE 2) revealed an area of strong homology to the μm sequence encoded by the μM1 exon. FIGURE 5 shows an alignment of μ and δ gene sequences in that area. In the 120 bp region coding for the most hydrophobic segments of the μ protein, the μ and δ nucleic acid sequences are over 60 percent homologous. Allowing for a two amino acid gap, 50 percent of the amino acids match and similar amino acids are substituted at corresponding positions. We conclude that this segment, which we term δM1, serves to bind IgD to the membrane. The acceptor RNA splice site that begins the δM1 exon is significantly upstream of the analogous site for μM1. Thus the amino acid sequence for δ is 16 residues longer than that for μ. This segment is not particularly hydrophobic and would likely lie on the outside of the membrane. The three glutamate residues conserved in the two structures may be important for stabilization of the membrane attachment, perhaps via an outer membrane protein interaction. It is also interesting to note that a cystine occurs in this portion of the IgD protein. This may serve in crosslinking IgD half monomers to one another on the membrane as was first suggested by Eidels.[33]

The δM1 exon is terminated by a concensus RNA splice site located in the exactly analogous position as observed for μM1. Hybridization results indicate that the next DNA transcribed is a region beginning 220 bp further downstream. This area is homologous to the μM2 exon and splicing to this acceptor would lead to a carboxyl terminal peptide consisting of just two residues, valine and lysine. These are precisely the same amino acids that are found in the membrane form of μ and would presumably lie on the inside of the B-cell membrane.

Using the DNA sequence and assumptions mentioned above, we predict a molecular weight of 45.2 kd for the unglycosylated δ_m chain. This estimate is within 6% of the estimate of 48.5 kd determined for the *in vitro* translation product of δm RNA.[28] McCune et al.[34] have recently reported that for the human membrane δ chain no large cytoplasmic domain could be demonstrated by proteolytic digestion of *in vitro* products translated in a microsomal system. This is also consistent with our proposal of a small cytoplasmic protrusion.

Is δm Protein Expressed in Multiple Forms?

Data presented in our previous paper, elsewhere,[9,21,22,28] and below confirm the existence of more than one form of δm mRNA in both tumor and B-normal cells. An important question is whether this multiplicity is reflected at the protein level. The published cell-free translation data[28,34] are consistent with only one δm form. However, we should point out that beyond δM1 there are about 15 potential RNA acceptor splice sites other than δM2. Any one of these, if used, would lead to a different carboxy terminal peptide sequence. Moreover, a donor splice site occurs at the end of the δM2 exon coinciding with the protein terminator codon so

FIRST MU MEMBRANE EXON:

```
                                                         \  G   E
TCTCCAGAACCATCAGGGCACCCCAACCCTTATGCAAATGCTCAGTCACCCCAGACTTGGCTTGACCCTCCCTCTGTGTCCCTTCATAGAGGGGGAG
TCT AG      C ACTA     CT G    CAA AC   C ACC       TG T     A GA GA
TCTGTAGGGTGGAAGCCTTCTCATGAGCACTAGTTCTTCCCTAGGCATAGTCAACACCATCCAACACTCGTGTATCATGGATGAGCAAAGTGACAGCTAC
FIRST DELTA MEMBRANE EXON:  / I V N T I Q H S C I M D E Q S D S Y
```

```
V N A E E G F E N L W T T A S T F I V L F L L S L F Y S T T V T L
GTGAATGCTGAGGAGGGAGAGGCTTTGAGAACCTGGACCACTGCTTCCCTCACTTCATCGTCCTTCTTCCTCTCAGCCTCTTCTACAGCACCACCGTCACCC
TG A   GAGGAGGA       A   CCTGTGG   CCAC    T CACTTC T G CCTCTTCCT CT A  CT  TCTACAG   C  CGTCACC
ATGGACTTAGAGGAGGA......GAACGGCCTGTGGCCCACAATGTCACCTTCGTGGCCCTTCTGCTCACTCTTGTTTCCGGCCTTCGTCACCT
M D L E E E            N G L W P T H C T F V A L F L T L L Y S G F V T F
```

```
F K /
TGTTCAAGGTAGTA.........
T  TCAAGGTAG
TCATCAAGGTAGGCCTCCTACCACCTCCTTCTGAACCCTTCCTGGCACATGTAAGATACCCTTCCAGGGGCATTTTGAAACCTCGGTACTTCTGGAG
I K /
```

```
.............TGGTTGTGGGGCTGAGGACACAGGGCTGGGACAGGAGGTCACCAGTCCTGCCTCTACCTCTACTCCCTACAAGTGGA
             T TTG G GGC   GG CAC G  G  C GGG   A    C CAC G CT T  CCT T   C ACAA  G
TGGCTAGGGAATGCACAGTAATTGGGAGGCCATGGTCACTGTTCAGCTCTGTTCGGGCCCTATGTAGCTCCACGGACTTTCCGTTTCTCAGACAACAGCC
```

```
MU CYTOPLASMIC EXON:    \V K
CAGCAATTCACACTGTCTCTGTCACCTGCAGGTGAAATGACTTCTCAGCATGGAAGGACAGCGAGACCAAGAGATCCTCCCACAGGGACACTACCTCTGG
AT  ACT       TC C GCAGGTGAA T   C   CA   A C GCA AC AGA A   C C   A T   C
TCTGTAT..GACTTCAGGGCTCTTCTGGCAGGTGAAGTAGACCAGGACAGCGAGAATCCTGCAACTACAGAGAAAAGTGCTTTCCCTCAACATGAAGCCAA
DELTA CYTOPLASMIC EXON:  /V K  .
```

FIGURE 5. Comparison of μ and δ chain membrane exons. The sequence of μ is shown on the bottom and that of δ on the top. Bases that match are repeated in the middle. Amino acids are aligned with the first base of the corresponding codon. Regions that were gapped to bring the sequences into translation register are shown with dotted lines. Acceptor (\) and donor (/) RNA splice sites that begin and end the M1 exon are shown.

that an array of additional peptides conceivably could be coded beyond the Val-Lys sequence. A direct analysis of the membrane δ carboxyl termini at the amino acid sequence level plus analysis of many cloned mRNAs will be needed to establish whether any of the alternative patterns is used. This may be quite difficult to detect if this occurs rarely or only during transient states of cellular differentiation.

Length Differences in δm mRNAs Probably Result from Alternative Polyadenylation-Termination

Downstream of the Val-Lys sequence are two positions at which poly(A) addition could signal the end of the mRNA. Hybridization studies reported in the previous paper show that the 3' ends of the two major δm RNAs are correlated with these two sites identified in the sequence. Therefore the simplest assumption that fits the majority of the data is that the length difference between the 2.1 kb and 2.9 kb mRNA species results from 3' untranslated sequence heterogeneity and that there is no difference in the δm protein encoded by these two transcripts. A similar 3' heterogeneity generates multiple mRNA which code for the same protein in the mouse dihydrofolate reductase gene.[35]

The Role of Secreted IgD

It is now clear from the protein data of Finkelman *et al.*[8] and the finding of a specific δS terminal exon in the mouse germline that secretion of IgD, albeit in small amounts, is not an artifactual phenomena but instead must have biological importance. The unique organization of the Cδ gene has led us through the following logic. Carboxyl terminal domains of all H chain classes (eg., Cδ3 for δ; Cμ4 for μ) have a conserved donor RNA splice site exactly 64 bp 3' of the second invariant Cys residue (FIGURE 4). A resting B-cell or memory cell uses this sequence to splice to downstream exons, but in plasma cells, it is not used; instead it is read through to transcribe the adjacently coded sequence. This results in expression of the membrane terminal exon in resting cells and the secreted terminus in plasma cells. IgD, however, is different from all other Ig classes in the distal location of both secreted and membrane exons. This arrangement suggests to us that IgD could also be secreted from the resting B-cell. Some efferent signal from the B-cell is needed to account for the observation that in B-cell deficient (anti-μ suppressed) animals, antigen and idiotypic specific Lyt 1 bearing T-helper cells fail to develop.[36] In this role, secretion of IgD could serve as an antigen specific signal to the immune network, indicating the B-cell population level that is expressing each V region. The loss of IgD synthesis when the B-cell differentiates to a plasma cell would then be logical. Continuation of IgD synthesis would account for the small number of IgD secreting plasma cells that have been observed.[37]

Do Membrane IgD and IgM Deliver Different Signals to the Inside of the Cell?

We expected the general principle of membrane attachment demonstrated for μ would apply also to δ, but we were surprised that the amino acids coded by δM2 are identical to those of μM2. This is the portion of the protein that would presumably extend into the cytoplasm and which could deliver a signal to the cell's interior. Thus, according to this theory, our data would predict that the signal delivered to the inside of the cell by IgD would be identical to that delivered by IgM—at least if the nature of the signal is determined by the terminal amino acid sequence exposed to the cytoplasm. However, it should be born in mind that the entire immunoglobulin may be internalized as a result of antigenic stimulation, or other surface proteins (eg., Fc receptors) may interact specifically with δ and not μ. In this case the two Igs could deliver different signals despite the identical nature of the carboxyl-terminal residues.

The Functional Contribution of the Flexible Regions of IgD

With completion of the DNA sequences of the carboxyl terminal exons, we have determined what we think to be the complete structure of murine IgD. Some

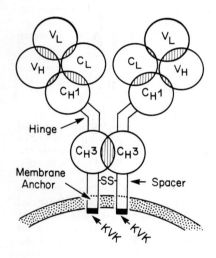

FIGURE 6. Schematic representation of cell surface IgD. Globular domains are drawn as circles and flexible regions as rectangles. Hatched areas denote major regions of non-covalent interaction between the chains. The 26 amino acid region proposed to lie between Cδ3 and the membrane is referred to as spacer. The transmembranal 26 residues are shown as the rectangle which passes through the lymphocyte membrane. The proposed short cytoplasmic protrusion (small black extension) has the sequence Lys-Val-Lys in both δ and μ chains.

of our present conclusions concerning the structure-function relationships of the sequence are illustrated in Figure 6. IgD is substantially different from all other mouse Igs in that the constant region has only two domains and a large part of the structure is contributed by flexible regions: the 35 amino acid hinge in both secreted and membrane forms, and a 26 amino acid "spacer" region that hypothetically separates the last domain from the transmembranal anchor.

The unusual δ hinge structure certainly correlates with the early suggestion[38] that proteolysis of this region plays a major role in B-cell triggering. The sequence is rich in tryptic-like cleavage sites which may be more exposed conformationally in the absence of inter-δ chain cysteine crosslinks. It may also be that these exposed amino acids would be involved in the instability of IgD in serum, a feature that would be crucial if the secreted molecule is to serve as an idiotype bearing chemical messenger. As shown in FIGURE 6, we predict that these same properties of the hinge in conjunction with its extended length allows the IgD molecule extreme flexibility. IgM, on the other hand, has restricted flexibility due to the lack of a hinge and the presence of two inter-μ chain disulfide bonds. These structural features correlate with the enhanced ability of surface IgD relative to IgM to bind pauci-valent antigens.[39]

The spacer segment of the membrane IgD molecule is far longer and shares little sequence homology with the corresponding segment of surface IgM. Perhaps this region serves as a target for some effector molecule interaction. In that regard, IgD is more effective than IgM in triggering B-cells by thymus-dependent antigens.[40] Regardless of the specific mechanism, the apparent identity of the internal amino acids makes it quite probable that the information pertinent to the differential roles of the IgD and IgM receptor resides on the outside of the B-cell membrane.

REFERENCES

1. COFFMAN, R. L. & M. COHN. 1977. J. Immunol. **118:** 806.
2. COZENZA, H. & H. KOHLER. 1972. Proc. Natl Acad. Sci. U.S.A. **69:** 2701.
3. EICHMAN, K. & K. RAJEWSKY. 1975. Eur. J. Immunol. **5:** 661.
4. VITETTA, E. S. & J. W. UHR. 1977. Immunol. Rev. **37:** 50.
5. BARGELLESI, A., G. CORTE, E. E. COSULICH & M. FERRARINI. 1979. Eur. J. Immunol. 490.
6. FINKELMAN, F. D., V. L. WOODS, A. BERNING & I. SCHER. 1979. J. Immunol. **123:** 1253.
7. VITETTA, E. S., E. PURÉ, P. C. ISAKSON, L. BUCK & J. W. UHR. 1980. Immunol. Rev. **52:** 211.
8. FINKELMAN, F. D., S. W. KESSLER, J. F. MUSHINSKI & M. POTTER. 1980. J. Immunol. **126:** 680.
9. MUSHINSKI, J. F., F. R. BLATTNER, J. D. OWENS, S. W. KESSLER, F. D. FINKELMAN, L. FITZMAURICE, M. POTTER & P. W. TUCKER. 1980. Proc. Natl. Acad. Sci. U.S.A. **77:** 7405.
10. TUCKER, P. W., C. P. LIU, J. F. MUSHINSKI & F. R. BLATTNER. 1980. Science **209:** 1353.
11. LIU, C. P., P. W. TUCKER, J. F. MUSHINSKI & F. R. BLATTNER 1980. Science **209:** 1348.
12. TUCKER, P. W., H-L. CHENG, J. F. MUSHINSKI, L. FITZMAURICE, C-P. LIU & F. R. BLATTNER. 1981. *In* B Lymphocytes in the Immune Response. N. KLINMAN, D. E. MOSIER, I. SCHER & E. S. VITETTA, Eds. **15:** 43. Elsevier/North Holland, the Netherlands.
13. FITZMAURICE, L., J. OWENS, H.-L. CHENG, P. W. TUCKER, C.-P. LIU, A. L. SHEN, F. R. BLATTNER & J. F. MUSHINSKI. 1981. *In* Immunoglobulins Idiotypes and Their Expression. C. JANEWAY, E. E. SERCARZ, H. WIGZELL & C. F. FOX, Eds. **1:** 263. Academic Press, N.Y.
14. TUCKER, P. W., R. ROBINSON, H-L. CHENG & F. R. BLATTNER. 1981. J. Supramol. Structure.
15. SPIEGELBERG, H. L. 1975. Nature **254:** 723.
16. LIN, L. C. & F. PUTMAN. 1979. Proc. Natl. Acad. Sci. U.S.A. **76:** 6572.
17. SIRE, J., G. ALCARAZ, A. BOURGOIS & B. JORDAN. 1981. Eur. J. Immunol. **11:** 632.
18. LIN, L.-C. & F. W. PUTNAM. 1981. Proc. Natl. Acad. Sci. U.S.A. **78:** 504.
19. PUTNAM, F. W., N. TAKAHASHI, D. TETAERT, B. DEBUIRE & L.-C. LIN. 1981. Proc. Natl. Acad. Sci. U.S.A. **78:** 6168.
20. CHENG, H.-L., F. R. BLATTNER, L. FITZMAURICE, J. F. MUSHINSKI & P. W. TUCKER. 1982. Nature. **296:** 410
21. FITZMAURICE, L., J. OWENS, F. R. BLATTNER, H.-L. CHENG, P. W. TUCKER & J. F. MUSHINSKI. 1982. Nature. **296:** 459.
22. Sequences of Immunoglobulin Chains. 1979. E. A. KABAT, T. T. WU & H. BILOFSKY. Eds. NIH Publication 80-2008; 138.
23. TUCKER, P. W., K. N. MARCU, N. NEWELL, J. E. RICHARDS & F. R. BLATTNER. 1979. Science **206:** 1303.
24. TUCKER, P. W., J. E. SLIGHTOM & F. R. BLATTNER. 1981. Proc. Natl. Acad. Sci. U.S.A. **78:** 7684.

25. ARNHEIM, N., P. SEPERACK, J. BANERJI, R. B. LANG, R. MIESFELD & K. N. MARCU. 1980. Cell **129:** 179.
26. DILDROP, R., & K. BEYREUTHER. 1981. Nature **292:** 61.
27. KEHRY, M., C. SIBLEY, C. FUHRMAN, J. SCHILLING & L. HOOD. 1979. Proc. Natl. Acad. Sci. U.S.A. **76:** 2932.
28. MAKI, R., W. ROEDER, A. TRAUNECKER, C. SIDMAN, M. WABL, W. RASCHKE & S. TONEGAWA. 1981. Cell **24:** 353.
29. GODING, J. W. & L. A. HERZENBERG. 1980. J. Immunol. **124:** 2540.
30. ROGERS, J., P. EARLY, C. CARTER, K. CALAME, M. BOND, L. HOOD & R. WALL. 1980. Cell **20:** 303.
31. EARLY, R., J. ROGERS, M. DAVIS, K. CALAME, M. BOND R. WALL & L. HOOD. 1980. Cell **20:** 313.
32. ALT, F. W., A. L. M. BOTHWELL, M. KNAPP, E. SIDEN, E. MATHER, M. KOSHLAND & D. BALTIMORE. 1980. Cell **20:** 293.
33. EIDELS, L. 1979. J. Immunol. **123:** 891.
34. MCCUNE, J. M., S. M. FU, H. C. KUNKEL & G. BLOBEL. 1981. Proc. Natl. Acad. Sci. U.S.A. **78:** 5127.
35. SETZER, D. R., M. MCGROGAN, J. H. NUNBERG & R. T. SCHIMKE. 1980. Cell **22:** 361.
36. JANEWAY, C. A., JR., R. A. MURGITA, F. I. WEINBAUM, R. ASOFSKY & H. WIGZELL. 1975. Proc. Natl. Acad. Sci. U.S.A. **74:** 4582.
37. BARGELLESI, A. G., G. CORTE, E. COSULICH & M. FERRARINI. 1979. Eur. J. Immunol. **9:** 490.
38. VITETTA, E. S. & J. W. UHR. 1975. Science **189:** 964.
39. PURÉ, E. & E. S. VITETTA. 1980. J. Immunol. **125:** 420.
40. SIDMAN, C. L. & E. R. UNANE. 1978. Proc. Natl. Acad. Sci. U.S.A. **75:** 2401.

———————◆———————

DISCUSSION OF THE THREE PRECEDING PAPERS

C. BRANT (Columbia University, New York, N.Y.): I'm curious about the inverted repeat structure found in portions of the DNA. Have you been able to relate those to any other repeated sequences?

F. R. BLATTNER: Julia Richards is giving a poster on this topic. However, we don't find these sequences involved. They tend to be very simple and many of them are dimers or repeating hexamers. There is a strong resemblance between one of the sequences and a sequence that is found in the ribosomal spacer, but that I think is CA to the Nth power so that's not too interesting.

F. D. FINKELMAN: There's a lot of interest in the idea that memory cells may exist which are, or could be, synthesizing RNA's for γ and δ or μ and γ or μ-γ and δ, all simultaneously using the same V region. Do any of these multiple splicer and acceptor sites found in the sequencing done so far provide any mechanism by which such a long mRNA could be processed to give rise to shorter mRNAs so that these three isotypes could simultaneously coexist?

P. W. TUCKER: My guess is that one might want to make a μ-γ memory type molecule by both mechanisms Fred Blattner discussed: that of deletion and that of multiple expression of two isotypes. In this case, the γ concentration would replace, possibly in the context of the DNA, the δ so there would be a deletion of δ, thus bringing gamma sequences closer to μ. There has been no proof of this. I think David Baltimore has observed a spontaneous switch in the Abelson system of a μ-γ 2b.

FINKELMAN: Any possible evidence for a δ-γ?

TUCKER: To my knowledge there's no evidence for it. However, it might require deletion of μ or possibly two deletions because one would have to move a γ. You'd have to get μ out of the way, too. I think there is a myeloma that was a δ-γ.

BLATTNER: I talked to Marty Weigart about the δ-γ myeloma. He said it is gone. Regarding your question of whether there's a sequence in front of delta that corresponds to so-called switch sequences in front of μ: All myeloma studies have shown, at the DNA level, that recombination occurs between the sequence right in front of μ, and a sequence 5', let's say to α, to produce an α secretor, and that is called the switch sequence. Honjo and Tonagawa have sequenced it. The sequence is a repeat of five bases.

TUCKER: The bases are: GAGCT.

BLATTNER: GAGCT and then also something like 4Gs with a T. In front of all of the immunoglobulin classes, except δ, there are similar sequences. Instead, δ has a six-base repeat that is completely different. We have proposed these repeat sequences might serve to recombine, in a different manner, not with the sequences in front of μ but in front of the γs so that by deleting at the B-cell level you can make a μ-$\times$ double producer. In order to secrete δ you would somehow have to get a recombination between these two nonhomologous switch sites. I would expect that to be rare, which would explain why TEPC-type tumors, delta secretion, and delta secretory cells are rare.

PARKHOUSE: I wonder if anyone can tell us whether there is anything different in the disposition of the DNA in cells that make μ but don't make δ, e.g., pre-B-cells or the early B-cells, and a variety of the B-cell IgM tumors and pre-B-cell tumors?

TUCKER: There has only been gross analysis of this at the level of doing a Southern blot. Generally, the conclusion is that the locus is not rearranged to the right. I think that it should be looked into in more detail because subtle changes in the δ locus would not be picked up at this level.

BLATTNER: If the analysis of the B-cell indicates that no change is taking place, then you have to assume that a pre-B-cell modification would have to be reversed.

M. D. COOPER: Considering the complexity of the δ gene, it's not too surprising that it takes developing B-cells some time to learn to use it and that very few plasma cells ever seem to get the message. But with regard to trying to understand some of the complexities at an expression level in B-cell differentiation, is there any information about how the messengers were used or, for example, is there any evidence on the relative stabilities of the message for δ and for μ and is there any evidence for translational control? For example, your BCL_1 makes very little δ relative to μ. Is that reflected by the level of the messages as well?

F. MUSHINSKI: We don't know as much about that as we would like. The problem is that it's so difficult to detect the δ messages in anything but the myelomas. It takes a lot of work and RNA to get a small amount of δ RNA from any other source. It is also difficult to detect δ on the surface of BCL_1. A colleague suggests that there is 100 times more μ than δ. In preliminary hybridization studies it appears that there is probably about 100th as much δ message as μ message in these cells. We are pursuing this question.

D. SIECKMANN: There was some data coming out of Ellen Vitetta's lab about a year ago showing the BCL_1 tumor could be stimulated by anti-immunoglobulin *in vitro*. Has anyone looked at changes in messages in the cells after activation as a result of such stimulation?

TUCKER: Yes, we have been doing some of that but primarily with LPS. The μ

gene is certainly under transcriptional control. When you add LPS you induce the secreted form of message, but if you don't do it in all or none fashion, there's still a lot of membrane mRNA formed and yet membrane IgM, based on peptide labeling the surface protein, is not present in the amount that would be dictated by the amount of membrane message. So overall RNA synthesis goes up, but the amount of surface IgM doesn't. In the case of IgD again working with the B-cell line, it's very difficult to follow. We don't see any evidence that IgD is induced by LPS.

E. VITETTA: I'd just like to reiterate that when you treat most tumors or most normal B-cells with mitogens IgD disappears so that's not a very good model to study induction of RNA. There is one model where it goes up and that is BCL_1 cultured in the absence of mitogens and anti-Igs and there the expression goes up considerably. I think that's the model one wants to use.

TUCKER: We haven't been able to demonstrate that the RNA goes up in those cells but again we are looking at an RNA species that is present in approximately 1/100 of the amount of the μ. I guess you are seeing three to fourfold increases at the surface. We may not even detect that, it's so low. It certainly doesn't go in a parallel fashion. It could be that this has something to do with the stabilization of the δ message.

THE LAST OF THE IMMUNOGLOBULINS: COMPLETE AMINO ACID SEQUENCE OF HUMAN IgD*

Frank W. Putnam, Nobuhiro Takahashi, Daniel Tetaert,
Lien-Ching Lin, and Brigitte Debuire

Department of Biology
Indiana University
Bloomington, Indiana 47405

INTRODUCTION

Since the first reports of the complete amino acid sequence of human κ and λ light chains[1,2] in 1966 and 1967, which led to the recognition of V and C regions, there has been great interest in the structure, genetic control and function of all classes of immunoglobulins. Though most attention was focussed on the genetic origin and structural diversity of the V regions and their relationship to the combining site of antibodies, there also was an intensive effort to establish the structure of the constant (C) regions of the heavy (H) chains of different classes of immunoglobulins and to relate their structure to individual biological effector functions.[3] Such an enormous body of structural data quickly developed so that it can now only be summarized by computer printouts in atlases of protein sequence.[4,5] In fact, even before the tide of DNA sequences of cloned genes for immunoglobulins began to sweep in beginning about 1978, already from one quarter to one third of all protein and peptide amino acid sequences were for immunoglobulins, largely for myeloma proteins from man and the mouse. FIGURE 1 illustrates the exponential increase in total amino acid sequence data for immunoglobulins of all species since our first report[6] of the partial sequence of a human κ Bence Jones protein in January of 1965, followed by the sequences of the κ, λ, and γ chains. With the development of automated protein sequencers, the complete structure of human IgM, IgE, and IgA (that is, the μ, ϵ, and α heavy chains in FIGURE 1) and also various subclasses and allotypes thereof soon followed.[3] But the structure of the fifth—and presumably the last—class of immunoglobulins remained elusive until this day. Why was this the case if IgD is so important as to be the focus of an entire conference of The New York Academy of Sciences?

Although IgD was discovered as a fifth class of human immunoglobulins more than 15 years ago, structural study of the IgD protein was greatly hindered by several factors. First, the low concentration of normal serum IgD, the rarity of IgD myeloma patients, and the uncertainty for a time as to whether a homologue of IgD existed in the mouse or other species. Second, the notorious susceptibility of IgD to "spontaneous" enzymatic degradation either in serum or during preparation. Third, the initial failure to identify significant biological functions for IgD. However, interest in the structure of IgD intensified after the evidence that IgD exists in two forms: sIgD secreted into serum and mIgD bound to the surface membrane of B-lymphocytes, where it functions as a receptor or recognition unit involved in B-cell differentiation and proliferation to produce antibody-forming

*This work was supported by Grants CA08497 from the National Cancer Institute and IM-2G from the American Cancer Society.

0077–8923/82/0399–0041$01.75/0 © 1982, NYAS

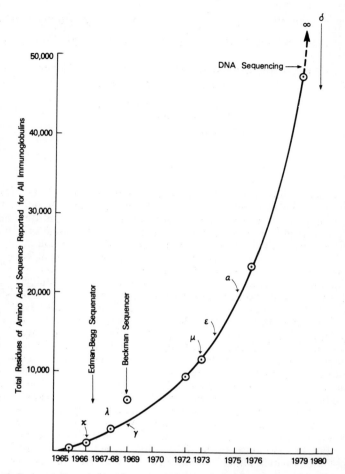

FIGURE 1. Increase in amino acid sequence data for immunoglobulins of all species since the first reports for the human κ chain in 1965 that revealed the existence of V and C regions.[1,6] The dates for the completion of the sequence of human κ, λ, γ, μ, ϵ, α, and δ chains are indicated.

cells.[7,8] The cloning and structural studies of the mouse δ chain reported by the preceding speakers,[9] as well as papers yet to come on its biological role, will focus interest on novel forms of IgD and raise questions about their number and role. It is our purpose here to present a definitive structure for human IgD; thus far this appears to be the only known structural form of human IgD, excluding δ chains that probably differ only in their tailpieces.

Structural Model of Human IgD

The structural model for human IgD was long in question because of ambiguity about the number of C region domains and the size of the human δ

chain. Probably because of effects due to its high carbohydrate content, earlier estimates of the size of the human δ chain ranged from 60,000 to 69,000 daltons; this led to suggestions that the δ chain, like μ and ε, might contain four C region domains.[7,8] By determination of the complete amino acid sequence of the δ heavy chain[10] and the λ light chain[11] of IgD myeloma protein WAH we have been able to construct a structural model for human IgD (FIGURE 2). The methods for the structural study are described elsewhere,[12-15] as well as the evidence that the partial sequence data for all other human IgD proteins thus far reported fits with our model. Our complete sequence data make it absolutely clear that the human δ chain has four domains: one V region domain (V$_H$) and three C region domains (Cδ1, Cδ2, and Cδ3), as well as an exceptionally long hinge region that adds to its length. The light chain is linked by a disulfide bond to Cys-C15 in the δ chain, and the two δ heavy chains are joined by a disulfide bridge at Cys-C161 to form a tetrachain monomeric molecule. Among human immunoglobulin classes, IgD is unique in having its two heavy chains linked by a single disulfide bridge. We have established the disulfide bridges and we have identified the carbohydrate at each site shown. Unreduced human IgD behaves as a monomer in gel filtration and in sedimentation studies, but, it is very susceptible to proteolytic degradation by trypsin, papain, and unknown serum proteases to yield a number of Fab and Fc fragments because of cleavage at several bonds in the hinge region. These and other less well characterized proteolytic fragments will not be described here; however, the unusual lability of IgD must be an important determinant in the regulation of and perhaps in the expression of its biological function.

   It is the extended length of the human δ chain hinge (64 residues) and the high content of carbohydrate in IgD (about 12%) that led to the misconception that IgD might have five domains. It is not human IgD that differs from the norm, but

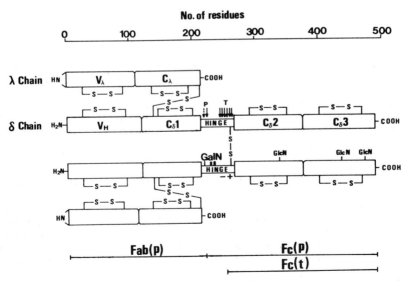

FIGURE 2. Schematic structural model for human IgD. (Modified from Lin and Putnam.)[12] GalN and GlcN denote oligosaccharides attached (galactosamine and glucosamine, respectively).

rather apparently it is mouse IgD. We have already heard that the DNA sequence of the mouse δ chain indicates the absence of the Cδ2 domain,[9] a deletion not yet reported, we believe, in any human immunoglobulin. Also, mouse IgD may exist on the surface of cells as a half molecule consisting of one δ chain linked to one light chain, and this accords with the absence in the mouse δ chain of the interchain disulfide bridge present at the end of the hinge of the human δ chain (FIGURE 2).

Amino Acid Sequence of the Human δ Chain

FIGURE 3 gives the complete amino acid sequence of the human δ chain WAH. This δ chain contains 512 amino acid residues; the molecular weight of the polypeptide chain portion is 56,213. The three GlcN glycans with $M_r \simeq 2,000$ and four or five GalN glycans each with $M_r \simeq 700$ would contribute about 9000 daltons for the carbohydrate portion yielding a total molecular weight of about 65,000. This accords well with the value of 66,000 $\pm$ 1,000 that we estimated[12] from electrophoresis in sodium dodecyl sulfate/polyacrylamide gel (SDS-PAGE). By determination of the complete amino acid sequence of the δ chain we have shown that there are only three C region domains (Cδ1, Cδ2, and Cδ3) but that the extended length of the δ hinge makes the δ chain intermediate in size between the μ and ϵ chains on one hand and the γ and α chains on the other.[10-15] To facilitate comparison, the principal characteristics of the five major classes and of some subclasses of the C regions of human heavy chains are listed in TABLE 1. In the following discussion we will consider the main characteristics of the human δ chain in their order from the amino terminus to the carboxyl terminus, namely the V region, the CDR3-J$_H$ region, the Cδ1 domain, the δ hinge, the Fc region, and the tailpiece.

The V Region and the CDR3 Segment

The WAH δ chain has the longest V region yet reported for human immunoglobulins, i.e., it has 129 amino acids compared to 126 in the Ou μ chain, the longest previously recorded.[16] It is difficult to compare V regions because of their differences in length. Therefore, we have used a double numbering system; one set of numbers represents the actual position beginning with the amino terminus, the other set accords with the computer-adjusted numbering system of Kabat et al.[4] In the latter case each of the framework (FR) sections and the complementarity determining regions (CDR) has a defined set of numbers for boundaries; insertions (extra residues), which occur most commonly in the CDR3 segment, are numbered 100A, 100B, as an example.

The V region of the WAH δ chain has a unique amino end group (arginine), a high concentration and clustering of aromatic amino acids, and exceptional length. However, it clearly belongs to heavy chain subgroup II because it has 37 of the 41 residues assigned as "invariant" in that subgroup.[4] The fact that the WAH δ chain has arginine as its amino end group instead of the blocked end group of pyrrolidone-carboxylic acid (hitherto almost invariant in subgroup II) simply shows the fallacy of classifying heavy chain V region subgroups just by the first few amino acids, as has often been done.

This δ chain is remarkable for the clustering of aromatic residues in the CDR1 region where the sequence Tyr-Tyr-Trp-Gly-Trp- occurs (see Tyr-34) and in

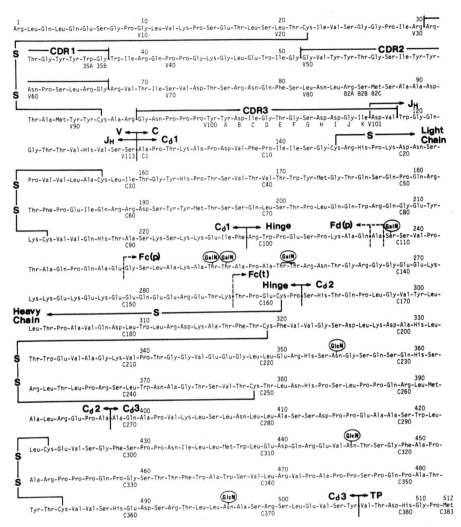

FIGURE 3. Complete amino acid sequence of the δ chain of human IgD WAH (from Takahashi *et al.*).[10] A double numbering system is used; the upper set represents the actual position beginning with the amino terminus. In the V region the lower set accords with the computer-adjusted system of Kabat *et al.*[4] which takes account of insertions (numbered, A, B, etc) in the complementarity determining regions (CDR). In the lower set the C region residues are designated C and are numbered consecutively beginning with Ala-C1. The hinge region has four (or five) GalN oligosaccharides attached, and the Fc region has three GlcN oligosaccharides. Points of limited cleavage by papain (p) or trypsin (t) are shown by dash lines. The probable boundaries of each domain, and of J_H, the hinge region, and the tailpiece (TP) are shown.

CDR2 where there are two Tyr-Tyr- sequences (see Tyr-54 and Tyr-60), as well as one Tyr-Tyr-sequence in CDR3 (see Tyr-105). There is a similar clustering of aromatic residues in CDR1 of the λ light chain of this IgD where the sequence Tyr-Val-Tyr-Trp-Tyr- occurs.[11] Thus, the CDR regions of this IgD protein epitomize the "ring-of-rings" discovered by Edmundson et al.[17] to be major determinants of combining specificity, especially for aromatic ligands.

The CDR3 segment, earlier called the third hypervariable region (HV3) or the hypervariable deletion region,[3] is known to be the major determinant of the size

TABLE 1

NUMBER OF AMINO ACID RESIDUES, DOMAINS, AND OLIGOSACCHARIDES IN THE C
REGIONS OF HUMAN HEAVY CHAINS

| Chain | C_H domains | Residues | | Oligosaccharides | |
		Hinge*	C region	GalN (hinge)	GlcN (domains)
δ	3	64	383	4 or 5	3
γ1	3	15	329	0	1
γ2	3	12	325	0	1
γ3	3	62	375	0	1
α1	3	26	353	5	2
α2	3	13	340	0	4,5†
μ‡	4		450		5
ε‡	4		420		6

*Estimates of the length of the human hinge regions are approximate. Lengths given for the γ3 and ε chains are estimates because the sequences are incomplete.

†The A2m(1) allotype of the α2 chain has four GlcN oligosaccharides, and the A2m(2) allotype has five.[26]

‡The μ and ε chains lack a hinge region but have an extra (fourth) C_H domain.

and shape of the antibody combining site and of idiotypic determinants. In a survey of human H chains we found[10] that the CDR3 segment varied from 7 to 17 residues and that differences in length of the V region are mainly manifested in CDR3. It is no surprise then that the exceptional length of the WAH V region is due to the fact that its CDR3 segment contains 19 residues and thus is the longest yet recorded for a human H chain. The CDR3 segment of the amino acid sequence essentially coincides with what is called the D or diversity segment in the DNA sequence, which is on the 5′ side of a separate exon that codes for the end of the V region. Potential germ-line sequences for the D segment are just beginning to be reported for human[18] and mouse[19] DNA. Their size is variable and is smaller than the usual CDR3 region, and their number in the germ line is unknown. Recent evidence suggests that the human D segments are encoded in tandem multigene families and that they may recombine and be read in different frames.[18]

In view of the unusual length of the CDR3 segment of the WAH δ chain we searched for homology with CDR3 in other human H chains and found none; each CDR3 sequence appeared to be unique. Accordingly, we asked Dr. Winona

C. Barker of the *Atlas of Protein Sequence and Structure* to make a computer search of their entire library of amino acid sequence of proteins of all kinds for homology to the 30-residue section of the WAH δ chain positions 100 to 129 that represent CDR3 and J_H. Of course, because of the variability of CDR3 we expected no identical sequence, and indeed there was none. Of almost 210,000 segments of length 30 compared, the first 41 that had nine or more identities included the CDR3-J_H area of the V region of immunoglobulin chains; most of the identities were in the J_H area and the sequences all terminated at the end of the V region. To our surprise, the highest score (14 identities) was for two mouse heavy chain V regions (FIGURE 4). Human and mouse H chain V regions were about equally represented for scores of 13 and 12, and dog and rabbit H chains were among those scoring 11. In fact, the degree of homology of the CDR3-J_H segment is unrelated to the species, class or subgroup of heavy chain. No significant relationship was found between the CDR3-J_H segment and the C region sequence of any immunoglobulin, nor was any important difference in the order found when the genetic code matrix was used in place of the unitary matrix. Hence, we conclude that neither CDR3 nor J_H have any evolutionary relationship to genes coding for the C region. However, from a separate computer search not described here, we have identified strong homologies in amino acid sequence that suggest that the J regions of all immunoglobulin chains of all species have a common evolutionary origin. Indeed, most of the homology shown in FIGURE 4 is in the J_H region in both species.

These results do pose a baffling question about the genetic control of CDR3 segments of amino acid sequence and about the number and the nature, and the kinds of interaction of the D segments of DNA that lie between the V genes and the J_H exons for heavy chains. A DNA exon codes precisely for every other discrete functional segment of immunoglobulin polypeptide chains (V, J_H, hinge, each C region domain, and the tailpiece), but the genetic control of the region most important in antibody specificity (CDR3) is still unknown.[18-20]

The Constant Region of the Human Delta Chain

Because mouse IgD lacks the Cδ2 domain,[9] we wish to emphasize that the C region domain structure of human IgD has no remarkable features or deletions. As has been found with other immunoglobulin classes,[3] each of the three C region domains of the δ chain is homologous to each other and each Cδ domain is also homologous to the corresponding C_H domain in other human heavy chains. FIGURE 5 illustrates the fact that the C_H1 domains of the five classes of human heavy chains have about the same degree of homology when compared pairwise to each other (≈30%). In fact, 55 residues in the Cδ1 domain, or about half, are identical to one or more residues at the same position in the C_H1 domain of the other four human heavy chains. Comparison of the sequence of the Fc regions of the five classes of heavy chains gave a similar result.[13,21] The overall homology of Fcδ to the Fc of the other four chains ranges from 22 to 25%.

Likewise, the human δ chain has the same pattern of internal homology that is exhibited by other heavy chains; this is a consequence of the fact that each domain has the three-dimensional structure of the immunoglobulin fold. This is illustrated in FIGURE 6 which shows the homology of the Cδ1, Cδ2, and Cδ3 domains using the three invariant cysteine and tryptophan positions as a register. The only unusual feature is the clustering of proline residues in Cδ3. Thus, except

FIGURE 4. Homology of the CDR3 and J_H segments of human and mouse immunoglobulin heavy chains as aligned by a computer comparison of the 30-residue sequence of the CDR3 and J_H segments of the WAH δ chain with the entire library of amino acid sequence data reported for all proteins. The score gives the number of identities with the CDR3-J_H sequence of IgD WAH. Sources of the immunoglobulin sequences are from standard atlases.[4,5]

	Heavy Chain		Score	Residues	
Hu	II	WAH δ	30	89	118
Mo	III	T601 α	14	107	136
Mo	I	MOPC315 α	14	88	117
Hu	II	Newm γ1	13	86	115
Hu	III	Til γ2,μ	13	93	122
Hu	III	Ga μ	13	88	117
Mo		X24	13	94	123
Mo	III	TEPC15* α	13	88	117
Mo	II	104E μ	13	90	119
Hu	II	Daw γ1	12	92	121
Hu	II	He γ1	12	92	121
Mo		MPC11	12	115	144
Mo		MOPC141#	12	95	124
Mo	III	MOPC511 α1	12	—	—

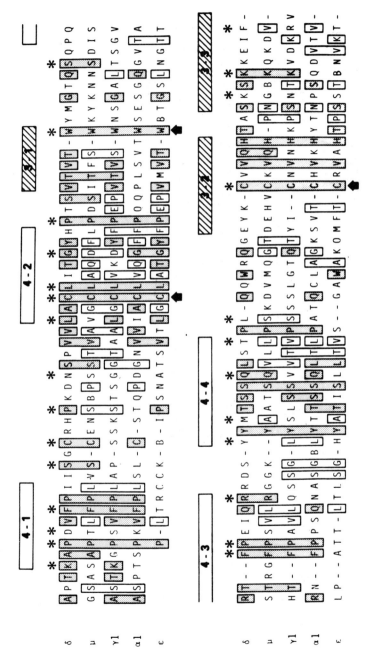

FIGURE 5. Comparison of the amino acid sequences of the C_H1 domains of the five classes of immunoglobulins. In this and in subsequent similar figures, the three invariant cysteine (C) and tryptophan (W) residues in each domain were used to place the alignment in register, and gaps were inserted to maximize the homology. Residues in the μ, γ, α, or ϵ sequences that share identity with the corresponding residues in the δ chain are outlined in shaded boxes; residues that are identical in sequences other than the delta chain are outlined in open boxes. The β-strands are numbered according to Edmundson *et al.*[17] with the four-stranded β-elements in open bars and the three-stranded β-sheets in hatched bars. Stars denote residues that are identical in the $C\delta1$ domains of human and mouse IgD. (Modified from Putnam *et al.*)[14]

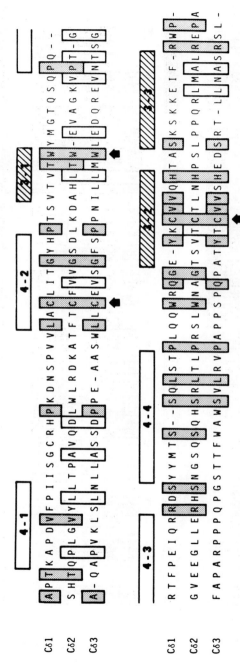

FIGURE 6.   Homology among the Cδ1, Cδ2, and Cδ3 domains of the human δ chain. The hinge region is not shown.

for its remarkable hinge region, the human δ chain has no exceptional features that cause it to deviate from the general principles established for heavy chains.

The Hinge Region

The hinge region is an unusual structure in the segment of the heavy chain that joins the Fd and Fc regions of immunoglobulin classes having only three C_H domains (IgG, IgA, and IgD) but is absent in IgM and IgE, which have four C_H domains (TABLE 1). The amino acid sequence of the hinge region is unique for each class, differs markedly even for subclasses, and appears to be unrelated to the rest of the H chain.[3] In γ and α chains the hinge region is rich in proline and cysteine; thus, it probably has a random flexible structure that pivots on multiple interchain disulfide bridges conveying a segmental flexibility that is thought to transduce a signal from the antibody combining site to the biological effector domains of Fc. The discovery that the hinge region of IgG is encoded precisely by a separate exon[20] helped explain the frequency of deletions and duplications in the hinge regions of IgG and IgA subclasses, but the γ and α hinge exons did not seem to fit into the evolutionary scheme linking all V and C region domains to a common ancestral gene. With this background we can now review the unusual features of the human δ chain hinge and its differences from that in the mouse.

The hinge of the human δ chain differs from the hinges in the γ and α chains of both man and animals in four critical characteristics: (1) its length (≈64 residues), which is about four times the length of the γ1, γ2, and α2 hinges and twice that of the α1 hinge though similar to that of the quadruplicated γ3 hinge (TABLE 1); 2) its division into two distinct segments (the GalN-rich NH_2-terminal half, which is very resistant to proteolytic enzymes, and the high-charge COOH-terminal half, which is very susceptible to proteases), 3) its dominant composition and repetitive pattern (alanine and threonine in the first half and glutamic acid and lysine in the second half versus cysteine and proline in the γ and α chains); and 4) the presence of only one half-cystine.

The human δ hinge is clearly divided into two parts (FIGURE 7). When we attempted to predict the conformation by the method of Chou and Fasman,[22] no clear result was obtained for the first half—the GalN-rich segment (~C99-C132) which appears to have a random structure. However, the high-charge region from Glu-C140 through Glu-C155 appears to form an ideal α-helical segment with four turns. It is this latter segment that is so suceptible to cleavage by trypsin and other serine proteases, presumably including those naturally present in blood. Thus, it was difficult to prepare the undegraded IgD that was necessary for structural study of this area. Since a well-defined α-helical structure is rare in immunoglobulins, we suppose the high-charge segment of the hinge is important in modulating the signal for conformational change that passes from the antibody site to the cell receptor size. The absence in the mouse δ hinge of the counterpart to the high-charge segment of the human δ hinge is puzzling and may reflect different biological functions for the two kinds of IgD.

The evolutionary origin of the hinge is unknown, and the hinge is the most mutable region in immunoglobulin chains, as shown by the frequency of deletions and duplications.[3] This caused us to search for homology in the C regions of other heavy chains, particularly in the μ chain which has an extra domain ($C\mu2$) where the hinge occurs in the δ chain. We searched the $C\mu2$ domain for possible homology to the δ chain hinge with the results shown in FIGURE 8. In

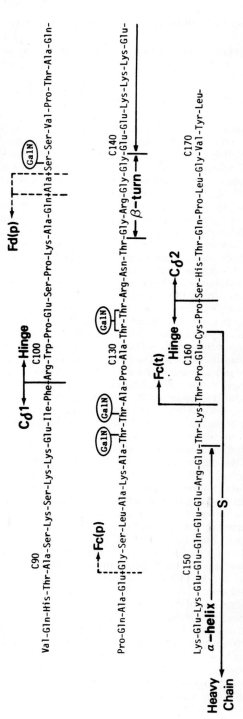

FIGURE 7. The hinge region of the human δ chain WAH. In the predicted conformation a β-turn separates the random structure of the GalN-rich region from the α-helical region, which is followed by the first β-sheet of the Cδ2 domain.

the GalN-rich segment of the human δ hinge, 12 of 36 successive residues are identical to a segment from the middle of the second C region domain (Cμ2) of the human μ chain except for uncertainty at Gln-C117 and Glu-C119. The same positions are identical in the dog μ chain, and most also are in the mouse μ chain. The 30-residue segment outlined in FIGURE 8 also scored highest in a computer search of about 180,000 segments of the same length in the data bank of the Atlas of Protein Sequence and Structure. A similar computer search using the genetic code matrix instead of the unitary matrix suggested that the first and second segments of the human δ hinge may have a common evolutionary relationship despite the fact that their primary and secondary structures are dissimilar. Thus, we have proposed that two human δ-hinge exons may have arisen by duplication and subsequent mutation of a common ancestral exon derived from the primordial gene for the Cμ2 domain, whereas evolutionary deletion of one hinge exon may have led to the half-size murine hinge.[10,14] This hypothesis fits with the evidence for the frequency of mutations, deletions, and duplications in the γ and α hinge regions.[3] If this hypothesis is correct, the hinge regions of human and mouse IgD may have acquired somewhat different biological functions, or there may be several forms of IgD in each species differentiated primarily by the site and extent of the deletions.

The Fc Region

Immunoglobulins of all classes in most species are subject to limited proteolytic cleavage to yield Fab and Fc fragments. However, the points of cleavage of the heavy chain, and the sizes and stability of the fragments vary greatly with the class and species of the immunoglobulin molecule. Human IgD is unique in its extreme susceptibility in vitro and presumably in vivo to various proteolytic enzymes. Indeed, the proclivity for spontaneous cleavage of human IgD by serum proteases during conventional isolation and storage procedures has hindered structural study because an intact δ chain is required to establish the complete primary structure. We were fortunate that a large amount of intact IgD WAH could be prepared with care in a simple two-step procedure. Also, we were able to obtain a stoichiometric yield of Fabδ(p) and Fcδ(p) after incubation of the intact IgD with papain for only 10 min at 37°C in the absence of cysteine. Brief treatment with trypsin of the Fcδ(p) fragment yielded a smaller Fcδ(t) fragment and several hinge peptides.

The complete amino acid sequence of the Fcδ(t) fragment was determined;[13] it is 226 residues long and includes three glucosamine-containing glycans, one in the Cδ2 domain and two in the Cδ3 domain. Shinoda et al.[21] obtained an identical sequence for the entire Fc region of another human IgD protein (NIG-65). Others have reported a similar amino-terminal sequence for various other human IgD proteins.[8] Hence, there can be no doubt that a Cδ2 domain is present in many, if not at all, human IgD proteins.

An alignment of the Fc sequences for the five classes of human immunoglobulins showed that the distribution of homologous residues is not random but can be characterized into several patterns that are revealed in the spatial model for IgD. FIGURE 9 illustrates this for the last domain of the five human heavy chains. Residues that are highly conserved tend to be clustered within segments of β-pleated sheet, especially around the two cysteines that form the intrachain disulfide bond and a tryptophan that is nearby in the three-dimensional structure.

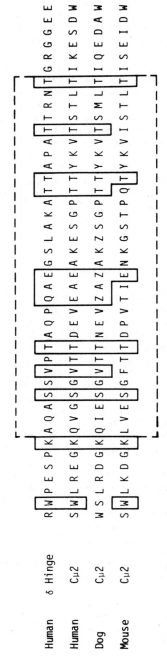

FIGURE 8. Identities in amino acid sequence of the Ga1N-rich segment of the hinge region of the human δ chain and the Cμ2 domain of human, dog, and mouse μ chains. Sequences aligned as having the highest identity in a computer search are enclosed by dashed lines. [From Putnam et al.][14]

Despite this common pattern, there are several areas where the δ chain diverges significantly from the other four heavy chains. Perhaps the most unique aspect of the δ chain is the large number of proline residues and their clustering at both the front and back ends of the Cδ3 domain (see FIGURE 9). Because proline residues tend to change the course of the polypeptide backbone, such clustering will necessarily affect the surface conformation of Cδ3, the very domain of IgD that is bound to the B-cell membrane. Two GlcN oligosaccharides are close to the back end of the Fc region and their polysaccharide chains probably spread over the outside surface of the Cδ3 domain. Counterparts of these two glycans are lacking in the last domain of other human heavy chains. Although there are differences from domain to domain, the overall homology of Fcδ to the Fc regions of the other four human heavy chains is about 25%; this is somewhat lower than the homology of other Fc pairs to each other and has led to the suggestion that the δ chain emerged early in evolution as an independent branch in the topology.[13,21]

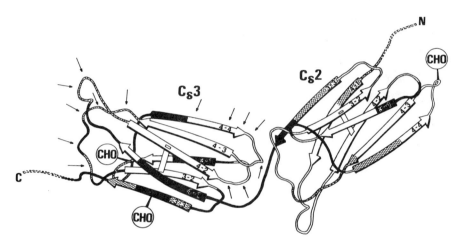

FIGURE 9. Spatial model of the IgD Fc region. The shading on the polypeptide backbone indicates the extent of sequence homology with the four other human heavy chains: open, highly conserved; cross-hatched, high divergence; solid, high homology among all except the δ chain. Arrows indicate the clustering of proline residues in Cδ3. (From Lin and Putnam.)[13]

The fact that a common framework structure is present in the C region of all heavy chains is illustrated by FIGURE 10, which compares only the carboxyl-terminal domain of the human δ, μ, γ, α, and ε chains. There are nine positions that appear invariant in the last domain in all five chains. It is noteworthy that eight of these are also identical in mouse Cδ3. Furthermore whereas Cδ3 is only 20–25% homologous to the last domains of the other four human chains, it is about 53% homologous to Cδ3 of the mouse (see starred positions in FIGURE 10). This is twice as great as the homology of Cδ1 of mouse and man (FIGURE 5). Thus, the domain that has the cytotropic function is most alike in the human and mouse δ chains.

Of course, binding to the cell membrane is thought to be vested in the tailpiece at the COOH-terminus of the heavy chain, and there is evidence that tailpieces of the secreted and membrane forms of IgD differ, just as they do for IgM.[9]

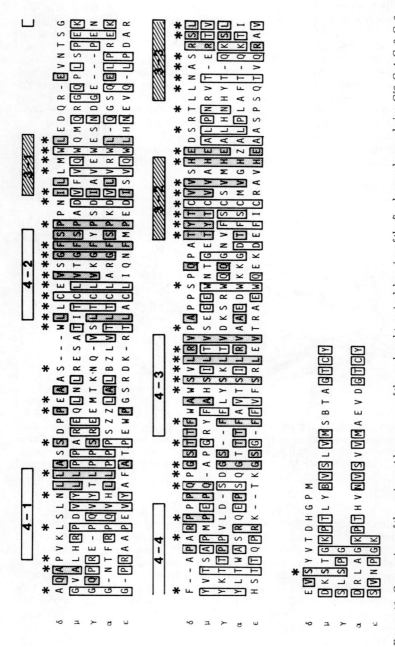

FIGURE 10. Comparison of the amino acid sequences of the carboxyl-terminal domains of the five human heavy chains: Cδ3, Cμ4, Cγ3, Cα3, and Cε4. Residues in the μ, γ, α, or ε chains that share identity with δ are outlined by shaded boxes; residues that show homology among sequences other than the δ chain are outlined in open boxes. Residues in the mouse Cδ3 that are identical with human Cδ3 are starred. (Modified from Lin and Putnam.)[13]

However, as seen in the next two sections, the tailpiece of the secreted human δ chain is unlike that of the human α and μ chains and, surprisingly, has no resemblance to the tailpiece of mouse δ.

The Oligosaccharides of Human IgD

The preceding sections have shown that except for the hinge region and the tailpiece, the polypeptide structure of the δ chain of human IgD conforms to the same general principles as the other four classes of human H chains. These principles are dictated by the common requirement for a series of contiguous domains, the conformation of each of which is molded into the immunoglobulin fold. However, all human H chains have at least one oligosaccharide attached, ranging from γ with one to $\alpha1$ with seven.[3] The human δ chain is rich in carbohydrate having three GlcN glycans and four or five GalN glycans. Determination of the number, nature, and location of the oligosaccharides was a difficult problem that is described elsewhere.[15] We acknowledge the help and advice of Dr. J. Baenziger who is determining the structure of each oligosaccharide in purified IgD glycopeptides we have given him.

Of most interest for the present conference is the comparison of the oligosaccharides of the five classes of human immunoglobulins, which is given in FIGURE 11, and also the comparison of the oligosaccharides in human and mouse IgD, which is discussed later. All human heavy chains contain at least one GlcN glycan which is N-linked to the asparagine in the tripeptide acceptor sequence Asn-X-Thr/Ser, where X can be any amino acid though usually not proline, and the third residue is either threonine or serine. Since this sequence dictates a β-turn, the GlcN glycans can be expected to be between domains or on a polypeptide turn at the surface of the molecule, which accords with their hydrophilicity. The GlcN glycans have molecular weights of about 2000 and may be complex heterosaccharides with di- and tri-branched structures or may be rich in mannose. In contrast, the GalN glycans are small and are usually di- or tri-saccharides; they are O-linked to threonine or serine but have no known peptide signal sequence and are rare in immunoglobulins. In fact, in the normal five human Ig classes, GalN glycans are found only in the $\alpha1$ hinge and in the δ hinge; however, since 4 or 5 are present, the function of the hinge is greatly affected.

The exact location and the kinds of oligosaccharides linked to the δ chain are given in the figure showing the complete amino acid sequence (FIGURE 3). It should be noted that the number of GalN glycans in human δ is still uncertain, being either four or five. The GalN carbohydrates contributed greatly to the extreme difficulty in determining the amino acid sequence of the hinge. It was necessary to remove them at least partially either by enzymatic digestion or by chemical cleavage with HF, and this left some uncertainty as to whether four or five are present.[15]

Three major points are made about the GlcN glycans by FIGURE 11. The first is that all three GlcN glycans of the human δ chain are in the Fc region, whereas the $\alpha2$, μ and ϵ chains have GlcN glycans in the Fd region, as does the mouse δ chain. The second point is that the first δ chain GlcN glycan is homologous to a similar oligosaccharide present in all heavy chains except the α chain in which the signal peptide is replaced by a Cys-Gly-Cys sequence involved in a surface interchain bridge in IgA. The third point is that the two GlcN glycans in the Cδ3 domain have no counterpart in the other human heavy chains. These last two oligosaccharides may thus be involved in the way in which the two Cδ3 domains of IgD are positioned on the surface of the B-cell membrane.

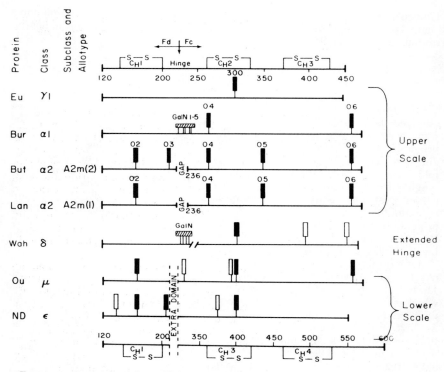

FIGURE 11. Location of the carbohydrate in human $\gamma 1$, $\alpha 1$, $\alpha 2$, δ, μ, and ϵ heavy chains. Vertical rectangles denote glucosamine oligosaccharides. Shading indicates that these have homologous positions in two or more chains. The numbers in the upper and lower scales give the residue positions in the chains, but the extra domain (Cμ2 and Cϵ2, respectively) has been omitted in the μ and ϵ chains.

The multiple GalN glycans of the $\alpha 1$ and δ hinges are attached to a random polypeptide chain structure projecting between the C$_H$1 and C$_H$2 domains.[26] The analogy between human $\alpha 1$ and human δ versus human $\alpha 2$ and mouse δ is interesting; the first two have multiple GalN glycans and also give evidence of a duplication in hinge structure, whereas the latter two lack GalN and give evidence of a deletion in structure. We know that the $\alpha 1$ and $\alpha 2$ chains have arisen late in primate evolution and that the deletion in the $\alpha 2$ hinge conveys resistance to cleavage by IgA1 proteases of pathogenic bacteria. Has a similar driving force resulted in the separate evolution of the hinge regions of human and mouse IgD?

Structural Comparison of Human and Mouse IgD

Although each of the three major classes of human immunoglobulins (IgG, IgA, and IgM) is very similar to domain structure and in amino acid sequence to its counterpart in the mouse, there is an unprecedented structural difference in human and mouse IgD. The most unexpected difference is the continuous deletion of 135 amino acids in the mouse δ chain corresponding to the absence of the Cδ2 domain and of the highly charged second half of the human δ hinge (FIGURE 12). In addition, the two δ chains differ in the number, kind, and location of their oligosaccharides and in the size and sequence of their tailpieces. The large deletion in mouse IgD must greatly affect its molecular conformation; not only is the δ chain shortened, but the cysteine that forms an inter-heavy-chain disulfide bridge in human IgD is missing. Hence, mouse IgD may exist as half-molecules. Thus, the absence of the Cδ2 domain and part of the hinge region must have a profound effect both on the molecular conformation of mouse IgD and on the interactions that may be transmitted between the antibody combining site in the V region to the cytotropic membrane binding site in the last domain.

Some unexpected differences in primary structure also exist between the undeleted portion of the mouse δ chain and the corresponding segments of the human δ chain. One surprising difference is the relatively low homology in amino acid sequence of the Cδ1 domains of the two δ chains (about 25%, see FIGURE 5) compared to the much greater degree of identity of the Cδ3 domains (see FIGURE 10). The homology of the human and mouse Cδ3 domains (about 53%) approaches the value expected for two heavy chains of the same class from different species.[3]

There is a greater similarity of the human and mouse δ hinge regions than may appear at first glance. This is shown in FIGURE 13, which gives an alignment of the GalN-rich half of the human δ hinge with the entire δ hinge region of mouse IgD. By inserting gaps through a visual comparison we obtained 17 identities in a 35-residue sequence, or about 50% identity. Although this may seem to be an arbitrary procedure, the computer search referred to earlier picked out the same segments for alignment and gave them a high score. This is one of the points that

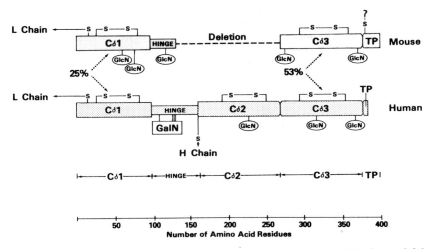

FIGURE 12. Structural models of the δ chains of human and mouse IgD. The model for human δ is from this work. The model for mouse δ is based on the updated DNA sequence of Tucker *et al.*[9] described in this conference[24] and the partial protein sequence of Dildrop and Beyreuther.[25] The Cδ1 domains of the two species have about 25% identity (see FIGURE 5) and the Cδ3 domains have about 53% identity (see FIGURE 10).

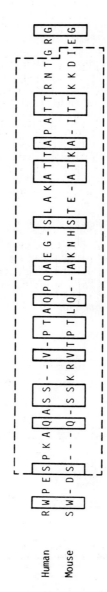

FIGURE 13. Similarity between the amino acid sequence of the Ga1N-rich segment of the hinge region of the human δ chain[14] and that of the entire hinge region of the mouse δ chain deduced from the DNA sequence.[9]

led to our hypothesis[10,14] that the 64-residue human δ hinge evolved by tandem duplication of a hinge exon coding for about 32 residues, whereas evolutionary deletion of one hinge exon may have led to the half-size murine hinge.

One of the most puzzling differences in the two δ chains is in the tailpiece. Whereas there are only two amino acid changes in the 20-residue tailpiece of the human and mouse μ chains of secreted IgM,[23] there is no structural relationship between the tailpieces of the secreted forms of human and mouse IgD. The S exon for the mouse δ chain codes for a 21-residue tailpiece which is identical to that determined from the protein sequence;[24] however, there are only seven residues in the tailpiece of the human δ chain, and they bear no resemblance to the mouse tailpiece.

Human and mouse IgD also differ from other classes of immunoglobulins such as IgG and IgM where the number and location of oligosaccharides is similar in the mouse and human homologues. Whereas human δ has four or five GalN glycans in the first half of the hinge, the mouse δ hinge has one GlcN glycan[25] with no report of any GalN (FIGURE 12). The apparent lack of GalN in the mouse δ hinge may be due to the absence of the characteristic GalN attachment sites of Ala-Thr-Thr and Ala-Ser-Ser present in the human δ hinge (see FIGURE 3) or of Pro-Ser, which is in the human α1 hinge. Seven Asn-X-Thr/Ser acceptor sites for GlcN were predicted from the preliminary DNA sequence for mouse δ, and six from the revised DNA sequence.[9,24] Of the latter, five are glycosylated in the IgD protein from mice of a different strain,[25] and the sixth has the unfavorable sequence of Asn-Pro-Thr. As seen from FIGURE 12, the distribution of the five GlcN oligosaccharides in the mouse δ chain is very different from that of the three in the longer δ chain. In fact, only one of the GlcN oligosaccharides in the human and mouse δ chains is at the same site, i.e., the one at the COOH-terminus.

Evolution, Structure, and Function of IgD

In attempting to trace the evolution of IgD as a separate class we used the homology alignments of the five human heavy chains (such as those given in FIGURES 5 and 10) to develop the topology of an evolutionary tree. As we earlier showed,[3] individual domains of the C regions of heavy chains must be compared rather than the whole chains; and this conclusion has been supported by the recent finding that exons code for individual domains as well as for linking segments such as J_H, the hinge, and the tailpiece.[18-20] Our results,[13,14] as well as those of Dayhoff and Barker (personal communication) suggested that the δ chain gene system originated early in evolution and branched off from the α chain shortly after the divergence of the gene systems for α and μ chains. Figure 14 shows two hypothetical pathways proposed by us for the genetic events leading to the origin of the δ chain. Shinoda et al.[21] have suggested a similar scheme. Although these pathways take account of current knowledge on the interrupted exon-intron structure for H chain genes, they do not explain the origin of the linking segments such as J_H, the hinge, and the tailpiece.

What have we learned from the structure of IgD that may be related to its function? One major point is that the exceptional lability of human IgD lies in its high charge region. When IgD is on the surface of the B-cell, this vulnerable helical segment may be protected by the galactosamine-rich hinge region (FIGURE 15-1). When membrane-bound IgD acts as a receptor, the high-charge region may be exposed to protease action because of a conformational change due to binding

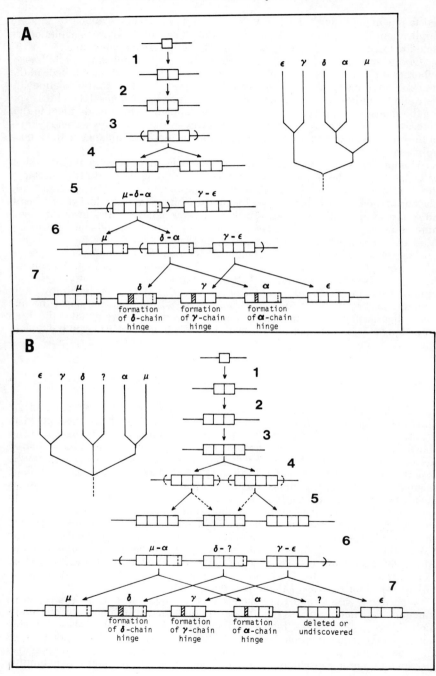

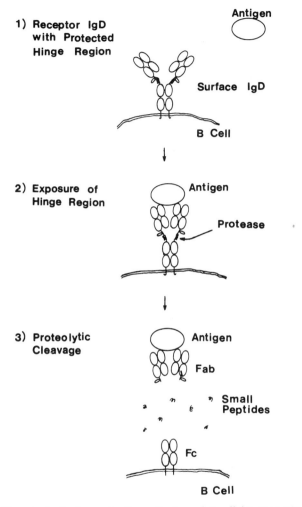

1) **Receptor IgD with Protected Hinge Region**

Antigen

Surface IgD

B Cell

2) **Exposure of Hinge Region**

Antigen

Protease

3) **Proteolytic Cleavage**

Antigen

Fab

Small Peptides

Fc

B Cell

FIGURE 15.   Hypothetical scheme for the activation of B-cell function triggered by the proteolytic cleavage of IgD. (For explanation, see the text.)

FIGURE 14. **A** and **B**: Two hypothetical pathways depicting the possible genetic events that might lead to the origin of the δ-chain gene. Exons coding for the immunoglobulin C (constant) domains are boxed, with the tailpiece separated from the last C domain by a broken line. The noncoding DNA segments are represented by a thin line. For simplicity, introns between the domain exons are deleted from the diagram. The hinge region for different heavy chains is assumed to have evolved independently from the second C domain by an unknown genetic mechanism. Unbranched arrows in the pathway represent events of internal duplication that lengthened the C gene; branched arrows represent events of discrete duplication that created new C genes (parentheses on the DNA segment cover the range of discrete duplication). The evolutionary tree depicted by each pathway is shown as an inset at the top. (Modified from Lin and Putnam.)[13]

of antigen (FIGURE 15-2). Proteolytic cleavage of the δ hinge could have three consequences (FIGURE 15-3). First, the release of Fab with more effective presentation of antigen to a nearby helper T-cell that would recognize the antigen and the idiotypic determinants of the Fab. This fits with recent findings that T-cells have CDR3 (D segments) similar to B-cells. Secondly, the various small highly charged peptides split out of the α-helical part of the hinge may exert a hormone-like or triggering effect on either the T- or B-cell. Thirdly, the conformational change in the Fc region will facilitate its endocytosis and engulfment and attachment to the cytoskeleton of the interior of the B-cell. This accords with the hypothesis of Bourgois et al.[27] who have proposed that the rapid enzymatic degradation of murine IgD elicits anti-idiotype responses that play a crucial role in initiating the immune response.

ACKNOWLEDGMENTS

We thank L.-C. Huang, J. Madison, S. Dorwin, P. H. Davidson, J. Dwulet, Y. Takahashi, and Drs. Y. and R. Kobayashi for valuable assistance, Dr. J. Baenziger for help in removal of sugar from the hinge glycopeptides, Dr. J. H. Keffer for the IgD plasma, and Dr. Winona C. Barker for computer analyses of protein sequences.

REFERENCES

1. PUTNAM, F. W., K. TITANI & E. WHITLEY, JR. 1966. Proc. R. Soc. London, Ser. B. **166:** 124–137.
2. PUTNAM, F. W., K. TITANI, M. WIKLER & T. SHINODA. 1967. Cold Spring Harbor Symp. Quant. Biol. **32:** 9–29.
3. PUTNAM, F. W. 1977. In The Plasma Proteins. F. W. Putnam, Ed. 2nd edit. **3:** 1–153. Academic Press. New York, N.Y.
4. KABAT, E. A., T. T. WU & H. BILOFSKY. 1979. Sequences of Immunoglobulin Chains. Publ. No. 80-2008. National Institutes of Health, Bethesda, Md.
5. DAYHOFF, M. O., Ed. 1978. Atlas of Protein Sequence and Structure. **5.** Suppl. 3: 73–93. Natl. Biomed: Res. Found. Washington, D.C.
6. TITANI, K. & F. W. PUTNAM. 1965. Science **147:** 1304–1305.
7. LESLIE, G. A. & L. N. MARTIN. 1978. Contemp. Top. Mol. Immunol. **7:** 1–49.
8. SPIEGELBERG, H. L. 1977. Immunol. Rev. **37:** 1–24.
9. TUCKER, P. W., C.-P. LIU, J. F. MUSHINSKI & F. R. BLATTNER. 1980. Science **209:** 1353–1360.
10. TAKAHASHI, N., D. TETAERT, L.-C. LIN, B. DEBUIRE & F. W. PUTNAM. 1982. Proc. Natl. Acad. Sci. U.S.A. **79:** 2850–2854.
11. TAKAHASHI, Y., N. TAKAHASHI, D. TETAERT & F. W. PUTNAM. To be published.
12. LIN, L.-C. & F. W. PUTNAM. 1979. Proc. Natl. Acad. Sci. U.S.A. **76:** 6572–6576.
13. LIN, L.-C. & F. W. PUTNAM. 1981. Proc. Natl. Acad. Sci. U.S.A. **78:** 504–508.
14. PUTNAM, F. W., N. TAKAHASHI, D. TETAERT, B. DEBUIRE & L.-C. LIN. 1981. Proc. Natl. Acad. Sci. U.S.A. **78:** 6168–6172.
15. TAKAHASHI, N., D. TETAERT & F. W. PUTNAM. 1982. In IV International Conference on Methods in Protein Sequence Analysis. Brookhaven National Laboratory. Sept. 21-25, 1981. M. Elzinga, Ed. Humana Press. Clifton, N.J. In press.
16. PUTNAM, F. W., G. FLORENT, C. PAUL, T. SHINODA & A. SHIMIZU. 1973. Science **182:** 287–290.
17. EDMUNDSON, A. B., K. R. ELY, E. E. ABOLA, M. SCHIFFER & N. PANAGIOTOPOULOS. 1975. Biochemistry **14:** 3953–3961.

18. SIEBENLIST, U., J. V. RAVETCH, S. KORSMEYER, T. WALDMANN & P. LEDER. 1981. Nature **294:** 631–635.
19. SAKANO, H., Y. KUROSAWA, M. WEIGERT & S. TONEGAWA. 1981. Nature (London) **290:** 562–565.
20. SAKANO, H., J. H. ROGERS, K. HUPPI, C. BRACK, A. TRAUENECKER, R. MAKI, R. WALL & S. TONEGAWA. 1979. Nature **277:** 627–633.
21. SHINODA, T., N. TAKAHASHI, T. TAKAYASU, T. OKUYAMA & A. SHIMIZU. 1981. Proc. Natl. Acad. Sci. U.S.A. **78:** 785–789.
22. CHOU, P. Y. & G. D. FASMAN. 1978. Annu. Rev. Biochem. **47:** 251–276.
23. RABBITTS, T. H., A. FORSTER & C. P. MILSTEIN. 1981. Nucleic Acids Res. **9:** 4509–4524.
24. TUCKER, P. W. 1982. N. Y. Acad. Sci. In press.
25. DILDROP, R. & K. BEYREUTHER. 1981. Nature **292:** 61–63.
26. TSUZUKIDA, Y., C.-C. WANG & F. W. PUTNAM. 1979. Proc. Natl. Acad. Sci. U.S.A. **76:** 1104–1108.
27. BOURGOIS, A., E. R. ABNEY & R. M. E. PARKHOUSE. 1977. Eur. J. Immunol. **7:** 210–213.

———————◆———————

DISCUSSION OF THE PAPER

L. M. SCHWARTZ (*Veterans Administration Medical Center, East Orange, N.J.*): I would like to know if there are pertinent changes between human and mouse IgD which can be ascribed to differences in the C-region and differences in the number and the location of carbohydrate?

F. W. PUTNAM: The differences in carbohydrate are purely secondary. They are not coded genetically as far as the sequence to which they are attached. We believe they have a function. The differences in mouse and humans I tried to emphasize relate to the shorter hinge in the mouse and the fact that that particular domain is missing. How that difference occurred may be a question of evolution in time so that there is a kind of domain skipping and a loss of the exon for that domain.

M. KLEIN (*Toronto, Canada*): What, if any, conformational changes take place in the Fc region upon cleavage of the IgD molecule on the surface of the cell?

My second question is regarding the $C\delta_2$ domain. Did you find the sequence that seems to be characteristic for C1 binding, which has to be a histidine followed by two lysines, that is present in all human IgG binding C1?

PUTNAM: I'd have to review to see whether that particular sequence is present. I have reviewed the binding sequence of C1q which has been published by Porter, and there is no clear relationship, it seems to me, to that particular sequence. I find it very hard to conceive something as big as C1q with a molecular weight of 340,000 is going to recognize just three or four amino acids. I think it's conformation and the carbohydrate present in that domain that is going to be extremely important.

KLEIN: Your speculation about the function of IgD is that, upon cleavage of the surface IgD, there would be some conformational changes occurring in the Fc portion down to the membrane. Why do you speculate this?

PUTNAM: We have done such conformational studies on IgM and we have done it on Fab, Fc, Fv and on individual domains and there is no question that there are conformational changes which you can detect by CD. Changes in the circular dichroism occur when you lop off the Fab portion of the molecule. There are also changes in the circular dicroism spectrum when you cleave between two domains. These differences probably reflect changes in the transverse and longitudinal interactions of domains.

KLEIN: This is the first evidence that cleavage can produce a change in the Fc portion. The crystallographic data do not support it.

PUTNAM: I think the conformational studies by CD are what you might call dynamic studies whereas those in the crystallographic state, beautiful as they are, to my knowledge are not at the high resolution for Fc as they are for Fab. Furthermore, the crystallographic studies that I am aware of, using intact Ig molecules have always been with molecules that lack a hinge. I don't believe anyone has ever obtained high resolution X-ray crystallographic results of molecules with a hinge. It certainly shows that the hinge has a very important function with respect to the conformation of the whole molecule.

F. D. FINKELMAN: There's an interesting report about rat IgD that makes one wonder whether that's a missing link between human and mouse IgD (δ chain).

PUTNAM: I haven't seen the second report. I understand there is one which indicates that rat IgD does have a domain missing. The first report was in error I think in terms of ascribing the relative relationships of the sequences that were given.

FINKELMAN: Dr. Bazin is here so maybe he can comment on it? I know that the sequence work on Dr. Bazin's myeloma protein showed a deletion that makes it very similar to a sequence for mouse δ chain.

BAZIN: Yes, but I have no data because the work has been done in Marseilles, not in my lab.

PUTNAM: I want to make one point about the missing domain. We know a number of other deletion proteins that have domains missing, for example the last domain is missing in some mouse α chains and some human α chains that we have. We know about the deletions of the hinge region, and of heavy chain disease proteins that have segments of the V-region all the way down to the hinge deleted, but to my knowledge there is no example in the literature other than the mouse IgD and possibly rat IgD for that particular second domain in the Fc to be missing. That is a unique event.

FINKELMAN: The other half of the story is the description of normal cell surface δ chain in the rat by Dr. Leslie and his collaborators which indicates it had a slower electrophoretic mobility than mouse δ chain, making it similar to human δ chain. I don't know if this has been repeated recently. One would wonder whether in the rat you are actually seeing this deletion process occuring from a normal state, like the human, to a mouse-like state as in Dr. Bazin's myeloma.

PUTNAM: I think it's an interesting point. I do want to remind everybody that the use of tunicamycin to prevent the synthesis of the oligosaccharide would give us clearer results of size based on electrophoretic mobility.

BLATTNER: I wonder if Dr. Leslie would like to comment on that last point? Is it true that rats are more like humans than mice at the level of electrophoretic mobility of δ?

G.A. LESLIE: We haven't done the tunicamycin experiments but we have done the cell surface studies using four different anti-rat δ reagents. The intact molecule has a molecular weight of about 180 to 185 thousand. The δ chain on the surface of the "normal" B-cell gives a two-shouldered peak of about 73,000 and 67,000 daltons and this has been done many times with various normal rat tissues. So it's real in our hands.

BLATTNER: In other words, it's bigger than mouse. Did you try mouse?

LESLIE: Yes, and it's bigger than mouse δ. Another point that was shown recently with Marvin Cuchens, Marvin Rittenberg and Hana Golding is, using anti-"normal" rat IgD, we can show antigenic cross-reactivity between human, mouse and rat δs.

BLATTNER: In the case of the mouse DNA sequence, there is a big intervening sequence between the hinge and the third domain that we had searched, possibly not with the sophistication of Margaret Dayhoff but we have not been able to find anything that looked faintly like the second domain of humans there.

TUCKER: My question was about your structure. Those proline clusters that you note toward each end of the third domain are, to my knowledge, unique as far as human heavy chains go. They do not seem to be there in other heavy chains, including the mouse. Would you like to speculate on their possible role in human IgD?

PUTNAM: The possible role that I can see is that whenever you have proline in a polypeptide chain you get a bend. When you have many such prolines you get quite a change in the conformation and so that represents a very unique area. Now, the fact that you have that change in the domain which is supposed to be close to the transmembrane piece and the fact that you also have the carbohydrates there, I feel, does have to do with the way this IgD sits down, or gets off the B-cell membrane, but that's all I can say in those terms.

VITETTA: Quite a bit of discussion occurred several years ago about the proteolytic model of cell surface IgD. We didn't pursue these studies but it seems to me that proof of that would be finding Fc fragments on the B-cell membrane following LPS treatment or something of that nature. Has anybody in this audience looked at that? If we can't find that, then I think the model rather dissolves.

R. M. E. PARKHOUSE (*National Institute for Medical Research, London, England*): Yes, we have and it's not there.

FINKELMAN: A similar experiment is one in which you try to cap with anti-κ and then look for the presence of δ Fc. And again, you don't find it. So there's no evidence that anti-κ makes the δ molecule break at the hinge.

J. C. CAMBIER (*Duke University Medical Center, Durham, N.C.*): We have attempted to approach this question by blocking the loss of δ following LPS stimulation with various protease inhibitors and have found virtually no effect of protease inhibitors on that loss. So that would suggest that the loss of δ is not mediated by protease.

H. L. SPIEGELBERG (*Scripps Clinic and Research Foundation, La Jolla, California*): The IgD δ chain of normal mouse B-cells migrated in our gel system just a little bit ahead of the μ chain and in no way as far down as the myeloma δ chain. Do you think that the mouse cell bound δ chain has that deletion, too?

BLATTNER: Absolutely, the mouse can't have a domain where there's no gene for it. We have sequenced the entire region and definitely feel that there's no domain in the normal situation.

TUCKER: Actually though it's not as big a difference as you think. If you make the computation based on the recent chain structure that we calculate for two domains and the hinge and you take the glycosylation sites that we observe in sequence of which there are about nine and make an average of maybe two to six thousand daltons, it quickly comes up to the right size. There have been other experiments in other labs using tunicamycin and also Goding has a result using enzymatic removal of carbohydrate that drops these large 70K proteins down to about 50K. So we feel very satisfied that the two domain model is normal for the mouse.

PUTNAM: One of the questions had to do with what happens to the Fc and is that proteolytic action really significant biologically? My suggestion was that the Fc disappears by endocytosis inside the cell and that is part of the biological function.

STUDIES OF HUMAN MYELOMA AND
CELL BOUND IgD*

Hans P. Kocher and Hans L. Spiegelberg

Department of Pathology
University of Geneva
Geneva, Switzerland
and
Department of Immunopathology
Research Insitute of Scripps Clinic
La Jolla, California 92037

INTRODUCTION

Although much has been learned about IgD since its discovery by Rowe and Fahey in 1965,[1,2] the function of both IgD antibodies and membrane bound IgD found on most mature B-lymphocytes remains unknown. Even the elucidation of the primary structure of IgD took much longer than that of the other Ig classes. The reasons for this were the low concentration of IgD in the serum, the difficulty to obtain IgD antibodies reacting to a given antigen and the rare occurrence of patients with IgD multiple myeloma having high concentrations of IgD in their sera allowing the isolation of large quantities of IgD for amino acid sequence analyses. An additional problem in obtaining isolated IgD is its great susceptibility to "spontaneous" degradation into heterogenous Fab and Fc fragments by serum enzymes such as plasmin.[3] Recently, the entire amino acid sequence of the constant region of the human δ chain has been reported.[4-6] Comparison to other Ig heavy chains showed no predominant homology to any one of the other four Ig classes. In previous studies we observed a similarity of IgD and IgE with respect to susceptibility of the Fab fragments to proteolysis.[7] In this paper, we present amino acid sequences of the variable-constant (V-C) switch region of three human δ chains, the structure of the terminal products of trypsin treated IgD Fab fragments and comparative analyses of Fc fragments of myeloma and cell bound IgD.

AMINO ACID SEQUENCE OF THE V-C SWITCH REGION
OF THREE HUMAN δ CHAINS

Heavy chains of three IgD myeloma proteins (Hu, Ac, Bu) were isolated[8] and fragmented with CNBr in 70% formic acid.[7] The resulting peptides were analyzed by sodium dodecyl sulfate polyacrylamide gel electrophoresis (SDS-PAGE) in reduced form (FIGURE 1). All three myeloma proteins, as well as an additional one (Di), showed one large peptide which was designated CB1. It was isolated by gel filtration on Sephadex G-100 columns equilibrated with 6 M guanidine HCl. The first peptide peak that eluted from the column represented

*This work was supported by UPHS Grant AI-15350 and Biomedical Research Support Program Grant RRO-5514. This is publication No. 2625 from the Research Institute of Scripps Clinic. Address reprint requests to Dr. H.L. Spiegelberg, Department of Immunopathology, Scripps Clinic and Research Foundation, 10666 North Torrey Pines Road, La Jolla, California 92037.

0077-8923/82/0399-0069$01.75/0 © 1982, NYAS

pure CB1. The CB1 peptides were applied to the sequencer and the cleaved residues were analyzed by gas chromatography[9] and by backhydrolysis with HI.[10] CB1 from proteins Hu and Ac were obtained in pure form, whereas that of Bu contained minor impurities because the patient had only 3 mg IgD/ml and only limited amounts of IgD were available that could not be further purified. Since only 80 nM of CB1 fragments of protein Hu and 40 mN of Ac and Bu were available for each of two duplicate analyses, the yields were low and some of the residues could not be clearly identified which is particularly true for the expected tryptophane residues. The N-terminal sequences of the three CB1 peptides are shown in FIGURE 2. It could clearly be established that all three δ chains must have had a cleavage in the third complementarity determining region, presumably

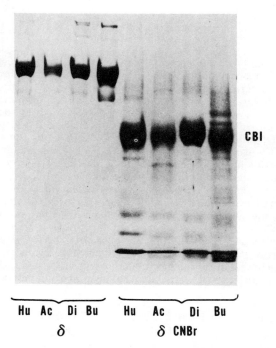

FIGURE 1. SDS-PAGE analysis of 4 δ chains (Hu, Ac, Di, Bu) before and after fragmentation with CNBr. CB1 marks the position of the CNBr fragments that were used for automated amino acid sequence analyses.

resulting from a methionine in this position. After 23, 14 and 13 residues, respectively, the constant amino acid sequence typical for δ chains was obtained. FIGURE 3 lists the amino acid sequences of the V-C switch region of the five known δ chains. All five δ chains show different amino acid sequences. Ravetch et al.[11] recently reported six different nucleotide sequences for the human J segment. Neither of the J region amino acid sequences of the five IgD myeloma proteins are identical to one of the reported prototype nucleotide sequences. The differences between the amino acid sequences and the reported nucleotide sequences may be the result of mutations and, in the case of the δ chain Hu, a

		Variable region											J region										
							100					105				110								
δ Hu	(M)	N	V	R	G	A	R	R	Y	A	F	D	D	X	G	Q	G	I	L	V	T	A	S
δ Bu									(M)	X	X	X	G	K	G	T	P	V	T	V	S	T	
δ Ac									(M)	I	X	G	Q	G	T	T	V	T	V	S	S		

Constant region

δ Hu	A	P	T	K	A	P	D	V	F	P				
δ Bu	A	P	T	K	A	P								
δ Ac	A	P	T	K	A	P	D	V	F	P	I	I	X	G	C

FIGURE 2. N-terminal amino acid sequences of the CB1 fragments from δ chains Hu, Bu and Ac. The sequences were aligned in a manner to demonstrate variable, J and constant region residues. X: unidentified residues.

deletion that occurred in one of the reported J sequences. Alternatively, they belong to as yet unrecognized J regions. In any event, δ chains do not appear to be associated with a particular J segment.

SUSCEPTIBILITY OF THE Cδ1 AND V_L DOMAINS OF IgD

Digestion of IgD with papain or trypsin, even for only short periods of time, results in the formation of Fab fragments differing in size and peptide structure. Since this was never observed in our laboratory when we prepared Fab fragments from IgG under the same conditions, we investigated the formation of IgD Fab fragments in detail.[7] First, Fab fragments of a human λIgD myeloma protein (Ac) were isolated by DEAE-cellulose chromatography after two min of digestion with trypsin. The Fab fragments were then incubated a second time with trypsin for one, two, four and eight hr. As shown in FIGURE 4, unreduced Fab fragments obtained after two min digestion with trypsin showed multiple bands indicating size heterogeneity. After reduction, they showed two major bands, one

δ CHAIN V–C SWITCH REGION

	100				105				110			
WAH	I	D	V	W	G	Q	G	T	T	V	H	V	S	S
ErI	(M)	———————	R	————————	T	———————	A
Hu	F	—— D	X	———————	I	L	—— T	A	S
Bu	(M)	X	X	X	—— K	————————	P	—— T	———————	T
Ac	(M)	I	X	—————————————————	T	———————

FIGURE 3. Comparison of the amino acid sequences of the V-C switch region of different δ chains. The sequences of δ chains Wah and ErI were taken from references 6 and 31, respectively.

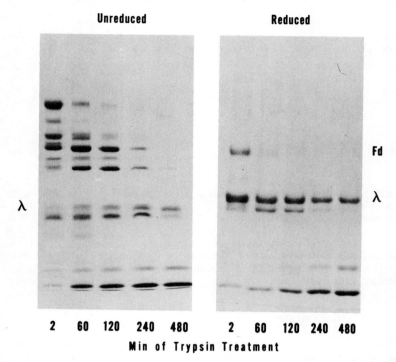

FIGURE 4. 10% SDS-PAGE analysis of native and reduced Fab fragments of IgD protein Ac isolated after two min of tryptic digestion and of the same preparation treated subsequently with trypsin for 60 to 480 min. Fd, marks the position of the Fd fragment; λ, that of the λ light chain.

corresponding to the Fd fragment and one to the λ chain. Digestion for 60-480 minutes resulted in disappearance of the Fd fragment and formation of peptides smaller than the λ chain. After 480 min of digestion, three major peptide bands were visible that remained essentially unchanged during further digestion for up to 48 hr. All three peptide bands showed the same mobility in reduced and unreduced preparations, indicating that they were not linked by disulfide bonds or consisted of yet smaller peptides which are linked by disulfide bridges. When a mixture of the three peptides was treated with CNBr, the fastest moving peptide disappeared, whereas the two slower ones remained unchanged, indicating that they did not contain methionine residues. The λ chains of protein Ac did not contain methionine and had a blocked N-terminus. Therefore, only the third and fastest moving band was likely to be derived from the δ chain. The three peptides remaining from IgD Fab fragments after eight hr digestion with trypsin were isolated by gel filtration and analyzed for their N-terminal amino acid sequences employing an automated Beckman Sequencer. The largest peptide which had the mobility of the λ chain did not yield an amino acid sequence that was compatible with being intact λ chain. The second largest peptide showed an N-terminal sequence identical to that of the constant domain of human λ chain beginning three amino acids C-terminal of the V-C switch. Therefore, this peptide could be identified as representing the C region of the λ chain. The third and smallest peptide had a blocked N-terminus, like the Ac δ chain, when subjected to amino acid sequence analysis. After treatment of the peptide with CNBr, a small fragment of 16 amino acids was isolated that did not contain homoserine and represented the C-terminal end. It had an amino acid composition compatible with the sequence at the V-C switch of the Ac heavy chain, ten amino acids belonging to the V and four to the C region. Therefore, we concluded that prolonged digestion of IgD Fab fragments results in the degradation of the Cδ1 and V_L region, leaving three stable peptides: λ chains, the Cλ chain region without the first three amino acids, and the Vδ region including the first four amino acids of the C region.[7]

Additional experiments on digestion of IgD myeloma proteins of both λ and κ light chain type revealed similar findings. They showed that even prolonged digestion with trypsin did not degrade the Fc fragment with the possible exception of the C-terminal area.[12]

To determine whether trypsin degrades Fab fragments of other Ig classes, Fab fragments of IgG1 to 4, IgA, IgM and IgE were treated with trypsin for eight hr and analyzed by SDS-PAGE. As shown in FIGURE 5, except for IgE, Fab fragments of all classes showed two peptides representing the Fd fragment and the light chain which did not change after trypsin treatment. IgE Fab fragments had become degraded before trypsin treatment, presumably because they were isolated after two hr of papain digestion. Bennich and Johansson[13] found that digestion of the IgE protein N.D. resulted in the formation of a fragment consisting of the Cλ domain. These authors suggested that their IgE myeloma protein (N.D.) might have an unusual light chain. However, this appears unlikely, since another IgE myeloma protein (Sha) used for our experiments showed the same phenomenon. Furthermore, six λIgD proteins digested with trypsin all showed the same terminal products after trypsin digestion. Therefore, it has to be concluded that the structure of Fab fragments of IgD and IgE proteins must be different from

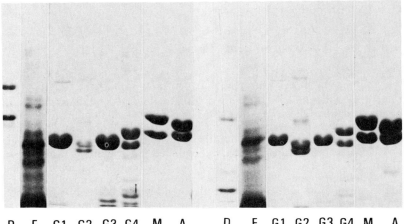

D E G1 G2 G3 G4 M A   D E G1 G2 G3 G4 M A

FIGURE 5. 10% SDS-PAGE analysis of reduced Fab fragments of IgD, IgE, the four IgG subclasses, IgM and IgA1 before trypsin treatment, left, and after trypsin treatment, right, for 8 hr.

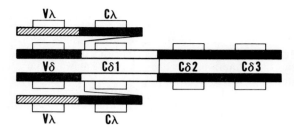

FIGURE 6. Areas of tryptic degradation of IgD: □, rapidly degradable region; ▨, region of intermediate susceptibility; and ■, trypsin-resistant region.

those of the other Ig classes and responsible for the degradation of CH1 and V_L domains by trypsin. Perhaps IgD and IgE Fab fragments have a less compact structure than those of the other classes that permits their proteolytic cleavage by enzymes such as trypsin.

The areas of degradation of IgD after incubation with trypsin for 8–24 hr are shown in FIGURE 6. The hinge and the Cδ1 region are rapidly and completely degraded after short incubation periods. The V_L region is digested in a fraction of the light chains, whereas the Vδ, the C_L and the Fc fragment remain intact. The reason why the V_L region is degraded is puzzling. There is no evidence to suggest that the V_L region of IgD does not combine with the V_H region differently from the Ig classes which form trypsin resistant Fab fragments. One explanation for this phenomenon may be that the Cl region of IgD and IgE have an entirely different tertiary structure than those of the other classes. This structure would allow access to proteolytic enzymes resulting in digestion of Cδ1 or Cε1 domain. After digestion of the CH1 domain, the light chains become free and degradable by trypsin in the V region before they can form dimers that are resistant to proteolysis. Whatever the explanation is, the susceptibility of Fab fragments to tryptic degradation is restricted to IgD and IgE Fab fragments.

COMPARISON OF MYELOMA AND MEMBRANE-BOUND Fc IgD FRAGMENTS

Comparison of ^{125}I-radiolabeled δ heavy chains from the sIgD(+) human lymphoblastoid cell line Wil-2WT and myeloma δ chains by SDS-PAGE indicated that membrane-bound δ chains are approximately 2500 daltons larger than myeloma δ chains.[3] These data suggested that cell-bound δ chains may have an additional structure necessary to anchor IgD in the cell membrane. To attempt to localize this structure, we either biosynthetically or cell surface labeled the IgD of Wil-2WT cells and compared the radiolabeled Fc fragments with those of myeloma IgD. Wil-2WT cells were radiolabeled by biosynthetic incorporation of ^{35}S-cysteine into proteins. The cells were cultured with the radioactive label in a cysteine free medium for two hr, centrifuged and lysed in 0.5% NP-40. To obtain Fc fragments, 150 μg of TPCK treated trypsin was added per ml cell lysate (20 × 10^6 cells/ml) and the mixture incubated for 10 min at room temperature. The reaction was terminated by addition of a twofold excess of soybean trypsin inhibitor. It had previously been shown that incubation with trypsin for 10 min effectively cleaves myeloma IgD molecules in the hinge region and degrades the Cδ1 domain, without destroying the Fc fragment.[7] Fc fragments generated in the cell lysates were immunoprecipitated with an antihuman δ chain antiserum and *Staphylococcus aureus*.

For comparison of molecular weights, Fc fragments from human IgD myeloma proteins were prepared as previously described.[8] The purified Fc fragments were mixed with the biosynthetically labeled immunoprecipitates and electrophoretically separated by SDS-PAGE on 10% gels under reducing conditions. Staining with Coomassie Blue revealed the myeloma Fc fragments, while autoradiography was used to detect the biosynthetically labeled material. FIGURE 7, part A shows the densitometric tracing of the autoradiography of the ^{35}S-cysteine labeled Fc fragments. Three peptide bands with m.w. between 25,000 and 30,000 could be distinguished. In FIGURE 7, part C the densitometric tracing of Coomassie Blue stained myeloma derived Fc fragments is shown. Fc fragments of myeloma IgD consistently display two peptide bands.

Comparison of the two densitometric tracings shown in FIGURE 7, part A and FIGURE 7, part C indicated that the two faster moving bands of the cysteine

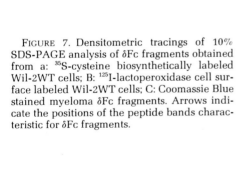

FIGURE 7. Densitometric tracings of 10% SDS-PAGE analysis of δFc fragments obtained from a: ^{35}S-cysteine biosynthetically labeled Wil-2WT cells; B: ^{125}I-lactoperoxidase cell surface labeled Wil-2WT cells; C: Coomassie Blue stained myeloma δFc fragments. Arrows indicate the positions of the peptide bands characteristic for δFc fragments.

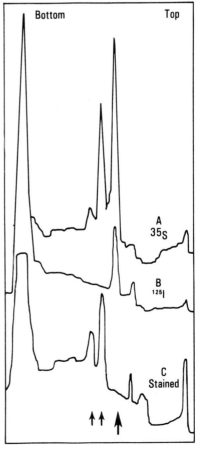

radiolabeled material comigrated with the two forms of myeloma Fc fragments. Therefore, we suspected that the immunoprecipitated band with the highest m.w. (FIGURE 7, part A) represented Fc fragments derived from membrane bound IgD. To check this assumption, Wil-2WT cell surface proteins were labeled by the lactoperoxidase-catalyzed iodination technique, lysed, subjected to tryptic digestion, immunoprecipiated and analyzed by SDS-PAGE on a slab gel in parallel with a cysteine ^{35}S biosynthetically labeled sample. The densitometric tracing of the surface labeled material is displayed in FIGURE 7, part B. As can be seen, there is indeed comigration of the biosynthetically labeled band with the highest m.w. and the cell surface labeled Fc fragment of Wil-2WT cells. We assume that the two smaller ^{35}S-labeled peptides comigrating with myeloma δ Fc fragments represent intracellular IgD.

The three bands obtained after biosynthetic labeling with ^{35}S-cysteine were cut out and eluted from the gel. The eluted material of each band was subjected to automated sequence analysis on a Beckman 890C Instrument and the radioactivity was determined in the first ten degradation steps. In all three instances radioactivity was recovered in degradation step 4, which indicates the presence of a cysteine residue in position 4 of the Fc fragments. This perfectly fits the amino acid sequence determined for the tryptic Fc fragment of human myeloma IgD where the cysteine in position 4 was shown to form the inter-heavy chain disulfide bond.[4,5,14] These results show that all three bands recovered from biosynthetically labeled Fc fragments display the same N-terminus, demonstrating that the multiple band formation observed by SDS-PAGE analysis is not the result of structural heterogeneity at the N-terminus of the Fc fragments. The reason why myeloma δFc fragments show two peptide bands in SDS-PAGE is unknown. It may reflect C-terminal[12] and/or carbohydrate heterogeneity.

Our results on human cell surface IgD (amino acid sequence and SDS-PAGE molecular weight determinations) and the amino acid sequence of myeloma IgD Fc fragments,[4,5] indicates the presence of two constant domains in the Fc fragment of lymphoblastoid cell surface-derived IgD and of human myeloma IgD. This is in contrast to recent reports of the nucleic acid sequences of cloned cDNA of mouse[15] and rat[16,17] δ chains that indicate a missing Cδ 2 exon in the myeloma δ chains of both species. In contrast, the molecular weights reported for both mouse[18] and rat[19] cell-bound δ chains suggest the presence of three constant domains in these species as in man.

The Fc fragment of human myeloma δ chains contain three methionine residues, one being the terminal residue.[4,5,12] In analogy to the structure of membrane bound μ chains,[20] one would expect membrane bound δ chains to have an additional peptide structure at the C-terminus. It was of interest to determine whether one could show a change in one of the three expected methionine-containing tryptic peptides, presumably the one which contains the methionine residue at the C-terminus. To attempt to show such a difference, we labeled Wil-2WT cells with ^{35}S-methionine, prepared Fc fragments as described above and applied them to SDS-PAGE. The three radioactive peptide bands shown in FIGURE 7, part A were observed. The three peptides were eluted from the gel and digested with trypsin. The cleavage products were then applied to a HPLC C18 column and eluted with a gradient of isopropanol. Only two peaks containing ^{35}S radioactivity eluted at similar positions from the column from digests of all three peptide bands. Since the two radioactive peptides from all three bands eluted at the same position, they were most likely derived from within the Fc fragments (positions 105 and 150 in reference 4). The failure to detect a third methionine containing peptide may be the result of irreversible attachment of the peptide to the HPLC column, C-terminal proteolytic degradation[12] or, in the case of cell surface IgD, of a C-terminal structure that does not contain methionine.

CONCLUDING REMARKS

The structural studies of human IgD myeloma proteins revealed some unique features. Trypsin degrades the Fab fragment and leaves the Vδ and the C_L regions as terminal products. In this respect, IgD resembles IgE whose Fab fragment is also rapidly degraded by conventional proteolytic digestion procedure used to prepare Fab and Fc fragments. In contrast to IgD and IgE, Fab fragments of IgG, IgM and IgA are resistant to tryptic digestion. Determination of the complete amino acid sequence of the constant region of the δ chain demonstrated greatest homology to the α chain;[4-6] however, the homology is not striking and not remarkably greater than that to other heavy chains. Therefore, it is not surprising that IgA differs from IgD in most of its features. IgA is the major secretory Ig,

TABLE 1

STRUCTURAL AND BIOLOGICAL SIMILARITIES BETWEEN IgD AND IgE

	IgD	IgE	IgG	IgA	IgM
Degradation of CH1 and V_L	+	+	−	−	−
C.D. spectra similarity	+	+	−	−	−
Heat and acid lability	+	+	−	−	−
Average concentration/ml serum	23 μg	0.1 μg	12 mg	2 mg	1 mg
Average half-life (days)	2.8	2.7	23	5.8	5.1
Extravascular catabolism	+	+	−	−	−
Half-life at elevated Ig conc.*	↑	↑	↓	=	=
Activation of classical C pathway	−	−	+	−	+
Activation of alternate C pathway	+	+	−	+	−
Effect of anti-δ in newborn rats on serum Ig levels	+	+	−	−	−

*↑: longer half-life; ↓: shorter half-life; =: unchanged.

forms dimers and combines with the secretory piece. Neither property is shared with IgD. In addition, IgA is very resistant to proteolytic degradation, whereas IgD is very susceptible. When we sequenced the N-terminal end of the IgD Fc fragment, we found greatest homology to the ε chain,[14] a homology which extends throughout the Cδ2 domain.[6] Therefore, we compared known biological properties of IgD with IgE[3] and found striking similarities which are summarized in TABLE 1. As mentioned above, conventional papain or trypsin digestion of IgD and IgE[7] results in the degradation of the first domain of the heavy chain and the variable domain of the light chain, which occurs only in these two Ig classes. The C.D. spectra pattern of intact IgD proteins contrasts markedly with that observed for IgG, IgA and IgM proteins but shows similarities with the spectra obtained for IgE.[21] Both IgD and IgE are relatively heat and acid labile.[22,23] The concentrations of IgD and IgE in the serum are much lower than those of the other Ig classes.[2] IgD and IgE have the fastest serum half-lives and the highest fractional turnover rates[24,25] and show a significant extravascular catabolism in contrast to the other three Ig classes. At elevated IgD and IgE serum concentrations, the turnover rate decreases for IgD and IgE, whereas it increases for IgG.[26] Increased IgM and IgA serum concentrations do not affect the IgM and IgA turnover. It has been reported that the submolecular sites governing the rate of IgG catabolism is located in the CH2 domain which is homologous to the CH2 domain of IgD and the CH3 domain of IgE.[27] It is interesting to note that IgD and IgE resemble each other most in this domain and both show similar rates of catabolism. Another biological function, namely complement activation, is attributed to a site in the CH2 domain of IgG.[27] Again, IgD resembles IgE with respect to complement activation. Neither activates the components of the classical pathway but activate those of the alternate pathway.[28] Another analogy between IgD and IgE has been reported by Bazin et al.[29] Injection of anti-δ chain specific antibodies into newborn rats results in a depression of predominantly IgD and IgE, whereas injection of anti-μ chain antisera affects all Ig classes. The great number of similarities between IgD and IgE suggests that these antibodies may have similar functions. IgE binds to high affinity Fc receptors on basophilic granulocytes and mast cells and after reaction with antigen induces the release of vasoactive substances from these cells. In the case of IgE, the function was known before the discovery of the class of antibodies that mediates it.[30] After its discovery, it was found that IgE is greatly elevated in parasitic disease and may be the immune system protecting the host from many parasites. Since parasitic infections are no longer common in developed countries, IgE levels are usually low, except for patients with allergic disease. Analogous to IgE, IgD antibodies may also be formed to selected, though as yet unknown, antigens and IgD cytophilically bound to Fc receptors rather than serum IgD may play an important role in the host's defense mechanism. The striking similarities between IgD and IgE warrant investigations searching for a cell type that has Fc receptors for IgD in the hope of finding the function of IgD serum antibodies.

The molecular weights of delta chains and δFc fragments of membrane bound IgD from the human lymphoblastoid cell line Wil-2WT is approximately 2500 daltons larger than those of their myeloma counterparts. The tryptic Fc fragments of membrane IgD had a half-cysteine residue in position 4 like myeloma IgD Fc fragments, indicating that Fc fragments of membrane bound IgD are structurally similar to myeloma IgD. Delta chains and δFc fragments obtained from myeloma proteins show two peptide bands in SDS-PAGE. Previously, we suggested that this may reflect C-terminal degradation because carboxypeptidase A released molar fractions of arginine and lysine residues from δ chains.[12] Carbohydrate heterogeneity of the δ chains could also be responsible for the multiple band formation and, at this time, this cannot be excluded. IgD Fc fragments obtained from cell surface labeled Wil-2WT cells showed only one peptide band, whereas Fc fragments obtained from biosynthetically labeled IgD show three bands. The largest band migrated identically to the cell surface labeled IgD. Therefore, the difference of 2500 daltons in molecular weight of membrane bound and secreted δ chains is most likely the result of an extension of the δ chain at the C-terminus of membrane bound δ chains. This would be analogous to the μ chain which has a hydrophobic peptide at the C-terminus allowing its anchorage in the cell membrane.

ACKNOWLEDGMENTS

The authors thank Professor P. Vassalli, chairman of the Department of Pathology, University of Geneva, for the encouragement and financial support that made part of this work possible. The excellent technical assistance of Mrs.

Chantal Dumais and secretarial help of Mrs. Margaret Stone are very much appreciated.

REFERENCES

1. ROWE, D. S. & J. L. FAHEY. 1965. A new class of human immunoglobulins. I. A unique myeloma protein. J. Exp. Med. **121:** 171–184.
2. ROWE, D. S. & J. L. FAHEY. 1965. A new class of human immunoglobulins. II. Normal serum IgD. J. Exp. Med. **121:** 185–199.
3. SPIEGELBERG, H. L. 1977. The structure and biology of human IgD. Immunol. Rev. **37:** 3–24.
4. LIN, L.-C. & F. W. PUTNAM. 1981. Primary structure of the Fc region of human immunoglobin D: Implications for evolutionary origin and biological function. Proc. Natl. Acad. Sci. USA **78:** 504–508.
5. SHINODA, T., N. TAKAHASHI, T. TAKAYASU, T. OKUYAMA & A. SHIMIZU. 1981. Complete amino acid sequence of the Fc region of a human δ chain. Proc. Natl. Acad. Sci. USA **78:** 785–789.
6. PUTNAM, F. W., N. TAKAHASHI, D. TETAERT, B. DEBUIRE & L.-C. LIN. 1981. Amino acid sequence of the first constant region domain and the hinge region of the δ heavy chain of human IgD. Proc. Natl. Acad. Sci. USA **78:** 6168–6172.
7. KOCHER, H. P. & H. L. SPIEGELBERG. 1979. Tryptic degradation of the CH1 and V_L regions of IgD and IgE. J. Immunol. **122:** 1190–1195.
8. SPIEGELBERG, H. L., J. W. PRAHL & H. M. GREY. 1970. Structural studies of human γD myeloma protein. Biochemistry **9:** 2115–2122.
9. PISANO, J. J. & T. J. BRONZERT. 1969. Analysis of amino acid phenylthiohydantoins by gas chromatography. J. Biol. Chem. **244:** 5597–5607.
10. SMITHIES, O., D. GIBSON, E. M. FANNING, R. M. GOODFLIESH, J. C. GILMAN & D. L. BALLANTYNE. 1971. Quantitative procedures for use with the Edman-Begg sequenator. Partial sequences of two unusual immunoglobulin light chains, RzF and Sac. Biochemistry **10:** 4912–4921.
11. RAVETCH, J. W., U. SIEBENLIST, S. Y. KORSMEYER, T. WALDMANN & P. LEDER. 1981. Structure of human immunoglobulin μ locus: Characterization of embryonic and rearranged J and D genes. Cell **27:** 583–591.
12. GOYERT, S. M., T. E. HUGLI & H. L. SPIEGELBERG. 1977. Sites of "spontaneous" degradation of IgD. J. Immunol. **118:** 2138–2144.
13. BENNICH, H. & S. G. O. JOHANSSON. 1971. Structure and function of immunoglobulin E. Adv. Immunol. **13:** 1–55.
14. SPIEGELBERG, H. L. 1975. NH_2-terminal amino acid sequence of the Fc fragment of IgD resembles IgE and IgG sequences. Nature **254:** 723–725.
15. TUCKER, P. W., C.-P. LIU, J. F. MUSHINSKI, & F. R. BLATTNER. 1980. Mouse immunoglobulin D: Messenger RNA and genomic DNA sequences. Science **209:** 1353–1360.
16. SIRE, J., G ALCARAZ, A. BOURGOIS & B. JORDAN. 1981. Rat IgD myeloma protein: cell-free translation of the δ mRNA and biochemical analysis of intracellular and membrane δ chain. Eur. J. Immunol. **11:** 632–636.
17. ALCARAZ, G., A. COLLE, A. BONED, B. KAHN-PERLES, J. SIRE, H. BAZIN & A. BOURGOIS. 1981. Tryptic and plasmic cleavage of a rat myeloma IgD. Mol. Immunol. **18:** 249–255.
18. GODING, J. W. & L. A. HERZENBERG. 1980. Biosynthesis of lymphocyte surface IgD in the mouse. J. Immunol. **124:** 2540–2547.
19. RUDDICK, J. H. & G. A. LESLIE. 1977. Structure and biologic functions of human IgD. XI. Identification and ontogeny of a rat lymphocyte immunoglobulin having antigenic crossreactivity with human IgD. J. Immunol. **118:** 1025–1031.
20. ROGERS, J., P. EARLY, C. CARTER, K. CALAME, M. BOND, L. HOOD & R. WALL. 1980. Two mRNAs with different 3' ends encode membrane-bound and secreted forms of immunoglobulin μ chain. Cell **20:** 303–312.
21. JEFFERIS, R. & J. B. MATTHEWS. 1977. Structural studies of human IgD paraproteins. Immunol Rev. **37:** 25–49.

22. HEINER, D. C., A. SAHA & B. ROSE. 1968. Lability of normal and myeloma IgD. Fed. Proc. **27:** 489.
23. DORRINGTON, K. & H. H. BENNICH. 1978. Structure-function relationships in human immunoglobulin E. Immunol. Rev. **41:** 3–25.
24. ROGENTINE, G. H., D. S. ROWE, J. BRADLEY, T. A. WALDMANN & J. L. FAHEY. 1966. Metabolism of human immunoglobulin D (IgD). J. Clin. Invest. **45:** 1467–1478.
25. IIO, A. W. STROBER, S. BRODER, S. H. POLMAR & T. A. WALDMANN. 1977. The metabolism of IgE in patients with immunodeficiency states and neoplastic conditions. J. Clin. Invest **59:** 743–755.
26. WALDMANN, T. A. & W. STROBER. 1969. Metabolism of immunoglobulins. Prog. Allergy **13:** 1–110.
27. YASMEEN, D., J. R. ELLERSON, K. J. DORRINGTON & R. H. PAINTER. 1976. The structure and function of immunoglobulin domains. IV. The distribution of some effector functions among the Cγ2 and Cγ3 homology regions of human immunoglobulin G. J. Immunol. **116:** 518–526.
28. SPIEGELBERG, H. L. & O. GOETZE. 1972. Conversion of C3 proactivator and activation of the alternate pathway of complement activation by different classes and subclasses of human immunoglobulins. Fed. Proc. **31:** 655.
29. BAZIN, H., B. PLATTEAU, A. BECKERS & R. PAUWELS. 1978. Differential effect of neonatal injections of anti-μ or anti-δ antibodies on the synthesis of IgM, IgD, IgE, IgA, IgG1, IgG2a, IgG2b, and IgG2c immunoglobulin classes. J. Immunol. **121:** 2083–2087.
30. ISHIZAKA, K. & T. ISHIZAKA. 1966. Physicochemical properties of human reaginic antibody. I. Association of reaginic activity with an immunoglobulin other than A or G globulin. J. Allergy **37:** 169–185.
31. MILSTEIN, C. P. & E. V. DEVERSON. 1980. J segment in human δ chains. Immunology **40:** 657–663.

◆

DISCUSSION OF THE PAPER

BLATTNER: Did you compare the proteolysis of the IgA-1 and IgA-2?

H. L. SPIEGELBERG: Yes, in the human the IgA-1 can be digested with streptococcal and pneumococcal bacterial enzymes. It is not easy to digest to make Fab. The IgA-2 to my knowledge cannot be digested. In the mouse it's different, mouse IgA is easy to digest.

BLATTNER: I have a feeling that neither of them is susceptible.

M. KLEIN: When you look at the proteolysis of your light chain it's probably secondary to the proteolysis of the Cδ1.

What do you mean that IgD and IgE activate the alternate pathway where Fc does not? Do you mean aggregated IgD?

SPIEGELBERG: The studies we did with Goetze and Eberhard used aggregated myeloma proteins and their Fc fragments. We then looked for conversion of the complement. Both activated the alternate C pathway.

KLEIN: We can show that aggregated IgD Fc and Fab can also activate the alternate pathway.

SPIEGELBERG: We couldn't show that.

PUTNAM: First I want to say that Dr. Spiegelberg's earlier work helped us very greatly in undertaking the study that we did and that there is virtual accordance in our work. Did you say that you had some data on the size of the mouse δ chain?

SPIEGELBERG: Yes. I put rat and mouse myeloma IgD on our gels together with human IgD. The human δ is just a little bit below the μ chain. But as you know, the slope is very different because of carbohydrate effects. Without extrapolation, the rat δ chain might be a little bit slower than γ chain (rat or human). The mouse was way down. It satisfied me that indeed the mouse and rat δ chains are quite different from the human.

D. S. ROWE (*World Health Organization, Geneva, Switzerland*): Could I comment on your suggestion that the IgD may be an anti-parasitic antibody? This idea occurred to us quite a long time ago and we looked at serum from Africans who had malaria and other parasites. The positive finding was that the serum IgD concentration prior to an age around puberty was very much higher, or at least had quite a different distribution with a tendency towards higher levels in that population. After that age the serum IgD concentration changed to the pattern which would become common among the Europeans and North Americans. When we came to look for specific antibodies, even among those high level individuals, we didn't find any. We didn't look very extensively for anti-parasite antibodies and I don't think the methods were very much available then. Moreover, when we immunized one or two of those people with tetanus toxoid we were not able to demonstrate antibodies in the IgD class although they were easily demonstrated in the IgD and IgM classes. So far as I'm aware very little work has been done on anti-parasite antibodies in this class. I'm personally not convinced that anybody in fact has isolated IgD and conclusively demonstrated antibody activity in serum IgD. The evidence seems to be mostly indirect for serum antibody activity in this class.

SPIEGELBERG: I did not want to say that IgD is an anti-parasite antibody, I just wanted to say by analogy maybe IgD is an anti-exotic viral or some unique class of antigen. The western world doesn't have many parasitic diseases anymore; therefore, we don't have much IgD because that class of antigen is not around anymore. Actually, what we see is some genetic variation in baseline IgD levels. I also don't think they are antiparasitic antibodies. It's just trying to find an explanation. In 1969 we studied about 600 children from a children's hospital in Los Angeles, and we also found an increase to the age of 15. Fifteen was the peak and then it went down. It happens in California as well as in Africa. But it didn't help us anyway to find a function because we have studied over 400 children with different diseases and there was absolutely no consistency.

VIOLATION OF SYMMETRY IN IMMUNOGLOBULINS: HYBRID MOLECULES ON THE SURFACE OF PLASMA CELLS*

James W. Goding

The Walter and Eliza Hall Institute of Medical Research
Royal Melbourne Hospital
Victoria 3050, Australia

The special structural features of membrane immunoglobulins are now reasonably well understood.[1-5] The membrane forms of each class of immunoglobulin possess a C-terminal extension containing three distinct regions (FIGURE 1). Adjoining the last regular domain is a short segment containing five–six acidic amino acids, and which might be considered a "membrane hinge." In membrane IgG[5,6] and IgD,[7] but not in membrane IgM, this region contains a cysteine residue. Immediately following is a segment of 20 or so uncharged and relatively hydrophobic amino acids. It is this region which is thought to span the lipid bilayer.[1] The final segment, which is presumably intracellular, consists of three amino acids (lysine, valine, lysine) in the case of IgM[1] and IgD,[7] and 28 amino acids in the case of IgG.[6]

The hydrophilic secretory C-terminus is encoded adjacent to the last regular domain.[1] In contrast, the membrane C-terminal segment is encoded by two exons which lie further downstream.[1] The first membrane exon encodes the "hinge" and transmembrane segments, and the second encodes the intracellular domain. The choice between production of secretory and membrane forms depends on alternate RNA splicing at the 3' end to generate mature messenger RNAs coding for proteins with different C-termini. Of particular relevance to this paper is the fact that the 5' ends of the RNAs encoding the remainder of the chains are shared,[6] and that apart from their C-termini the amino acid sequences of membrane and secreted immunoglobulins are identical.[3]

While the elucidation of those mechanisms has helped the understanding of how these proteins reach their correct destinations, an interesting new question arises. If one cell produces both membrane and secretory forms of immunoglobulin, do special mechanisms, such as different hinge regions[8] or physical sequestration, exist to prevent the formation of hybrid molecules?

If such mechanisms exist, the prediction is clear. Hybrid molecules will not be seen. On the other hand, if special mechanisms do not exist, pairing would be expected to depend on random collision. In other words, the formation of IgG molecules would depend on the law of mass action, and the extent of hybrid formation would depend on the relative rates of synthesis of the two forms. This simplest formulation would have to be slightly modified to take into account the fact that the two types of heavy chain are in separate phases. Phase separation would favor homologous pairing. Accordingly, in cells in which the rate of synthesis of secretory forms is relatively low, most membrane forms would pair with a membrane-heavy chain. In plasma cells, where the rate of synthesis of secretory forms might be as much as one thousand times that of membrane forms,

*This work was supported by the National Health and Medical Research Council of Australia.

it would be predicted that most membrane forms would pair with a secretory form, resulting in asymmetrical hybrid molecules (FIGURE 1).

A further prediction of the "random pairing" model would be that if the cysteine residues in the C-terminal extension[5,6] were normally disulfide-bonded to the homologous membrane heavy chain, in asymmetrical hybrid IgG these cysteines would be unpaired (FIGURE 1). Alternatively, they might pair with the membrane-heavy chain of another hybrid, resulting in 8-chain IgG dimers.

One of the most characteristic features of immunoglobulins is their twofold axial symmetry. In any one molecule, it has been a general rule that the two light chains are identical to each other, and that the two heavy chains are also identical. In this paper, an exception to this rule will be presented. It will be shown that the great majority of membrane IgG on the plasma cell MOPC-21 consists of hybrids between secretory and membrane-heavy chains. Although the exceptional case has only been demonstrated in one myeloma cell line, the logic used strongly suggests that whenever membrane-heavy chains are synthesized by plasma cells, they will pair with a secretory heavy chain to generate hybrid molecules.

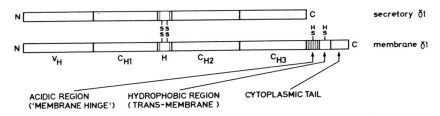

FIGURE 1. Structure of secretory and membrane forms of murine γ1 heavy chains. The vertical lines in the segments labeled "H" and "membrane hinge" denote acidic amino acids.

MATERIALS AND METHODS

Cell Lines

The B-lymphoma lines WEHI-231[9] and 2PK3[10] and the plasmacytoma lines MPC-11,[11] MOPC-21[12] and its nonsecreting variant NS-1[13] were maintained in exponential growth in Dulbecco's modified Eagle's medium with 10% fetal calf serum and 5×10^{-5} M 2-mercaptoethanol.

Cell Surface Radioiodination and Electrophoretic Analysis

Cells were harvested, washed extensively in phosphate-buffered saline, and radioiodinated by the lactoperoxidase method as previously described.[14] The viability,[15] as assessed by the acridine orange/ethidium bromide method was always greater than 98%, both before and after iodination. After two more washes, cells were lysed in a buffer containing 100 mM tris-HCl, pH 7.4, 1 mM N-ethylmaleimide, 1 mM phenylmethylsulfonyl fluoride, 1 mM ethylenediamine tetra-acetic acid and 0.5% Triton X-100.[16] After 15 min at 4°C, nuclei were removed by centrifugation at 2,000 × g for 10 min, and an equal volume of 5% sodium dodecyl sulfate (SDS) in H_2O plus 15% glycerol was added. The sample was placed in a boiling water bath for 5 min, and then subjected to two-dimensional (nonreduced, reduced) polyacrylamide gel electrophoresis in the presence of SDS (2-D PAGE) as described.[16,17] The first dimension contained 5% acrylamide, and the second dimension 7.5% acrylamide. The upper tank buffer in the second dimension always contained 5 mM sodium thioglycolate to prevent reoxidation during electrophoresis. Further details are given elsewhere.[16,17]

Gels were stained with Coomassie blue, destained and dried.[14] Staining allowed the detection of cytoplasmic IgG and nonradioactive molecular weight standards myosin (Mr = 200,000) (Mr; relative molecular mass), β-galactosidase (Mr = 116,000), phosphorylase (Mr = 95,000), bovine serum albumin (Mr = 68,000) and ovalbumin (Mr = 43,000). Accurate alignment of the gel with the autoradiograph was facilitated by marking the gel at several points with ink containing ^{35}S-methionine.

Immunoprecipitation

This was carried out by standard procedures.[14]

Peptide Mapping

Peptide mapping by partial proteolysis was carried out as described by Cleveland et al.[18] with slight modifications.[17,19] Staphylococcal V8 protease was used at 50 μg/ml for one hour at room temperature. In some experiments, 4 M urea was incorporated in the stacking gel.[19] Undigested MOPC-21 IgG was used as a standard.

RESULTS

Disulfide Bonding in ^{125}I-labeled Membrane Proteins of the B-Lymphomas WEHI-231 and 2PK3

The B-lymphomas WEHI-231 and 2PK3 were radioiodinated, and their membranes solubilized and analyzed by 2-D PAGE. Results are shown in FIGURE 2. It is very surprising how few heavily labeled proteins are made up of disulfide-bonded chains.[16] This is probably not because of selective labeling, because the lactoperoxidase technique is thought to be the least selective of all available cell surface labeling methods.[20,21] Even more remarkably, most of the disulfide-bonded structures seen can be tentatively or positively identified.

As previously reported,[16] the surface IgM of WEHI-231 was extremely prominent in the whole extract. Its chain composition and disulfide bonding was consistent with the expected μ_2K_2 structure. In this experiment, higher molecular weight polymeric forms were not seen. Similarly, the surface IgG2a of 2PK3 was clearly visible in the whole extract. The identity of these chains was confirmed by immunoprecipitation (data not shown). It should be noted that the Mr of the membrane γ2a chain was approximately 60,000, compared to approximately 50,000 for secretory γ2a chains in the same gel. These size estimates are in reasonable agreement with those of Oi et al.[8] The intact Mr of membrane IgG2a of 2PK3 was slightly greater than that of secretory IgG2a, consistent with a 4-chain structure.

Polypeptides A and B

Polypeptide A (Mr 200,000 intact and 116,000 reduced) was present in 2PK3 but absent in WEHI-231 (FIGURE 2). It was also present in the plasmacytomas MPC-11, MOPC-21 and NS-1 (FIGURE 3 and see below), but was not detectable in thymus, nor in any of the T-lymphomas WEHI-7, WEHI-22, WEHI-222, WEHI-242 or ST-4. Very small amounts were sometimes detectable in spleen. The

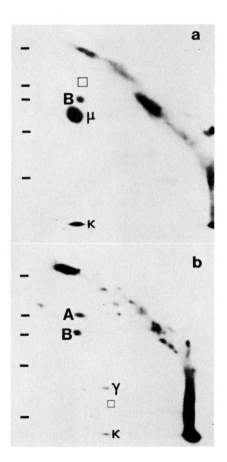

FIGURE 2. Two-dimensional analysis of membrane proteins of the B-lymphomas WEHI-231 (panel a) and 2PK3 (panel b). Electrophoresis proceeds from left to right (intact; 5% acrylamide) and then from top to bottom (reduced; 7.5% acrylamide). The square in panel "a" indicates the expected position of polypeptide A seen in panel "b." The square in panel "b" indicates the position of γ2a chains from nonradioactive MOPC-173 protein run in the same gel. Polypeptide B is the transferrin receptor. The horizontal bars indicate the positions of molecular weight standards. From top to bottom: 200,000; 116,000; 95,000; 68,000; 43,000.

reduced Mr of polypeptide A is similar to that reported for the plasma cell alloantigen PC-1.[22] It is therefore interesting to note that 2PK3 secretes small amounts of IgG2a[8,10] while IgM secretion is virtually undetectable in unstimulated WEHI-231 cells.[23] Antibodies to PC-1 precipitated polypeptide A (data not shown).

Polypeptide B (Mr 200,000 intact and 95,000 reduced) has previously been demonstrated to be the receptor for the iron transport protein transferrin.[16,17]

A third disulfide-bonded membrane protein (Mr 135,000 reduced and approx-

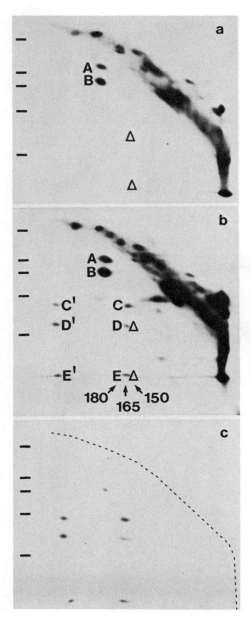

FIGURE 3. Two-dimensional analysis of membrane proteins of myeloma cells. Conditions of electrophoresis and molecular weight standards as for FIGURE 2. Panel a: MPC-11, panel b: MOPC-21, and panel c: immunoglobulin from MOPC-21. The dotted line indicates the mobility of proteins which are not made up of disulfide bonded subunits. The triangles indicate the positions of nonradioactive stained cytoplasmic γ and light chains.

imately 300,000–400,000 intact) was seen in 2PK3 extracts (FIGURE 2). This protein shares some properties with the insulin receptor,[24] although it has not been formally identified as such.

Disulfide Bonding in ^{125}I-labeled Membrane Proteins of the Plasmacytomas MPC-11 and MOPC-21

The IgG2b-secreting line MPC-11 did not possess detectable amounts of membrane immunoglobulin (FIGURE 3), although cytoplasmic IgG was readily detected in the same gel by staining. This result gives confidence that the ^{125}I labeling was confined to the plasma membrane, and is consistent with reports that IgG2-secreting plasmacytomas do not possess easily detectable membrane immunoglobulin.[25]

In contrast to MPC-11, the plasmacytoma MOPC-21 revealed a somewhat complex, and initially puzzling, surface immunoglobulin pattern (FIGURE 3). Two heavy chain spots were observed, of Mr 65,000 (C) and 55,000 (D). These spots lay on the same vertical line as the light chain spot E, and corresponded to an intact Mr of about 165,000. A similar triad of spots (C', D' and E') were also present at a position corresponding to an intact Mr of about 250,000. All six polypeptides were precipitated by anti-IgG1 antibodies (FIGURE 3). Traces of polypeptide B precipitated by anti-IgG1 may be due to contaminating antibodies to transferrin, as previously discussed.[17] Examination of the nonsecreting variant NS-1 showed an identical pattern to that of MOPC-21 except that spots C, C', D, D', E and E' were all absent (data not shown).

The unreduced mobility of spots C, D and E was consistently less than that of cytoplasmic IgG in the same gel (FIGURE 3). The mobility of ^{35}S-labeled secreted MOPC-21 IgG was not detectably different from that of the stained cytoplasmic IgG (data not shown). There was no detectable radioactivity over the stained cytoplasmic γ or light chain spots, indicating that the label was confined to the cell surface. The possibility that spot C consisted of partially reduced IgG containing one secretory heavy chain and one light chain was ruled out, because examination of gels in which nonradioactive MOPC-21 IgG had been added revealed complete reduction.

Peptide Mapping

By analogy with 2PK3 (reference 8 and FIGURE 2), it seemed possible that spots C and D represented membrane and secretory γ1 chains, respectively. In an attempt to clarify their identity, spots C, C', D, D', E and E' were cut out of the dried gel, rehydrated and subjected to peptide mapping using staphylococcal V8 protease. Results are shown in FIGURE 4.

Surprisingly few cleavages occurred, in spite of the fact that the proteins had been previously boiled in SDS, fixed, stained, destained, dried, rehydrated and the digestion occurred in SDS. It is clear, however, that polypeptides C' and C were very similar, as were D' and D, E' and E. Moreover, the cleavage patterns of C and C' were virtually identical to those of D and D', except that C and C' were seen to possess an extra peptide (FIGURE 4). Polypeptide C was thus identified as membrane γ1 chain (see DISCUSSION).

Peptide mapping was also carried out in the presence of 4 M urea (FIGURE 5). A much larger number of cleavages were seen, consistent with more extensive

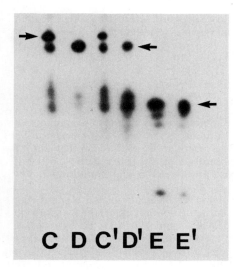

FIGURE 4. Peptide maps of polypeptides from FIGURE 3. Spots were cut out, rehydrated, placed in the sample well of a 15% acrylamide gel and overlaid with staphylococcal V8 protease. Current was stopped for one hour when the dye marker approached the main gel. The arrow pointing to the right indicates the position of undigested membrane γ1 chains. The arrow pointing to the left in lane D' indicates the mobility of undigested secretory γ1 chains, while the arrow pointing to the left in lane E' indicates the position of undigested light chains.

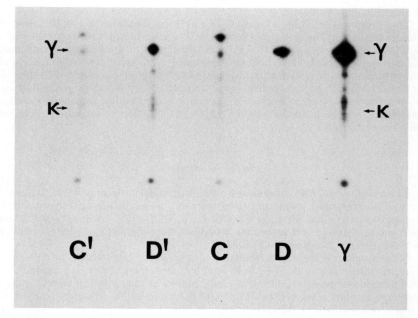

FIGURE 5. Peptide maps of polypeptides from FIGURE 3. Conditions were as described in the legend to FIGURE 4, except that the stacking gel included 4M urea. The lane on the extreme right shows a map of ^{125}I-labeled secretory γ1 chains from purified MOPC-21 IgG.

unfolding. Homology of C, C', D and D' to each other was confirmed, and all four were homologous to authentic $\gamma1$ chains.

Reproducibility

The results reported here were consistently obtained in numerous experiments. Work was always performed rapidly, and the time between addition of Triton X-100 and loading the gels did not usually exceed 30 min. The ratio of the intensities of spots C:D and C':D' was not altered when the Triton lysate was held at 37°C for one hour prior to addition of SDS and electrophoretic analysis (data not shown).

DISCUSSION

Polypeptide A

Polypeptide A (intact Mr 200,000; reduced Mr 116,000) was very prominent in the plasmacytomas MOPC-21, NS-1 and MPC-11. It was also present in the secretory B-lymphoma 2PK3, but was absent from the nonsecretory B-lymphoma WEHI-231. It was undetectable in thymus, while traces were present in spleen.

Polypeptide A has the same reduced Mr as the plasma cell alloantigen PC-1.[22] The unreduced Mr of PC-1 has not been published to my knowledge. The data therefore suggest that PC-1 is a disulfide-bonded homodimer.

The PC-1 alloantigen is not confined to lymphoid cells. It is also found on brain, liver and kidney,[22] all of which may be considered secretory organs. If polypeptide A and PC-1 are identical, the question arises whether it is a component of the secretory apparatus. A likely candidate would be one of the Mr 100,000 polypeptides associated with coated vesicles.[26]

Polypeptide A shows a number of interesting parallels to the transferrin receptor (polypeptide B). Both appear to be disulfide-bonded homodimers. Both appear to be developmentally regulated (associated with secretion and cell proliferation, respectively). Both may have a transport function (exocytosis and endocytosis,[27] respectively).

These considerations indicate that polypeptides A and B may have a common evolutionary origin, and suggest a series of experiments. Can polypeptide A be induced in spleen cells by lipopolysaccharide? Does polypeptide A contain covalently attached lipid, as has been recently shown for the transferrin receptor?[28] Can sequence homology be detected by peptide mapping or gene sequencing?

Peptide Mapping of $\gamma1$ Chains

The limited number of cleavages of $\gamma1$ chains by staphylococcal V8 protease (FIGURE 4) was surprising. It appears that a considerable degree of domain structure is preserved in the presence of SDS. Oi and Herzenberg were able to generate large fragments of $\gamma2a$ chains under very similar conditions.[29]

Staphylococcal V8 protease cleaves at glutamic and aspartic acid residues.[30] The size of the largest fragment of membrane $\gamma1$ chains was virtually identical to the size of intact secretory $\gamma1$ chains (FIGURE 4), consistent with cleavage at the "membrane hinge" where there is a short stretch of six acidic amino acids (see FIGURE 1). A second cleavage, which occurred in all heavy chains, resulted in two fragments each about the size of light chains. A likely site of cleavage is the two acidic residues in the middle of the first hinge (FIGURE 1). In the presence of 4M urea, cleavage was much less selective (FIGURE 5).

Subunit Structure of Surface IgG on MOPC-21

Several recent reports have shown that the membrane form of γ chains has an Mr of approximately 10,000 larger than the secretory form.[4,8] The size, surface location, antigenic properties and homology with secretory $\gamma1$ chains clearly identify polypeptides C and C' as membrane forms of $\gamma1$ chain. Polypeptides E and E' are identified as light chains on the basis of their size and disulfide bonding to heavy chains.

Interpretation of the data is crucially dependent on the identity of spots D and D'. One possibility would be that spots C, D, and E represent a simple mixture of conventional secretory and membrane IgG. This possibility is unlikely for several reasons. The unreduced mobility of these two forms should be different, because there is a difference of about 20,000 ($2 \times 10,000$) in the Mr of the heavy chains. This difference in unreduced Mr (170,000 versus 150,000, or more than 10%) is well within the resolving power of the gels. Moreover, the mobility of unreduced secretory and cytoplasmic IgG was clearly faster than the mobility of spots C, D and E in the same gel (FIGURE 3). Finally, it appears that all three are part of an integral membrane protein, because all were recovered from the detergent phase when analyzed by the method of Bordier,[31] while secretory MOPC-21 IgG was recovered exclusively in the aqueous phase (manuscript in preparation).

Spot D might possibly have represented a breakdown product of membrane $\gamma1$ chains. This possibility is unlikely for several reasons. Inhibitors of thiol, metallo- and serine proteases were included during solubilization, which was performed rapidly and in the cold. Prolonged incubations at 37° did not alter the relative amounts of these chains. Proteolytic breakdown of membrane IgG is totally unable to explain the presence of spots C', D and D'. Finally, proteolysis is not tenable as an explanation because it would have to be partial, and partial proteolysis would cause heterogeneity of the unreduced size, resulting in three distinct entities (both heavy chains intact; one heavy chain cleaved; both heavy chains cleaved). This form of heterogeneity was not observed.

Spots D and D' are certainly not cytoplasmic $\gamma1$ chains, because the mobility of the latter was clearly distinct (FIGURE 3). Could they have represented differently glycosylated forms of membrane $\gamma1$ chains? Asymmetry of glycosylation of rabbit γ chains was observed by Fanger and Smyth.[32] Secretory $\gamma1$ chains have only one glycosylation site, and the $\gamma1$ membrane C-terminal extension does not contain potential glycosylation sites for N-linked sugars.[5,6] Moreover, the polypeptide sequence predicted by cDNA clones indicates that the membrane $\gamma1$ polypeptide backbone must be 7,000 daltons larger than secretory $\gamma1$ polypeptide.[6] The contribution of carbohydrate is only around 2,000 daltons.[33] Thus, even completely unglycosylated membrane $\gamma1$ chains would be expected to have an apparent Mr substantially greater than that of secretory $\gamma1$ chains. Finally, there is no way that asymmetry of glycosylation could generate spots C', D' and E'.

Spots C', D' and E' could have represented noncovalent aggregates. This is rendered highly unlikely by the fact that they ran as a tight band approximately 10 mm from the end of the gel, and were not polydisperse. The dismissal of spots C′, D′ and E′ as random noncovalent aggregates would still require that a second unlikely event (e.g., asymmetrical glycosylation) also took place.

All of these inconsistencies can be resolved by postulating that C, D and E are subunits of a hybrid IgG molecule consisting of one membrane heavy chain, one secretory heavy chain and two light chains, and that this hybrid molecule is capable of forming disulfide-bonded dimers. This postulate is consistent with current knowledge of the synthesis of membrane and secretory proteins. Apart from its simplicity and compelling logic, it is the only explanation that fits all the data.

In a cell producing both secretory and membrane IgG1, both nascent γ1 chains must be transported across the membrane of the rough endoplasmic reticulum. After removal of their leader sequences, the secretory chains lie free in the lumen, while the membrane chains remain attached to the membrane via their hydrophobic C-termini (FIGURE 6). Shortly after synthesis, interchain disulfide bonds begin to form. In IgG1-secreting cells, the interheavy chain bonds form first.[34] Unless there are special mechanisms to prevent the formation of hybrid molecules,[8,35] the pairing of closely related heavy chains would be expected to follow the law of mass action. Thus, in a cell in which the rate of synthesis of secretory γ1 chains is greatly in excess of that of membrane γ1 chains, virtually all membrane γ1 chains would be disulfide-bonded to a secretory γ1 chain (FIGURE 6). This is precisely what is observed (FIGURE 3).

If such a simple and obvious explanation of surface immunoglobulin on MOPC-21 is correct, why has it not been seen until now? There are probably several reasons. First, many investigators may have felt reluctant to examine the surface of plasma cells because of the difficulty in deciding what is "true" membrane IgG versus what is "on the way out." However, the greatly improved understanding of membrane insertion and secretion in recent years makes it clear that secretory IgG "on the way out" would be immediately washed away both before and after iodination. Only firmly attached IgG would remain. Secondly, it is only recently that it has become clear that membrane and secretory γ chains can be distinguished structurally.[4,8] Thirdly, any labeling of "secretory-size" γ chains may have been incorrectly dismissed as indicating cytoplasmic labeling. Only in a two-dimensional system can this possibility be ruled out.

The literature on the biochemical characterization of surface immunoglobulin on secretory cells is quite difficult to evaluate.[25] Here, I will describe two examples where the data may have been incorrectly interpreted.

Singer and Williamson[4] examined surface immunoglobulin on human lymphoblastoid cell lines. The lines which expressed both forms of immunoglobulin (BTAB and BEC-11) incorporated 1.1% and 2.1% respectively of TCA-precipitable ^{35}S-methionine counts into cytoplasmic immunoglobulin over a one-hour period. In contrast, the corresponding mean incorporation into cytoplasmic immunoglobulin for murine plasmacytomas was 30% over a 30 minute period.[34] Close inspection of the data on surface IgG of BEC-11 shows that small amounts of secretory-size γ chains were labeled in addition to membrane-size γ. The data concerning BJAB was difficult to evaluate because the difference in mobility between secretory and membrane μ was much less that the width of the ^{125}I-labeled μ chain peak. Thus, the data of Singer and Williamson are not incompatible with the data presented here.

Oi et al.[8] examined the surface IgG on the B-lymphoma 2PK3. Surface labeling with ^{125}I revealed heavily labeled Mr 65,000 γ2a chains and lightly labeled Mr 55,000 γ2a chains. The latter were dismissed as being due to cytoplasmic labeling of dead cells, or secretory γ2a chains "on the way out." They proposed that membrane and secreted immunoglobulins may have different hinge regions to prevent incorrect pairing. However, the nucleotide sequence of the hinge region of a cDNA clone of membrane γ1 RNA is identical to that of secretory γ1 chains.[6]

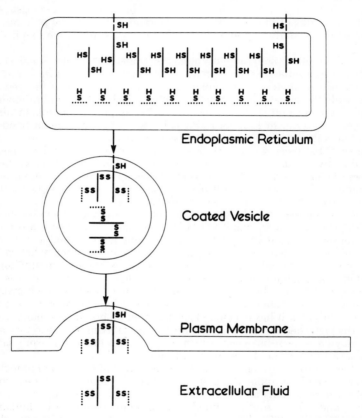

FIGURE 6. Assembly and transport of membrane and secretory IgG in plasma cells. The hydrophobic C-terminal extension of membrane γ1 chains is shown as a dashed line. For simplicity, the Golgi complex has been omitted, and it is assumed that membrane and secretory γ1 chains travel to the surface in the same coated vesicle.

Similarly, the amino acid sequence of secretory and membrane forms of μ chains (which do not possess a hinge) differ only at their C-terminus.[3] It is therefore very unlikely that hinge region differences are a general mechanism for the prevention of pairing of membrane and secretory heavy chains.

Thus, the data of Singer and Williamson,[4] and that of Oi et al.[8] may be explained by the fact that in both cases the rate of secretion was much less than that of plasmacytomas, and the selective partitioning of membrane heavy chains in the membrane would favor homologous pairing. Only in plasmacytomas would the vast excess of secretory chains force the formation of hybrids.

The formation of dimeric forms of surface IgG1 (FIGURE 3) is also simply explained by a "random collision" model. The nucleotide sequence for the C-terminal extension of membrane γ1 chains contains codons for two cysteine residues[5,6] (FIGURE 1). One of these lies in a hydrophilic segment which probably lies outside the cell,[5,6] while the other is probably situated within the lipid bilayer.[5,6] The location of these cysteine residues is such that it is most unlikely that they would pair with each other. In a conventional surface IgG1 molecule, they would presumably pair with the homologous membrane heavy chain. In a hybrid IgG1 molecule they might be unpaired (FIGURE 1), or might pair with the corresponding cysteine residues in another hybrid IgG1 molecule, resulting in hybrid IgG dimers, as seen in FIGURE 3.

The sulfhydryl-blocking reagent N-ethylmaleimide was included in the solubilization buffer to prevent the formation of artifactual disulfide bonds and disulfide bond interchange. It therefore seems likely that the dimers of IgG actually exist on the cell surface.

What is the biological significance of hybrid IgG1 molecules on the surface of MOPC-21 cells? Is it a mere "curiosity"? Nossal and Lewis[36] found that a large proportion of both IgM and IgG plaque-forming cells had detectable surface immunoglobulin as late as 10 days after primary immunization and four days after secondary challenge, with decreasing amounts thereafter. Even by day eight in the secondary response, surface immunoglobulin was detectable on some plaque-forming cells. Thus, the potential of antibody-forming cells to respond to antigen may be preserved until a very late stage in B-cell differentiation.

In a fully developed plasma cell, the rate of synthesis of secretory immunoglobulin is more than one hundred-fold that of membrane immunoglobulin.[33] What would be the biological consequences of heavy chain pairing driven only by the law of mass action? Secretion would be unimpaired because less than 1% of secretory γ1 chains would be diverted to the membrane. The fact that the monomeric hybrid IgG molecules remained in the membrane during multiple washes indicates that only one hydrophobic tail is sufficient for membrane anchoring. The biological function of membrane immunoglobulin on plasma cells is not known, although it may transmit a negative signal in some circumstances.[37] The effect of a single hydrophobic tail on transmembrane signalling is hard to predict.

Many plasmacytomas do not possess detectable amounts of membrane immunoglobulin.[25] MOPC-21 may thus represent an unusual case. Nonetheless, the results obtained here can tell us a number of things about the biosynthesis and assembly of immunoglobulins in general. The synthetic and assembly mechanisms of membrane and secretory immunoglobulins are shared. There do not appear to be special mechanisms to prevent pairing of membrane and secretory heavy chains, apart from simple diffusion. However, the biological cost of the resulting hybrid molecules is probably very small. The presence of only one hydrophobic tail is evidently sufficient for retention of IgG1 in the membrane. The C-terminal extension cysteine residues of membrane γ1 chains in hybrid IgG1 molecules are either unpaired or may allow the formation of hybrid IgG dimers. Finally, if the reasoning presented in this paper is correct, it would appear that whenever high-rate antibody secreting cells make membrane forms, their surface immunoglobulins will be asymmetrical.

ACKNOWLEDGMENTS

I thank Rod Mitchell for excellent technical assistance and Brett Tyler for discussions and communication of unpublished data.

REFERENCES

1. ROGERS, J., P. EARLY, C. CARTER, K. CALAME, M. BOND, L. HOOD & R. WALL. 1980. Two mRNAs with different 3′ ends encode membrane-bound and secreted forms of immunoglobulin μ chain. Cell **20:** 303–312.
2. ALT, F. W., A. L. M. BOTHWELL, M. KNAPP, E. SIDEN, E. MATHER, M. KOSHLAND & D. BALTIMORE. 1980. Synthesis of secreted and membrane-bound immunoglobulin μ heavy chains is directed by mRNAs that differ at their 3′ ends. Cell **20:** 293–301.
3. KEHRY, M., S. EWALD, R. DOUGLAS, C. SIBLEY, W. RASCHKE, D. FAMBROUGH & L. HOOD. 1980. The immunoglobulin μ chains of membrane-bound and secreted IgM molecules differ in their C-terminal segments. Cell **21:** 393–406.
4. SINGER, P. A. & A. R. WILLIAMSON. 1980. Cell surface immunoglobulin μ and γ chains of human lymphoid cells are of higher apparent molecular weight than their secreted counterparts. Eur. J. Immunol. **10:** 180–186.
5. ROGERS, J., E. CHOI, L. SOUZA, C. CARTER, C. WORD, M. KUEHL, D. EISENBERG & R. WALL. 1981. Gene segments encoding transmembrane carboxy-termini of immunoglobulin γ chains. Cell **26:** 19–27.
6. TYLER, B. M., A. F. COWMAN, S. D. GERONDAKIS, J. M. ADAMS & O. BERNARD. 1982. Messenger RNA for surface immunoglobulin γ chains encodes a highly conserved transmembrane sequence and a 28-residue intracellular domain. Proc. Natl. Acad. Sci. U.S.A. **79:** 2008–2012.
7. BLATTNER, F. T. 1982. Genetic aspects of IgD expression. Ann. N.Y. Acad. Sci. This volume.
8. OI, V. T., V. M. BRYAN, L. A. HERZENBERG & L. A. HERZENBERG. 1980. Lymphocyte membrane IgG and secreted IgG are structurally and allotypically distinct. J. Exp. Med. **151:** 1260–1274.
9. WARNER, N. L., A. W. HARRIS & G. A. GUTMAN. 1975. Membrane immunoglobulin and Fc receptors of murine T and B lymphomas. In Membrane Receptors of Lymphocytes. M. Seligmann, J. L. Preud'homme and F. M. Kourilsky, Eds.: 203–216. North-Holland/American Elsevier.
10. WARNER, N. L., M. J. DALEY, J. RICHEY & C. SPELLMAN. 1979. Flow cytometry analysis of murine B cell lymphoma differentiation. Immunol. Rev. **48:** 197–243.
11. LASKOV, R. & M. D. SCHARFF. 1970. Synthesis, assembly and secretion of gamma globulin by mouse myeloma cells. J. Exp. Med. **131:** 515–541.
12. HORIBATA, K. & A. W. HARRIS. 1970. Mouse myelomas and lymphomas in culture. Exp. Cell. Res. **60:** 61–77.
13. KÖHLER, G., S. C. HOWE & C. MILSTEIN. 1976. Fusion between immunoglobulin-secreting and non-secreting myeloma cell lines. Eur. J. Immunol. **6:** 292–295.
14. GODING, J. W. 1980. Structural studies of lymphocyte surface IgD. J. Immunol. **124:** 2082–2088.
15. LEE, S-K. J. SINGH & R. B. TAYLOR. 1975. Subclasses of T cells with differing sensitivities to cytotoxic antibody in the presence of anesthetics. Eur. J. Immunol. **5:** 259–262.
16. GODING, J. W. & A. W. HARRIS. 1981. Subunit structure of cell surface proteins: Disulfide bonding in antigen receptors, Ly-2/3 antigens, and transferrin receptors of murine T and B lymphocytes. Proc. Natl. Acad. Sci. U.S.A. **78:** 4530–4539.
17. GODING, J. W., & G. F. BURNS. 1981. Monoclonal antibody OKT-9 recognizes the receptor for transferrin on human acute lymphocytic leukemia cells. J. Immunol. **127:** 1256–1258.
18. CLEVELAND, D. W., S. G. FISHER, M. W. KIRSCHNER & U. K. LAEMMLI. 1977. Peptide

mapping by limited proteolysis in sodium dodecyl sulfate and analysis by gel electrophoresis. J. Biol. Chem **252:** 1102–1106.

19. HANDMAN, E., G. F. MITCHELL & J. W. GODING. 1981. Identification and characterization of protein antigens of *Leishmania Tropica* isolates. J. Immunol **126:** 508–512.

20. HUBBARD, A. L. & Z. A. COHN. 1976. Specific labels for cell surfaces. In Biochemical Analysis of Membranes. A. H. Maddy, Ed.: 427–501. John Wiley and Sons. New York, N.Y.

21. KAPLAN, G., H. PLUTNER, I. MELLMAN & J. C. UNKELESS. 1981. Studies on externally disposed plasma membrane proteins. Trinitrobenzene sulfonic acid derivatization and immune precipitation. Exp. Cell. Res. **133:** 103–114.

22. TUNG, J-S., F. W. SHEN, E. A. BOYSE & E. FLEISSNER. 1978. Properties of the PC-1 molecule. Immunogenetics **6:** 101–105.

23. BOYD, A. W., J. W. GODING & J. W. SCHRADER. 1981. Regulation of growth and differentiation of a murine B cell lymphoma. I. Lipopolysaccharide-induced differentiation. J. Immunol. **126:** 2461–2465.

24. SIEGEL, T. W., S. GANDULY, S. JACOBS, O. M. ROSEN & C. RUBIN. 1981. Purification and properties of the human placental insulin receptor. J. Biol. Chem. **256:** 9266–9273.

25. STALL, A. M. & P. K. KNOPF. 1978. The effect of inhibitors of protein synthesis on the re-expression of surface immunoglobulin following antigenic modulation. Cell **14:** 33–42.

26. RUBENSTEIN, J. R. L., R. E. FINE, B. D. LUSKEY & J. E. ROTHMAN. 1981. Purification of coated vesicles by agarose gel electrophoresis. J. Cell Biol. **89:** 357–361.

27. KARIN, M. & B. MINTZ. 1981. Receptor-mediated endocytosis of transferrin in developmentally totipotent mouse teratocarcinoma stem cells. J. Biol. Chem. **256:** 3245–3252.

28. OMARY, M. B. & I. S. TROWBRIDGE. 1981. Covalent binding of fatty acid to the transferrin receptor in cultured human cells. J. Biol. Chem. **256:** 4715–4718.

29. OI, V. T. & L. A. HERZENBERG. 1979. Localization of allotypic determinants on mouse immunoglobulin. Mol. Immunol. **16:** 1005–1017.

30. DRAPEAU, G. R. 1976. Protease from *Staphylococcus aureus*. Meth. Enzymol. **45:** 469–475.

31. BORDIER, C. 1981. Phase separation of integral membrane proteins in Triton X-114 solution. J. Biol. Chem. **256:** 1604–1607.

32. FANGER, M. W. & D. G. SMYTH. 1972. The oligosaccharide units of rabbit immunoglobulin G, asymmetric attachment of C2-oligosaccharide. Biochem. J. **127:** 767–774.

33. WORD, C. J. & W. M. KUEHL. 1981. Expression of surface and secreted IgG2a by a murine B-lymphoma before and after hybridization to myeloma cells. Mol. Immunol. **18:** 311–322.

34. BAUMAL, R. & M. D. SCHARFF. 1973. Synthesis, assembly and secretion of mouse immunoglobulin. Transplant Rev. **14:** 163–183.

35. KÖHLER, G., H. HENGARTNER & M. J. SHULMAN. 1978. Immunoglobulin production by lymphocyte hybridomas. Eur. J. Immunol. **8:** 82–88.

36. NOSSAL, G. J. V. & H. LEWIS. 1972. Variation in accessible cell surface immunoglobulin among antibody-forming cells. J. Exp. Med. **135:** 1416.

37. BOYD, A. W. & J. W. SCHRADER. 1980. Mechanism of effector-cell blockade. I. Antigen-induced suppression of Ig synthesis in a hybridoma cell line, and correlation with cell-associated antigen. J. Exp. Med. **151:** 1436–1451.

DISCUSSION OF THE PAPER

D. S. ROWE: Have you studied capping in this particular tumor cell line. If it only has one instead of two hydrophobic tails sticking through, it makes no difference to the one transmembrane function that one can study?

J. W. GODING: I think that there is evidence to show that the membrane Ig on plasma cells can transmit at least a negative signal in some circumstances. The work of John Schrader and his colleagues on effector cell blockade and also others have shown that membrane Ig can mediate turning off secretion under some circumstances. We have not studied capping in this cell line, but the issue is discussed in detail in reference 25.

IgD: A COMPONENT OF THE SECRETORY IMMUNE SYSTEM?*

Joan C. Olson and Gerrie A. Leslie

Department of Microbiology and Immunology
The Oregon Health Sciences University
Portland, Oregon 97201

INTRODUCTION

IgD, identified by Rowe and Fahey in 1965,[1] remains the only class of serum immunoglobulin whose function is unknown. Its usually low concentration in human serum yet frequent presence on the surface of B-cells has led many investigators to examine the possible role of IgD as a B-cell surface antigen receptor. However, no one has succeeded in identifying a function for the IgD-receptor that is not also associated with the IgM-surface receptor. Thus, it has been proposed that the IgD-receptor serves as a "filler" immunoglobulin, possibly buffering the cell from the limited diversification associated with IgM only bearing lymphocytes and IgM secreting plasma cells.[2,3]

Arguments that favor a unique role for IgD include its phylogenetic conservation. In addition to humans, IgD has been identified in nonhuman primates,[4,5] mice,[6,7] rats,[8,9] rabbits[10] and chickens.[11] In each of these species, however, the serum concentration is low, and there is no evidence, except in the human, of an antibody function. Evidence supporting the importance of IgD was revealed in recent studies of Metcalf et al.[12] They observed that IgD-suppressed mice succumbed to an infectious dose of *Salmonella typhimurium*, whereas control animals recovered. Their inability to cope with a challenge by this live organism emphasized that the immune system of the anti-δ treated animals was functionally impaired; however, by all other criteria studied these animals appeared normal.

This paper reports the observation that high concentrations of IgD exist in rat milk. The known similarities in physicochemical and regulatory properties of IgD as compared to the secretory immunoglobulins, IgA and IgE, and the now recognized prevalence of IgD in milk may provide some of the missing links to the IgD mystery.

MATERIALS AND METHODS

Animals

The animals used in these studies were the F22 generation of HPR (high precipitin responder) strain of rats, which had been selectively brother-sister inbred in our laboratory for the production of high concentrations of precipitating anti-group A streptococcal carbohydrate (anti-SACHO) antibodies.[13]

*This investigation was supported by grants from the National Institute of Child Health and Human Development (HD 12381), The Medical Research Foundation of Oregon, a Biomedical Research Support grant from OHSU, and the N.L. Tartar Research Fund.

97

Immunizations

When indicated, animals were immunized with group A streptococcal vaccine (GASV), prepared as previously described.[13] The standard immunization protocol requires the injection of 1 mg of GASV intravenously (iv) three times a week for three weeks. However, in these studies some animals were given antigen via the same protocol intragastrically (ig).

Milking Protocol

Seventeen female HPR rats were each milked four separate times during their nursing period. The actual times of milking varied with the individual rats but ranged from within a few hours after birth of progeny until progeny were 27 days of age. No milk could be obtained from the females after day 27. Prior to milking, each female was anesthetized I.M. with 0.25 ml of a mixture containing ketamine HCl (100 mg/ml), xylazine HCl (20 mg/ml), acepromazine (10 mg/ml) and saline in a ratio of 1:0.5:0.2:0.3, respectively. Approximately 10 minutes later, when the effects of the anesthetic became apparent, animals were injected iv with 0.25 units of oxytocin. Using a suction apparatus, each nipple was then sequentially milked. Depending upon the time during the nursing period from 0.5–7.0 ml of milk could be obtained from each mother. The highest yields were obtained from days 12–20 after birth of progeny.

Antisera

Anti-rat IgD was prepared in our laboratory by four different techniques. The preparation and specificity of the sheep and the rabbit anti-membrane IgD antisera have been previously reported.[14,15] In addition, an anti-rat serum IgD reagent was prepared using as immunogen an eluate from a rabbit anti-rat membrane IgD coupled immunoadsorbent (IA) column over which a large pool of rat serum had been passaged. This antiserum was extensively absorbed to assure its δ specificity. A fourth antiserum was similarly prepared but the IgD was isolated from the serum of a single rat that had a high level of IgD. Other class and subclass specific antisera were prepared as previously described.[16]

Analysis of Colostrum and Milk

Methods for Ouchterlony analysis, radial immunodiffusion assays, gel filtration, and the preparation and elution of affinity IA columns have been previously described. Our standard in the IgD assays was quantified through the kindness of Dr. Herve Bazin.

RESULTS

The Identification of IgD in Rat Milk

During an extensive screening program designed to detect conditions under which IgD concentrations were elevated in rats, we consistently observed that milk obtained from several strains of rats contained very high concentrations of IgD. The presence of IgD within rat milk was confirmed by Ouchterlony analysis using three different approaches. Firstly, a reaction of identity was observed when four different anti-rat δ preparations were reacted against rat milk. These included separate sheep and rabbit reagents prepared against rat membrane associated IgD, a reagent prepared against pooled rat serum IgD and one prepared against the IgD of a single rat having hyper-IgD in its serum. Secondly, reactions of nonidentity were observed when anti-rat δ, μ, α and γ antisera were reacted against rat milk, while a reaction of partial identity occurred when anti-rat δ and Fab' antisera were reacted against rat milk (FIGURE 1, upper gel diffusion). Thirdly, a reaction of identity was observed between a hyper-IgD rat

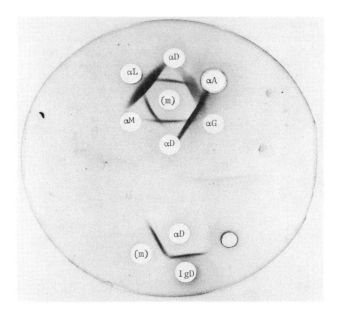

FIGURE 1. Upper: Gel diffusion analysis of rat milk (m) with anti-IgD (αD), anti-IgA (αA), anti-IgG2a, 2b (αG), anti-IgM (αM) and anti-Fab' (αL). Lower: Gel diffusion analysis of rat milk (m) and a rat serum containing a high level of IgD with anti-IgD (αD). The unmarked well contained a mixture of three parts milk: one part serum.

serum and rat milk when reacted with anti-rat serum IgD (FIGURE 1, lower gel diffusion). We also observed that milk obtained from the same or different females at different times during the nursing period all contained an antigen which gave a reaction of identity with anti-rat IgD. In contrast, maternal or neonatal serum obtained at the same time from the respective rats showed no detectable IgD by gel diffusion analysis.

Interestingly, as shown in FIGURE 1, (lower gel diffusion) rat milk diluted 3:1 in normal rat serum appeared to lose much of its IgD reactivity as assessed by Ouchterlony analysis. Diluting the milk sample 3:1 in buffer does not produce as significant a loss of activity. This implies that a normal serum component(s) is either breaking down or masking the IgD specific-antigenic determinants.

The Concentration of IgD in Rat Milk

In order to analyze the kinetics of IgD production in rat milk, a total of 17 GASV-immune or nonimmune HPR female rats were bred to nonimmune males of the same strain. After the birth of progeny each female was repeatedly milked. Two age groups of mothers were included, three months and seven months old, respectively. In order to determine if different routes of immunization would alter the concentrations of IgD in milk, one group of females was fed GASV and another group was injected with GASV iv. Both groups received GASV via the same hyperimmunization schedule. Concomitant with the milkings, the mothers and newborns were bled which enabled a direct comparison to be made of immunoglobulin and antibody concentrations in maternal and pup sera with that in milk.

The concentrations of IgD in milk at various times after the birth of progeny are shown in Figure 2 (upper graph). Regardless of the route of immunization, all animals exposed to GASV via the standard immunization schedule had comparable concentrations of IgD in their milk and were thus grouped together.

There is a consistent trend in all three groups of animals for milk obtained early and late in the nursing period to contain higher concentrations of IgD than

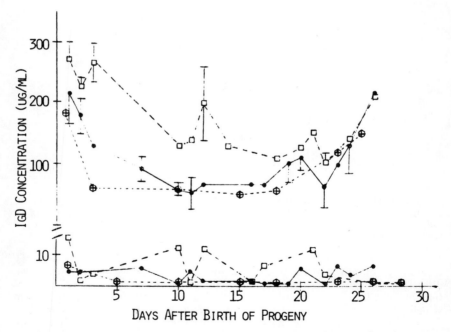

FIGURE 2. The concentration of IgD in HPR rat milk (upper part of graph) compared to the concentration in maternal serum (lower part of graph). IgD levels in milk or sera obtained from six GASV-immune mothers 7 months of age = □; nine GASV-immune mothers 3 months of age ●; two nonimmune mothers 3 months of age. Bars represent the standard error of the mean and indicate that more than one female of the specific group was sampled on that date.

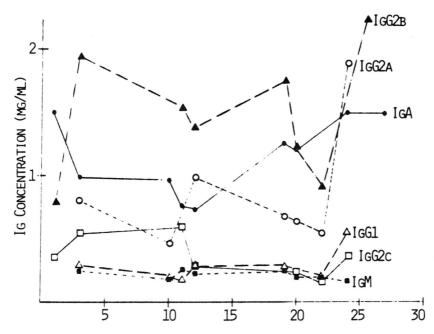

FIGURE 3. The concentration of immunoglobulin classes and subclasses in the milk of four different GASV-immunized HPR females at various times after parturition.

milk obtained during the interim. The higher IgD levels correspond to the periods of low milk volume output. Also noted is the consistent tendency for seven-month-old mothers to produce milk containing higher IgD concentrations than three-month-old mothers. Three-month-old immune females appeared to have slightly higher milk IgD concentrations than did nonimmune three-month-old females; however, the significance of this difference requires further studies.

FIGURE 2 (lower graph) compares the concentrations of IgD in the sera of the various mothers used in these milking experiments. The different groups of females showed the same relative concentrations of IgD as did their milk samples, but the concentration of IgD in the mother's serum was 10–30 times less than that found within the respective female's milk. IgD was detectable in the serum of only three of the 46 babies analyzed. The IgD concentration in these samples was <10 μg/ml, and all positive sera were obtained from pups less than seven days old.

Mean concentrations of IgA, IgM, IgG1, 2a, 2b, 2c in rat milk samples obtained from four GASV-immune females are shown in FIGURE 3. Two points should be emphasized: 1) with the exception of IgM, whose concentration did not change appreciably, all classes and subclasses showed increased concentrations in milk towards the end of the nursing period, similar to that seen for IgD, and 2) although the concentration of IgA in milk approached that found in maternal serum, contrary to that observed for IgD, the concentration of the other immunoglobulins in milk remained only a fraction of that found in the mother's serum. When the concentration of immunoglobulins in the milk obtained from immune and nonimmune females was compared, milk from immune mothers consistently contained higher concentrations of IgA, IgG2a, IgG2b and IgG2c. The concentration of IgM remained comparable in immune vs nonimmune milk, and interestingly the concentration of IgG1 in milk from nonimmune females appeared elevated.

The Molecular Weight of IgD in Rat Milk

In order to estimate the molecular weight of rat milk IgD, milk obtained from HPR mothers 18–22 days after parturition was pooled and passaged over a Sephacryl S-300 gel filtration column. The majority of the IgD was eluted from the column in peak I, which is comparable to the elution volumes of high molecular weight IgM and IgA. A small amount of IgD was also present in peak II, very close to the elution volume of rat IgG. This implies that some heterogeneity exists in the molecular weight of milk IgD, but that the majority of the IgD is most likely in a polymeric form.

DISCUSSION

These studies demonstrate the presence of surprisingly high concentrations of IgD in rat milk. Why the high concentration of IgD in milk and from where it is derived remain questions to be answered. In this regard, Brandtzaeg has shown that significant numbers of IgD-containing plasma cells are present in human mammary tissue.[17]

Kinetic studies indicate that IgD concentrations within rat milk vary with the age of the mother. One would expect, therefore, that if IgD had an immunoregulatory role in the neonate, subtle differences in immune responsiveness would be observed between progeny born to younger vs older mothers. Such studies are in progress. In addition, our suggestive evidence that immunization of mothers may have some effect on milk IgD concentrations could indicate that maternally derived IgD has the potential to function in an antigen dependent manner.

The molecular weight of IgD in rat milk as assessed by gel filtration, suggests the presence of high molecular weight polymers. This observation is consistent with that of Bazin et al. who observed polymeric IgD in rat serum.[18]

In addition to its presence in rat milk, others have shown IgD to be present in human milk.[19,20] Our preliminary studies confirm the presence of IgD in human milk, and also show IgD to be in mouse milk. Unlike the rats, the concentration of IgD in human milk is relatively low. We have not yet quantified the concentration of IgD in mouse milk. The lower IgD levels in human milk may be related to the larger volume of milk produced by humans compared to that of rats, or to differences in species specific needs. Regarding the latter, it is known that rats receive very little maternally derived immunity via transplacental transfer. Such animals might require increased concentrations of IgD neonatally in order to intensify their acquisition of a protective immunity. In any event, knowing that interspecies differences in both the concentrations and structure of IgD do exist, it is highly conceivable that an increased understanding of these differences will add further clarification to the role of IgD.

Previous studies provide evidence for an interregulatory link between IgD, IgA and IgE synthesis.[21,22] The fact that maternally derived IgD is exposed to gut associated lymphoid tissue early in development may implicate the involvement of soluble IgD in the development of gut-associated immunity during ontogeny. A question posed by this hypothesis is that if milk derived IgD has an immunoregulatory effect on gut-associated lymphoid tissue, how does this compare to the function of IgD on the surface of B-cells and/or in the serum? It is known that patients who have IgD myeloma also acquire heptomegaly, splenomegaly and lymphadenopathies. These conditions are all reflective of increased lymphoid or cellular proliferation. High IgD concentrations may be directly, indirectly or possibly only circumstantially related to this proliferative signal. The prognosis of IgD myeloma patients is much worse than that for myelomas associated with any other immunoglobulin classes. Although no definitive conclusions can be drawn, these observations, do provide clues as to why the body has devised efficient mechanisms for maintaining low concentrations of IgD in serum and may allude to the role of IgD in milk during development.

In conclusion, we have observed high concentrations of IgD in rat milk. Although the function of this IgD is unknown, indirect evidence suggests that it may deliver a lymphoproliferative signal to gut associated lymphoid tissue. The lack of this signal could lead to an immunodeficiency in mucosal immunity and/or possibly to inadequate protection following challenge of the systemic immune system. The breeding of anti-δ suppressed animals and subsequent analysis of secretory and systemic immune responsiveness of progeny should test this hypothesis. These studies support the idea that soluble IgD has a legitimate antibody function.

ACKNOWLEDGMENT

We wish to thank Dr. Herve Bazin for quantifying IgD in our standard and for his kind gift of rat myeloma sera.

REFERENCES

1. ROWE, D. S. & J. L. FAHEY. 1965. A new class of human immunoglobulin. I. A unique myeloma protein. J. Exp. Med. **121:** 171.
2. VITETTA, E. S. & J. W. UHR. 1975. Immunoglobulin receptors revisited. Science **189:** 964.
3. VITETTA, E. S., J. C. CAMBIER, F. S. LIGLER, J. R. KETTMAN & J. W. UHR. 1977. B-cell tolerance. IV. Differential role of surface IgM and IgD in determining tolerance susceptibility of muring B cells. J. Exp. Med. **146:** 1804.
4. LESLIE, G. A. & R. C. ARMEN. 1974. Structure and biological functions of human IgD. III. Phylogenetic studies of IgD. Int. Arch. Allergy **46:** 191.
5. MARTIN, L. N., G. A. LESLIE & R. HINDES. 1976. Lymphocyte surface IgD and IgM in non-human primates. Int. Arch. Allergy **51:** 320.
6. ABNEY, E. R. & R. M. E. PARKHOUSE. 1974. Candidate for immunoglobulin D present on murine B lymphocytes. Nature **252:** 600.
7. MELCHER, U., E. S. VITETTA, M. McWILLIAMS, M. E. LAMM, J. M. PHILLIPS-QUAGLIATA & J. W. UHR. 1974. Cell surface immunoglobulin. X. Identification of an IgD like molecule on the surface of murine splenocytes. J. Exp. Med. **140:** 1427.
8. RUDDICK, J. H. & G. A. LESLIE. 1977. Structure and biological function of human IgD. XI. Identification and ontogeny of a rat lymphocyte immunoglobulin having antigenic cross-reactivity with human IgD. J. Immun. **118:** 1025.
9. BAZIN, H., B. PLATTEAU, A. BECKERS & R. PAUWELS. 1978. Differential effect of neonatal injections of anti-μ or anti-δ antibodies on the synthesis of IgM, IgD, IgE, IgA, IgG1, IgG2a, IgG2b and IgG2c immunoglobulin classes. J. Immunol. **121:** 2083.

10. SIRE, J. A., A. COLLE & A. BOURGOIS. 1979. Identification of an IgD like surface immunoglobulin on rabbit lymphocytes. Eur. J. Immunol. **9:** 13.

11. LESLIE, G. A. 1980. Idiotypy and IgD isotypy of chicken immunoglobulins. *In* Phylogeny of Immunological Memory. M. J. MANNING, Ed.: 253. Elsevier/North-Holland Biomedical Press. Amsterdam, the Netherlands.

12. METCALF, E. S., J. J. MOND, I. SCHUR, M. A. LAVECK & F. D. FINKELMAN. 1982. B-cell function in mice treated with anti-IgD from birth. Ann. N.Y. Acad. Sci. In press.

13. STANKUS, R. P. & G. A. LESLIE. 1975. Genetic influences on the immune response of rats to streptococcal A carbohydrate. Immunogen **2:** 29.

14. CUCHENS, M. A., L. N. MARTIN & G. A. LESLIE. 1978. The effects of anti-IgD on serum immunoglobulins, antibody production and immunoglobulin bearing cells in adult rats. J. Immunol. **121:** 2257.

15. GOLDING, H., M. A. CUCHENS, G. A. LESLIE & M. B. RITTENBERG. 1979. Cross-reactivity of rat, mouse and human IgD. J. Immunol. **123:** 2751.

16. LESLIE, G. A. 1979. Expression of a cross-reactive idiotype on the IgG2c subclass of rat anti-streptococcal carbohydrate antibody. Mol. Immunol. **16:** 285.

17. BRANDTZAEG, P. 1982. The secretory immune system of lactating human mammary glands compared with other exocrine organs. Ann. N.Y. Acad. Sci. In press.

18. BAZIN, H., A. BECKERS, G. URBAIN-VANSANTEN, R. PAUWELS, C. BRUYNS, A. F. TILKEN, B. PLATTEAU & J. URBAIN. 1978. Transplantable IgD immunoglobulin-secreting tumors in rat. J. Immunol. **121:** 2077.

19. DUNNETTE, S. L., G. J. GLEICH, R. D. MILLER & R. A. KYLE. 1977. Measurement of IgD by a double antibody radioimmunoassay: Demonstration of an apparent trimodal distribution of IgD levels in normal human sera. J. Immunol. **119:** 1727.

20. SEWELL, H. J., J. B. MATTHEWS, V. FLACK & R. JEFFERIS. 1979. Human immunoglobulin D in colostrum, saliva and amniotic fluid. Clin. Exp. Immunol. **36:** 183.

21. BUCKLEY, R. H. & S. F. FISCUS. Serum IgD and IgE concentrations in immunodeficiency diseases. J. Clin. Invest. **55:** 157.

22. REISFELD, R. A., F. P. INMAN, Eds. 1978. Contemporary Topics in Molecular Immunology. Plenum Press **7:** 1.

LONG TERM GROWTH OF B-LYMPHOCYTES

William E. Paul, Anthony DeFranco, Benjamin Sredni, and
Maureen Howard

Laboratory of Immunology
National Institute of Allergy and Infectious Diseases
National Institutes of Health
Bethesda, Maryland 20205

INTRODUCTION

The great heterogeneity displayed by cells of the immune system presents formidable obstacles to those who wish to study the mechanisms that regulate activation, proliferation and differentiation of lymphocytes. In general, immunologists have employed indirect techniques in which "read outs" with large amplification factors are used to detect the outcome or have used model systems, such as those provided by the action of polyclonal activators on partially purified lymphocyte populations. Both approaches have yielded valuable information concerning lymphocyte biology but our inability to directly apply the techniques of cellular and molecular biology to antigen-driven immune phenomena have given a tentative character to many of our conclusions.

One solution to these problems has been to find and study tumors of lymphocytes which can be propagated in tissue culture and which retain certain features of normal cellular regulation. Such tumor cell lines have many advantages, not the least of which is that they can be obtained in very large quantities. Their main disadvantage is that they are rarely capable of more than a very limited degree of *in vitro* differentiation.

A second solution to this problem has been to develop long term lines of nontransformed lymphocytes. Techniques to propagate several important functional types of T-lymphocytes, and for cloning these cells have been developed and are now in wide use.[1] Many perplexing problems in T-lymphocyte biology have been clarified through the study of these cells. Until recently, no such progress in the propagation of nontransformed B-lymphocytes had been made. Our group has been interested in the development of long term B-lymphocyte lines and has had success in culturing both human and mouse B-lymphocytes over extended periods.[2,3] In this communication, we will discuss our current concepts of the growth factors important in B-cell proliferation and the strategies which we have employed in long-term culturing of B-cells.

REGULATION OF B-LYMPHOCYTE PROLIFERATION

One convenient model system for the determination of B-lymphocyte growth requirements has been the study of the proliferation of these cells in response to anti-immunoglobulin (Ig) antibody. Since anti-Ig antibody reacts with the antigen-binding receptor of B-lymphocytes, we regard it as an antigen analog and assume that the lessons learned by the study of lymphocyte activation in response to this stimulant have physiologic relevance. It has been known since the work of Sell and Gell that anti-Ig antibodies could cause lymphocyte activation.[4] In the last five years, this system has been the subject of renewed attention.[5-8]

0077–8923/82/0399–0105 $01.75/0 © 1982, NYAS

Purified goat anti-IgM (anti-μ) antibodies are powerful stimulants of B-cell proliferation. Indeed, it is now clear that all B-cells from mature donors are stimulated to enter and progress through the G_1 phase of the cell cycle by exposure to anti-μ.[9,10] Thus, all small B-cells synthesize RNA within 24 of continued exposure to anti-μ. A more sensitive measure of the response of B-cells to anti-μ is size enlargement. Resting B-cells, isolated by Percoll density gradient centrifugation, are a homogeneous cell population with a mean volume of ~110μ.[3] The entire population of these cells increases in size within one hour of addition of anti-μ and this enlargement progresses for the initial 24 hr of culture, when the cells have a volume approximately twice that of resting cells. Removal of anti-μ at any time during this phase of G_1 causes the cells to halt and to remain "frozen" in their position in the activation process.

The regulation of B-cell proliferation, in contrast to B-cell activation, appears more complex. Thus, although all B-cells enter G_1 in response to anti-μ, only approximately 50% enter S phase. Furthermore, entry into S phase requires much higher concentrations of anti-μ than does entry into G_1. Even more strikingly, entry into S phase appears to be very cell-density dependent. This latter observation raises the question of whether "co-stimulants" or growth factors are required for stimulation of B-cell proliferation by anti-μ.

Our group[11,12] had concluded that B-cell proliferation to anti-μ was independent of T-cells and, if 2-mercaptoethanol was present, of macrophages. The conclusion that T-cells were not required was based on the capacity of B-cells purified by treatment with an anti-T-cell antibody and complement and then by cell sorting on the basis of presence of membrane Ig to synthesize DNA upon stimulation with anti-μ or anti-δ antibody. The conclusion that macrophages were not required was based on extensive depletion by adherence to plastic dishes and by treatment with carbonyl iron and exposure to a magnetic field.

Recent studies have led us to reexamine these conclusions. We have now made use of a B-cell purification technique recently introduced by Leibson et al.[13] Donors are pretreated with an anti-thymocyte serum. Spleens are obtained two days later and cell suspensions prepared from them passed over Sephadex G-10 and then subjected to two rounds of treatment with complement and a "cocktail" of monoclonal antibodies specific for T-cell and null cell determinants. The resulting cell population is capable of entering S phase in response to anti-μ if cultured at high cell density (5 × 10^5 cells/0.2 ml) in the presence of high concentrations of anti-μ (50 μg/ml). However, if cell density or anti-μ concentration is diminished, the response diminishes strikingly. Indeed, a plot of log cell density versus log ^{3}H-thymidine uptake in response to anti-μ has a slope that is approximately three. This is consistent with the response to anti-μ requiring three limiting elements that are diluted together in the process of diluting the responding cells.

Thus, it was obvious that by selecting appropriate culture conditions, it might be possible to identify the elements, other than B-lymphocytes and anti-μ, which were needed for the response. Initially, we utilized a density of 5 × 10^4 cells/0.2 ml and an anti-μ concentration of 10 μg/ml. Under these conditions, only a modest incorporation of ^{3}H-thymidine was observed. A supernatant prepared from the mouse T-cell lymphoma, EL-4, by stimulation with phorbol myristate acetate (PMA), caused a very substantial enhancement of the uptake of ^{3}H-thymidine in response to anti-μ, although it had virtually no activity in the absence of anti-μ. In collaborative experiments with Drs. John Farrar and Mary Hilfiker, we characterized the component within EL-4 supernatant that contained this co-stimulatory activity.[14] The material has an apparent molecular weight (M_r)

of 18,000 by gel filtration on ACA 54, and is well separated from interleukin-2 (IL-2), which has a M_r of 30,000 by this technique. It is also clearly separated from colony stimulating factor as well as IL-2 by phenylsepharose chromatography; the B-cell co-stimulator elutes between the former and the latter with a gradient of ethanediol. Furthermore, cytotoxic T-lymphocyte lines, which bear receptors for IL-2, fail to absorb this material from EL-4 supernatant. This factor may also be distinguished from the late acting "T-cell replacing factor" [TRF] since EL-4 supernatant has no TRF activity and the supernatant of B151K12, a T-cell hybridoma which secretes TRF[15] has no B-cell co-stimulator activity. We have designated this new T-cell factor which regulates B-cell proliferation as B-cell growth factor [BCGF].[14]

Although BCGF has a powerful co-stimulator activity in the proliferation of B-cells in response to anti-μ, it appears not to be the only required factor. This may be observed by examining the thymidine incorporation of purified B-cells stimulated with anti-μ at still lower cell density ($10^4/0.2$ ml). Even in the presence of a source of BCGF, a very meager response is obtained. We tested the supernatant of the macrophage line P388D$_1$, induced with PMA, for co-stimulating activity under these culture conditions. The unfractionated supernatant was highly inhibitory. However, when separated by gel filtration, a fraction with a M_r between 10,000 and 20,000 proved to have substantial co-stimulatory capacity. Whether this entity is interleukin 1 is now being actively studied in collaborative experiments with Dr. S. Mizel.

We have reexamined the relationship between log cell density and log ^{3}H-thymidine uptake in the presence of anti-μ, BCGF, and the 15,000 M_r P388D$_1$ material and have obtained a slope of 1.2 over the range between 10^3 and 10^5 cells/0.2 ml. This suggests that BCGF and the macrophage factor are the principal co-factors involved in regulation of the growth of those B-cells which can be stimulated to enter S phase in response to anti-μ. Studies of the phase in the cell cycle of which the growth factors operate, and of the regulation of growth control of those B-cells which do not proliferate in response to anti-μ are now in progress. However, the information now available should be important in clarifying both the physiologic regulation of B-cell growth and the best approaches to long term propagation of B-cells.

Long Term Growth of B-Lymphocytes

Our efforts to grow B-lymphocytes in long term culture began in 1979 and the strategies initially evolved do not take full advantage of recent progress in our understanding of the requirements for B-cell growth. The results described here are similar to those which have appeared in our publications on long term propagation of human and mouse B-lymphocyte lines.[2,3] Efforts to improve these techniques based on the use of better characterized growth factors, are now in progress.

Human B-lymphocyte lines have been established from soft agar colonies. Our techniques utilize a B-lymphocyte enriched population of human peripheral cells which are cultured, in suspension, for three days in the presence of phytohemagglutinin (PHA), pokeweed mitogen (PWM), or staphyloccal protein A. This initial three day culture is required in order to prepare B-cells to form soft agar colonies. T-lymphocytes have a role in this initial step; if they are rigorously depleted from the starting cell population, then cells with colony forming capacity do not appear. The activity of T-lymphocytes in endowing B-lymphocytes with colony forming ability may be replaced with irradiated T-cells or with a growth-factor containing supernatant prepared by incubating human peripheral blood mononuclear cells with PHA for more than 3 days. Cells prepared in this way will form colonies if seeded into the upper layer of a two-layer soft agar system. The lower layer must contain either the mitogenic agent used in the initial suspension culture or a growth-factor containing supernatant, prepared as described above. Under these conditions approximately 200–400 colonies per 10^6 seeded cells form. The colonies may be picked from the soft agar and placed in round bottom microtiter culture wells, together with irradiated peripheral blood mononuclear cells and a source of growth factor. A substantial percentage of such wells will undergo cell growth and it is generally possible to transfer these cells to flat bottom microtiter culture wells and thence to larger wells (i.e., 24-well Costar plates). During this period, and indeed for the life of the cultures, feeding with growth-factor containing supernatant approximately every three days is important. Generally, when the cells are transferred to the larger culture wells, they enter a period of crisis. During this period, they require irradiated peripheral blood mononuclear cells, as well as growth factor. One-third to ¼ of the initial lines survive the "crisis" period and may be propagated for extended times. Such lines have the following characteristics. Most (~80%) of the cells express membrane Ig. They fail to form rosettes with sheep erythrocytes or to ingest latex particles. Their growth is dependent upon the addition of growth factor. Indeed, if growth factor is removed, the cells will generally die within 48 hours. The cells have 46 chromosomes as their modal number and a diploid amount of DNA. They are negative when tested by immunofluorescence for the Epstein-Barr nuclear antigen (EBNA).

Lines grown in this manner may or may not secrete immunoglobulin, depending on the growth factor preparation in which they are maintained. Thus, a line grown in one growth factor preparation may contain fewer than 100 "reverse" plaque-forming cells (PFC) per 10^6 cells; upon transfer to another preparation, 20,000 to 40,000 reverse PFC per 10^6 cells can appear within 4 days.[2]

The nature of the human growth factor required for propagating B-cells and for induction of Ig synthesis have not yet been elucidated. However, the supernatant obtained from human peripheral blood mononuclear cells cultured for more than three days in PHA have essentially no IL-2 activity. It seems likely that they provide a source of human BCGF. Whether a human analog of the macrophage-derived growth factor is also present in these supernatants has not been established.

Cells from long term B-cell lines can be grown in limiting dilution culture, using 0.05% sheep erythrocytes as a filler population. Plots of the log of the fraction of negative wells against the log of the number of cells plated suggest that single element is limiting; cloning efficiencies up to now have been approximately 1 in 3.

Mouse B-lymphocyte lines have been grown by an entirely different initial strategy.[3] Highly purified mouse B-cells are cultured, at relatively high density, for one to two weeks, in the presence of lipopolysaccharide. At the end of this initial culture period, a growth factor-containing supernatant—generally from PMA stimulated EL-4 cells is added. Cells from such cultures will generally proliferate, although at a rather slow rate. Cell lines may be propagated for periods up to 10 months by feeding them every three days with growth factor containing supernatant, and splitting as necessary. These long term cell lines consist of cells bearing membrane (m) IgM but lacking mIgD. They express Ia antigens and lack Thy1 markers. They secrete little or no antibody spontaneously but, in the presence of supernatants obtained from concanavalin-A stimulated spleen cells, they can be induced to produce Ig.

Our current efforts center about the use of more highly defined growth factors in the long term propagation of B-cells coupled with efforts to speed the proliferation rate and increase the viability of the cultured cells. At the same time, we wish to develop an understanding of how growth factors regulate cell growth with emphasis on the sequence of action of the various stimulants. An important long term goal is to develop lines of cloned antigen-specific B-cells. These should be critically important tools in the examination of B-lymphocyte physiology.

REFERENCES

1. PAUL, W. E., B. SREDNI & R. H. SCHWARTZ. 1981. Nature **294:** 697–699.
2. SREDNI, B., D. G. SIECKMANN, S. H. KUMAGAI, I. GREEN & W. E. PAUL. 1981. J. Exp. Med. **154:** 1500–1516.
3. HOWARD, M., S. KESSLER, T. CHUSED & W. E. PAUL. 1981. Proc. Natl. Acad. Sci. USA **78:** 5788–5792.
4. SELL, S. & P. G. H. GELL. 1965. J. Exp. Med. **122:** 423–440.
5. PARKER, D. C. 1975. Nature **258:** 361–363.
6. WIENER, H. L., J. W. MOOREHEAD & H. CLAMAN. 1976. J. Immunol. **116:** 1656–1661.
7. SIECKMANN, D. G., R. ASOFSKY, D. E. MOSIER, I. ZITRON & W. E. PAUL. 1978. J. Exp. Med. **147:** 814–829.
8. SIDMAN, C. L. & E. R. UNANUE. 1978. Proc. Natl. Acad. Sci. USA **75:** 2401–2405.
9. DEFRANCO, A. L., E. S. RAVECHE, R. ASOFSKY & W. E. PAUL. 1982. J. Exp. Med. **155:** 1523–1536.
10. DEFRANCO, A. L., J. T. KUNG & W. E. PAUL. 1982. Immunological Rev. **64:** 269–290.
11. SIECKMANN, D. G., R. HABBERSETT, I. SCHER & W. E. PAUL. 1981. J. Immunol. **127:** 205–211.
12. SIECKMANN, D. G., I. SCHER, R. ASOFSKY, D. E. MOSIER & W. E. PAUL. 1978. J. Exp. Med. **148:** 1628–1643.
13. LEIBSON, H., P. MARRACK & J. KAPPLER. 1981. J. Exp. Med. **154:** 1681–1688.
14. HOWARD, M., J. FARRAR, M. HILFIKER, B. JOHNSON, K. TAKATSU, T. HAMAOKA & W. E. PAUL. 1982. J. Exp. Med. **155:** 914–923.
15. TAKATSU, K., K. TANAKA, A. TOMINAGA, Y. KUHARA & T. HAMAOKA. 1980. J. Immunol. **125:** 2646–2653.

DISCUSSION OF THE PAPER

J. J. MOND: If you deplete only for T-cells or only for macrophages, do you then change the slope from three to two?

W. E. PAUL: It's our general experience that if you simply dilute the unseparated spleen cells the slopes are closer to two. If there are three elements and all are limiting, the slope should come out to three but it does come out closer to two.

MOND: And I was wondering why EL-4 reconstituted the most dilute cells best.

PAUL: My interpretation of that would be that these B-cell preparations despite the efforts we've put in are not really completely pure. They contain small numbers of T-cells that will produce small amounts of growth factor endogenously. If this is a bimolecular reaction, the likelihood of going forward is in a sense going to be predicted by the products of the concentrations of the two reactants. If you dilute each of the reactants twofold the likelihood of the reaction going forward is one-fourth as likely. So of course you'll see the effect much more clearly as you dilute.

C. PARKER (Grafton, Mass.): In my experiments with anti-immunoglobulin and various sources of factors, I find a difference in looking at thymidine incorporation at two and three days and at total cell recoveries at four days. Some factors help the thymidine incorporation, but don't lead to an actual accumulation of increased numbers of B-cells in culture. I'm wondering if you looked at the assay?

PAUL: We haven't used that as a routine assay. On the other hand we've looked in selective instances at cell expansion, and I think we would say that in the presence of the 15,000 M_r fraction of P388D1 supernatant and B-cell growth factor we get substantial proliferation of the cells in culture. So that it is not simply an enhanced thymidine incorporation.

PARKER: What we find is that we absolutely need IL-2, at least with the FS-6 hybridoma supernate, in order to get increases in cell number. Absorption with IL-2 dependent cell lines removes the effect and adding back purified human T-cell growth factor restores it.

PAUL: As I showed you in our hands both IL-2 and B-cell growth factor were required for a PFC response and I concluded that the IL-2 worked on T-cells, but that's not based on evidence only on surmise. I wouldn't rule out the possibility that IL-2 works on B-cells also, but I would be surprised considering Ken Smith not being able to show IL2 receptors on B-cells.

PARKER: We've looked for IL2 receptors in B-cell cultures and we find them, but they're at fairly low levels.

D. E. MOSIER (Institute For Cancer Research, Philadelphia, Pa.): We've been doing similar experiments in a slightly different system. We have collected all the factors that we can find and have done limiting dilution experiments in a serum free system, either using purified B-cells or in fact totally unpurified mouse spleen cells. The basic finding is that, although we can add all of these factors in saturating amounts, we can never get a limiting dilution curve with a slope of one. We can never get B-cells to keep growing without putting in some cell other than a B-cell. What this leads me to conclude is that there is still a requirement for a cell to cell contact and that this event cannot be replaced by any soluble factor.

PAUL: I should say that we can also get a slope of one with certain fillers. Recently Bona and Mond have created a congenic line of nude mice which are unresponsive to LPS and virtually all mitogenic agents and anti-μ. Cells from these mice cannot respond to these stimulants, but when they are used as fillers, they will give a slope of one in the anti-μ response of other cells; whereas, with the factors we're adding we get a slope of 1.2 but not 1.0. I also should say that the B-cell lines we have grow very slowly and there's a very substantial amount of cell death in those cultures. So we don't really claim that we have achieved what's needed to grow mouse B-cells in large numbers.

G. J. THORBECKE: In studying the enhancing effect of a lymphocyte-rich supernatant on the PFC response in vitro to TNP-polyacrylamide, we also find that IL-2 is an essential component. Removing the T-cells from the assay spleen cells enhances the effectiveness of the IL-2. We also find that it still has a large effect when added late during the culture period. I am therefore persuaded that IL2 works possibly directly on B-cells at a certain stage of maturation.

PAUL: We really believed that we wouldn't need IL2 and we did the experiment over and over again, but B-cell growth factor plus TRF doesn't work. I should say IL2 on the other hand plus TRF doesn't work either. We needed all three. However, I'm very troubled by the need for so many factors after the one cell. It seems to me to be a rather inelegant system and I would like to believe that the IL2 is acting on a residual T-cell. Also we can't dilute the cells out: if we go below 5×10^5 cell per well in the sheep cell response, even with the growth factors, we lose the response completely.

THORBECKE: But you don't get away from the fact that you would still need a third factor to act on the B-cell even if the IL-2 works via T-cells. Then the T-cell is making your third factor.

PAUL: Yes that's quite true. The question was whether indeed there is still a role for a histocompatability-restricted T-cell, which could be the cell IL2 is acting upon.

D. G. SIECKMANN: I was just wondering if the cells which turn on with anti-μ alone are the same B-cell sub-set as those that turn on with the T-cell factor and anti-μ? Are they present in NzB mice?

PAUL: We have concluded that the proliferative responses are T-dependent because at low cell density we need factors. We really haven't proven that the response at high cell density is, in fact, T-dependent. There may well be a subset of B-cells which can proliferate without such factors. I would have to say, due to the difficulty involved in purifying these cells completely of T-cells, that I would regard that as an open question. Cells from CBA/N mice do not proliferate to anti-μ even in the presence of EL4 supernate. So the defect is in fact preserved even when the cell growth factor is given to those cultures.

B-CELL SUBPOPULATIONS IDENTIFIABLE
BY TWO-COLOR FLUORESCENCE ANALYSIS
USING A DUAL-LASER FACS*

R. R. Hardy, K. Hayakawa, J. Haaijman,† and L. A. Herzenberg

Department of Genetics
Stanford University School of Medicine
Stanford, California 94305

†Institute of Experimental Gerontology
Health Organization TNO
Rijswijk, the Netherlands

Two-color immunofluorescence studies using monoclonal antibodies specific for IgM[1] and IgD,[2] labeled respectively with fluorescein and "Texas Red" (a new red-fluorescent dye), reveal several previously unrecognized B-cell subpopulations in spleen and lymph node. Measured individually, these surface markers (IgM and IgD) show only that B-cells are broadly heterogenous with respect to the amount of surface Ig expressed; however, measured simultaneously with a dual-laser Fluorescence Activated Cell Sorter (FACS) the correlated expression of these B-cell surface markers defines three B-cell subpopulations.

FIGURE 1 compares two displays of the IgM-IgD staining pattern for spleen cells from a one month old NZB/J mouse. Panel (a) shows a linear-linear display of the data while panel (b) presents data from the same cells analyzed instead with logarithmic amplifiers. The log-log display shows clearly that the brightest IgM⁺ cells include many IgD⁺ cells and that the bright IgD⁺ population is IgM⁺. For the linear illustration if we chose a gain for Texas Red low enough to keep most of the brighter IgD⁺ cells on scale, then the majority of IgM⁺ cells appear to be IgD⁻, whereas at a higher linear gain (not illustrated) many of these can be seen to be IgD⁺. Similarly, if the fluorescein-IgM gain is chosen so as to keep most of the IgM⁺ cells on scale, then this gives the impression of a large IgD⁺, IgM⁻ population which again is an artifact of the particular linear gain settings employed. Careful analysis by specialists of data taken at several pairs of linear gains would be required to reach conclusions that are obvious to the uninitiated from the log-log display.

The IgM-IgD subpopulations defined by our studies are diagrammed schematically in FIGURE 2a. One of these populations (I), which is predominant in spleen and constitutes the overwhelming majority of B-cells in lymph nodes, is missing in CBA/N (Xid) mice known to be deficient with respect to their B-cell immune responses.[3] This population, which is relatively low in IgM and intermediate in IgD, clearly shows a positively correlated expression of these markers. The other population is high in IgM but quite heterogeneous with respect to IgD levels. It appears that this latter population is further divided into bright and dull IgD subpopulations (II and III) on the basis of differences between spleen and lymph nodes.

We have carried out an extensive IgM-IgD staining survey of mouse lymphoid cell populations from different strains, ages, and organs. We will describe the

*This work was supported in part by NIH Grants AI-01287, CA-04681 and GM-17367.

0077-8923/82/0399-0112 $01.75/0 © 1982, NYAS

studies in detail elsewhere; however, the highlights are summarized in FIGURES 2, 3 and 4. FIGURE 3 presents the organ distribution of the three subpopulations and simultaneously illustrates the CBA/N defect. FIGURE 4 shows that population I is the last subpopulation to appear during ontogeny in the spleen. Finally, FIGURE 2 (b-f) demonstrates that there are genetically controlled differences in the mature levels of population II with BALB/c showing the low phenotype and CBA (characteristic of the high) showing approximately twice the number in this subpopulation. Organ and strain variation of the three populations are summarized in TABLE 1.

Two-color staining with monoclonal antibodies specific for ThB[4] and for a subset of splenic B-cells has yielded further information regarding the subpopula-

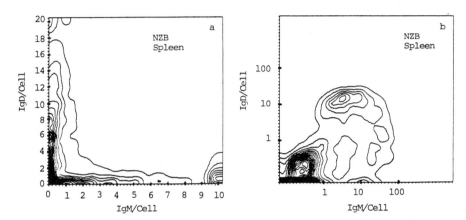

FIGURE 1. A comparison of IgM-IgD two-color immunofluorescence displayed as linear-linear (a) or log-log (b) contour plots. One month NZB/J spleen cells (10[6]) were stained with 0.5 micrograms of fluorescein-labeled monoclonal rat anti-IgM[1] and 0.5 micrograms of biotinated monoclonal mouse anti-IgD[2] in 100 microliters of biotin-free RPMI-1640 containing 10 mM HEPES buffer, 0.1% sodium azide, and 3% newborn calf serum for 30 minutes of 0° C. Cells were washed three times with RPMI and stained with one microgram of Texas Red-avidin in 50 microliters of RPMI for 30 minutes at 0° C. Cells were washed three times with RPMI, resuspended in 300 microliters of the same buffer and analyzed on the dual-laser FACS equipped with both linear and logarithmic amplifiers. To permit subsequent analyses, "list-mode" data recording the scatter and two fluorescence measurements for each cell were collected on 30,000 cells using a VAX 11/780 computer.

tions described above. Previous single parameter staining with the monoclonal anti-ThB divided mouse strains into bright (or "high") and dull (or "low") for this marker.[5] Furthermore, ThB expression on B-cells was shown to be under autosomal co-dominant control so that an F1 hybrid of a "high" and a "low" was "intermediate." Two parameter staining of ThB and IgM illustrated in FIGURE 5 (a and b) shows that most of this variation occurs in the IgM dull population (I) with the IgM bright populations remaining uniformly high for ThB. Another monoclonal antibody previously shown to stain spleen cells weakly ("E2")[6] stains only the high IgM populations (II and III) as shown in FIGURE 5 (c and d).

FIGURE 6 presents Ia expression on these populations which was examined

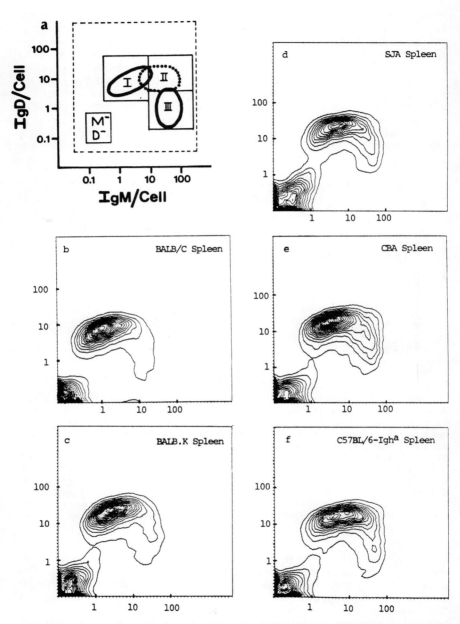

FIGURE 2. (a) A schematic diagram of the B-cell subpopulations defined by IgM-IgD immunofluorescence staining. (b-f) There are two levels at which population II occurs depending on strain. BALB/c and BALB.K are low (b, c), while SJA, CBA and C57BL/6 are high (d-f).

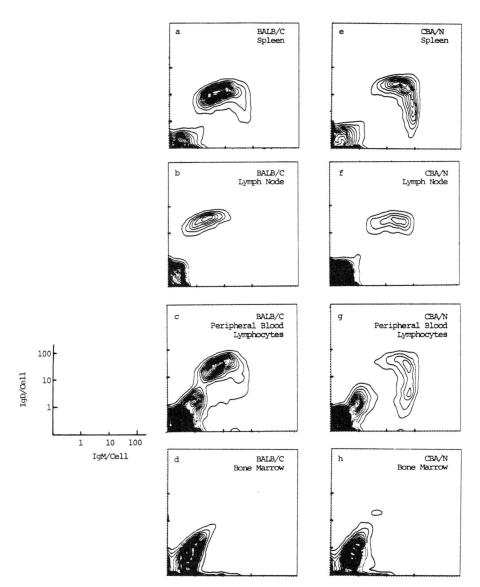

FIGURE 3. Variation of the three populations with lymphoid organ both in normal (BALB/c) and defective (CBA/N) mice. Spleen, lymph node, peripheral blood lymphocytes and bone marrow of BALB/c: a–d, of CBA/N: e–h.

using a monoclonal antibody specific for Ia of k, specificity 2.[2] Staining Balb.K spleen showed only slight variation of Ia density among the three populations with greater heterogeneity in the high-IgM populations. Staining CBA/N spleen simplified the situation by eliminating population I (high-Ia) and clearly showed that population III expresses reduced amounts of Ia compared to the other two

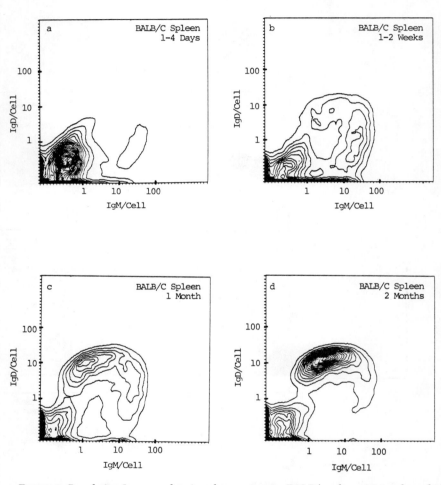

FIGURE 4. Population I appears late in spleen ontogeny. BALB/c spleen: (a) 1-4 days; (b) 1-2 weeks; (c) 1 month; (d) 2 months or older.

populations. The relative expression of several surface antigens on the three populations is summarized in TABLE 2.

Functional distinctions of these three subpopulations are at present unknown, but the immune defects of CBA/N mice certainly suggest that they may be functionally distinguishable. CBA/N mice (which lack population I) have low

TABLE 1

PERCENTAGES OF CELLS IN IgM/IgD-DEFINED B-CELL SUBPOPULATIONS*

Strain	Organ	I	II	III
BALB/c	Spleen	40	8	2
	Lymph node	20	2	<1
CBA	Spleen	30	17	3
	Lymph node	18	5	<1
CBA/N	Spleen	4†	16	8
	Lymph node	<1	4	<1
NZB/N	Spleen	27	9	7
	Lymph node	15	2	<1

*CBA/N mice lack the major B-cell subpopulation found in spleen and lymph nodes in normal mice. NZB mice, on the other hand have an elevated level of population III compared to normal mice. Data show the percentages of total spleen or lymph node cells present in the B-cell subpopulations shown in FIGURE 2a. Percentages for populations I and II may be in error by as much as five percent in the BALB/c, CBA and NZB determinations due to overlap between these populations. Subpopulations defined by 2-color FACS analysis shown in FIGURE 2.

†This figure (4%) is attributable to overlap from population II.

serum levels of IgM and IgG3,[7] have reduced numbers of splenic B-cells,[8] are unable to respond to type II thymus independent antigens (eg., TNP-ficoll),[9] and lack a B-cell surface antigen known as Lyb-3.[10] It is tempting to speculate that these deficiencies are all due to the lack of population I, however preliminary data indicate that the CBA/N B-cells in populations II and III are defective in some respects compared to cells in these populations from normal mice. This points out a clear danger in considering CBA/N B-cells as normal CBA B-cells minus a subpopulation of cells.

Population III is very unusual because at least some cells in this subpopulation express the T-cell antigen Lyt-1 (see FIGURE 1). One of us (K.H.) previously detected a cell with this phenotype (Ig+,Lyt-1+) in an *in vitro* antibody formation assay[11] and previous single fluorescence staining has demonstrated mouse B-

TABLE 2

LEVEL OF EXPRESSION OF SEVERAL CELL SURFACE ANTIGENS
ON THE IgM-IgD DEFINED SUBPOPULATIONS*

Surface Marker	I	II	III
IgM	1–50	100	100
IgD	50–100	100	10
Ia	100	100	50
ThB	1–50;50‡	100	100
E2	<10	100	100
Lyt-1†	<1	<1	10

*The three populations are quite heterogenous in their surface phenotypes for a number of cell surface antigens. The surface densities are normalized separately for each antigen.

†Density relative to average Lyt-1 density on T-cells.

‡Depending on ThB(low) or ThB(high) strain.

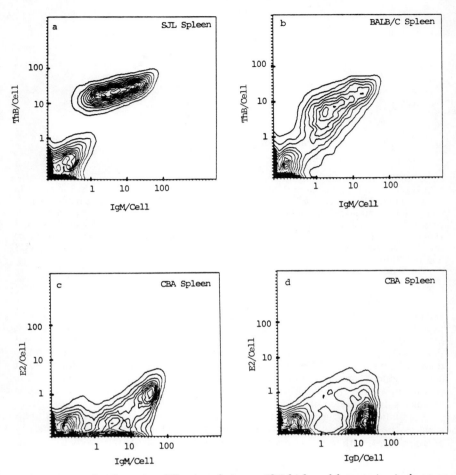

FIGURE 5. (a–b) The major differences between ThB high and low strains is due to a difference in surface density on population I. SJL is a high strain (a) and BALB/c is a low strain (b). (c–d) E2 is a surface antigen found only on populations II and III; that is, it is found on all bright-IgM cells (c), but on IgD cells with widely varying surface density (d).

lymphomas expressing Lyt-1 and IgM.[12] Two-color staining of a number of different mouse strains consistently showed 1–2% of spleen cells with this phenotype, but the most impressive demonstration of its presence is in NZB mice which have 5–10%. These mice also have an unusual IgM/IgD profile with many more population III cells and many fewer population II cells compared to similar high-IgM strains. The cells lack Thy-1 and Lyt-2 which is consistent with the phenotype described in the *in vitro* assay (K. Okumura, K. Hayakawa and T. Tada, manuscript in preparation). Whatever role these cells might play in the well-known autoimmune disorder of NZB mice[13] is speculative at present and can be investigated using sorted cells.

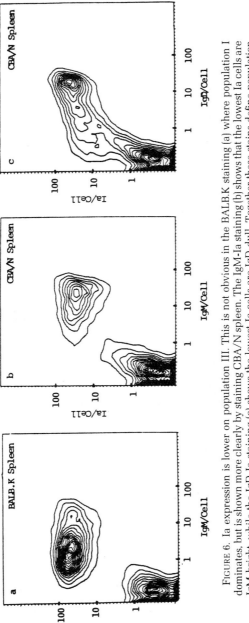

FIGURE 6. Ia expression is lower on population III. This is not obvious in the BALB.K staining (a) where population I dominates, but is shown more clearly by staining CBA/N spleen. The IgM-Ia staining (b) shows that the lowest Ia cells are IgM-bright, while the IgD-Ia staining (c) shows the lowest Ia cells are IgD-dull. Together these stains define population III.

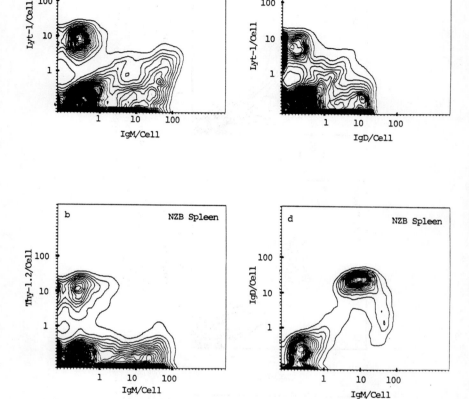

FIGURE 7. The NZB mouse spleen contains elevated amounts of a cell expressing both IgM and the T cell antigen Lyt-1 (a). These cells do not express Thy-1 (b), but do express low amounts of IgD (c). This places the cells in the IgM-IgD pattern as population III and indeed the IgM-IgD staining profile(d) is unusual with increased population III and decreased population II compared to other strains tested.

ACKNOWLEDGMENTS

We acknowledge the Institute of Experimental Gerontology, Health Organization TNO, Rijswijk, the Netherlands, for providing the CBA/N mice used in these studies. We thank Dr. P. Kincade for the monoclonal rat anti-IgM, Dr. D. Parks for invaluable assistance with the dual-laser FACS and Mr. W. Moore for writing the VAX data handling programs.

REFERENCES

1. KINCADE, P. W., G. LEE, L. SUN & T. WATANABE. 1981. J. Immunol. Meth. **42:** 17–26.
2. OI, V. T., P. P. JONES, J. W. GODING, L. A. HERZENBERG & L. A. HERZENBERG. 1978. Curr. Top. Microbiol. Immunol. **81:** 115–129.
3. SCHER, I., M. M. FRANTZ & A. D. STEINBERG. 1973. J. Immunol. **110:** 1396–1401.
4. YUTOKU, M., A. L. GROSSBERG & D. PRESSMAN. 1974. J. Immunol. **112:** 1774–1781.
5. ECKHARDT, L. A. & L. A. HERZENBERG. 1980. Immunogenetics **11:** 275–291.
6. LEDBETTER, J. A. & L. A. HERZENBERG. 1979. Immunol. Rev. **47:** 63–90.
7. PERLMUTTER, R. M., M. NAHM, K. E. STEIN, J. SLACK, I. ZITRON & W. E. PAUL. 1979. J. Exp. Med. **149:** 993–998.
8. FINKELMAN, F. D., A. H. SMITH, I. SCHER & W. E. PAUL. 1975. J. Exp. Med. **142:** 1316–1321.
9. MOSIER, D. E., J. J. MOND & E. A. GOLDINGS. 1977. J. Immunol. **119:** 1874–1878.
10. HUBER, B., R. K. GERSHON & H. CANTOR. 1977. J. Exp. Med. **145:** 10–20.
11. OKUMURA, K., K. HAYAKAWA & T. TADA. J. Exp. Med. In press.
12. LANIER, L. L., N. L. WARNER, J. A. LEDBETTER & L. A. HERZENBERG. 1981. J. Immunol. **127:** 1691–1691.
13. WARNER, N. 1979. *In* Autoimmunity, N. Talal, Ed.: 33–62. Academic Press. New York, N.Y.

DISCUSSION OF THE PAPER

C. MILCAREK (*Columbia University*): What influence on affinity, if any, does the deletion in CH1 of the γ 2A have on antigen binding?

LEN HERZENBERG: Precise affinity measurements have not been done, but I think there is certainly no large difference.

MILCAREK: So you do make H2L2?

HERZENBERG: Yes, we do. The heavy-light chain disulphide is not formed so if you prepare an SDS gel without reduction you get free light chains and a heavy chain dimer. But in nondenaturing solvents we get a four chain molecule.

C. BONA: Do your results show that the cells switch independently of antigen stimulation?

HERZENBERG: Yes, but these variants occur in frequencies around 1 in 10^5–10^7, and this is therefore not normal B-cell differentiation. I wouldn't want to say that this has anything to do with the mechanism involved in normal B-cell switching, where for example you don't go from γ 1 to γ 2b.

M. KLEIN: I really appreciated your study on the segmental flexibility, for it goes well with complement binding, which we know is linked to the length of the hinge region. How do you visualize in three dimensions the binding of the light chain to VHC γ 2 which still binds complement? Do you think that it's a VLVH which is leading to self assembly?

HERZENBERG: I have to say something of that sort because I know that CH1 and C κ are supposed to associate very nicely and yet there's no CH1 for C κ to bind to. It's a nice molecule for a crystallographer or chemists to look at and you are welcome to have it.

THE EFFECT OF THE *IN VIVO* PASSAGE ON sIg EXPRESSION OF BALB/c B-CELL LINES

K. J. Kim, C. B. Evans, B. J. Fowlkes, William M. Leiserson, and
R. Asofsky

Laboratory of Microbial Immunity
National Institute of Allergy and Infectious Diseases
National Institutes of Health
Bethesda, Maryland 20205

INTRODUCTION

The switching of the expression of sIg isotype on B-cells has been a controversial issue for a long time. Recently, Abney *et al*[1] suggested the following model for early B-cell development from their ontogeny studies:

$$M^+ \Big\backslash \begin{array}{l} \diagup M^+ \to M^+D^+ \to M^+ \text{ PFC} \\ \diagdown M^+G^+(A^+) \to M^+D^+, G^+(A^+) \to G^+(A^+) \text{ PFC} \end{array}$$

The development of mature B-cells bearing M^+D^+ and those bearing $M^+G^+(A^+)$ on the cell membrane from immature B-cells bearing M^+, was suggested to be a simultaneous but independent phenomenon. Furthermore, it was suggested that B-cells expressing M^+G^+ differentiated eventually into G-secreting plasma cells via the stage of $M^+D^+G^+$. However, there was no direct proof for the changes occuring on the lineage of B-cells bearing M^+G^+. It is difficult to demonstrate the presence of triple isotypes or switching of Ig isotypes on a single cell. Therefore, a cell line which bears triple isotypes or switches isotypes would be ideal for analyzing B-cell differentiation. In some cases, tumor cells were shown to have kept properties of normal cells. For instance, the switching of Ig isotypes in myeloma cells has been reported.[2] Further, MOPC-315 plasmacytoma was shown to differentiate from M315 producing, nonsecreting, lymphoid cells to large M315-secreting plasma cells during *in vivo* growth.[3]

Several BALB/c B-cell lines bearing sIgM and sIgD were reported previously.[4] However, the expression of heavy chain on A20, one of those B-cell lines, was difficult to detect even though the kappa light chain was readily detectable on the cell membrane. In addition, it was often noticed that B-cell lines bearing sIg became sIg negative after prolonged culture *in vitro*. The gradual loss of sIg during *in vitro* cultivation may be due to the rapid proliferation and/or the lack of *in vivo* regulatory mechanisms that influence the maturation of these cells. Therefore, in the present study, we have compared the expression of surface sIg on these B-cell lines before and after *in vivo* passage, using microfluorometric analysis. It was shown that A20.3 tumor cells began to express sIgM and sIgG2, only after *in vivo* passage. We also examined the effect of lipopolysaccharide (LPS) on X16C 8.5 bearing sIgM and sIgD, in an attempt to induce the differentiation of these tumor cells. It was found that LPS enhanced the expression of sIgM on X16C 8.5 but decreased the expression of sIgD.

0077-8923/82/0399-0122 $01.75/0 © 1982, NYAS

Tumors and Cell Lines

Tumors developed spontaneously in aged BALB/c mice (more than 15 months), were adapted *in vitro* several years ago.[4] For *in vivo* passage, $1-2 \times 10^6$ tumor cells were injected i.p. into BALB/c mice obtained from the Small Animal Section, NIH, Bethesda, Maryland 20205. Long term B-cell lines, X16C 8.5, K46R, L10A 6.2, BALENLM 17.7.2, and A20.3, were routinely transferred in Click's medium containing 10% fetal calf serum (FCS) at 37°C in an atmosphere containing 5% CO_2 as described earlier.[4]

Analysis of Surface Immunoglobulin (sIg)

The expression of sIg on the tumor cells was examined by direct immuno-fluorescence (IF) staining. IF staining was carried out by using fluoresceinated F(ab')$_2$ fragments of goat anti-mouse M (F-GαMμ), goat anti-mouse G1 (F-GαMγ1), goat anti-mouse G2 (F-GαMγ2) and goat anti-mouse K (F-GαMκ). In order to detect surface D, a fluoresceinated hybridoma 10-4.22, anti-mouse D (F-4.22αMδ)[5] was used. The level of fluorescence staining was determined by flow microfluor-ometry (FMF) analysis using a fluorescence-activated cell sorter II (FACS II, Becton, Dickinson, Mountain View, California).[6] Since the fluorescence emission detected on the FACS II was shown to be linearly related to the number of Ig molecules bound per cell,[7] and the staining profiles of tumor cells gave a single peak, the levels of fluorescence staining were expressed as mean fluorescence units per cell (MFU) at fluorescence gain 20 (MFU20). MFU was obtained from the following formula:

$$\text{MFU 20} = \text{MFU at gain A} \times \frac{\text{gain 20}}{\text{gain A}}$$

Since the ratio of the number of fluorescein isothiocyanate molecules per the number of protein molecules (F/P ratio) was different among different reagents, one should not compare the MFU20 among different staining reagents.

The Expression of sIgM and sIgD on Several B-cell Lines

Several BALB/c B-cell lines have been adapted *in vitro* previously. The expression of sIgM and sIgD on these tumors has been demonstrated by the incorporation of ^{3}H-amino acids[8] as well as by ^{125}I-surface labeling techniques.[9] The expression of sIgM, sIgD, sIgG1, and sIgG2 on several B-cell lines was examined by FMF analysis (TABLE 1). Normal spleen cells were included as controls for the positive staining. The level of fluorescence staining was expressed as MFU20. BALB/c spleen cells are known to have approximately the same amount of sIgD and sIgM by ^{125}I-surface labeling techniques.[10] However, F-GαMμ gave much brighter staining than F-4.22αMδ. This could be due to the difference in the affinity of the antibodies used. Further, MFU20 for the unstained control of tumor cells was much higher than that of normal spleen cells

TABLE 1

THE EXPRESSION OF SIG OF B-CELL LINES IN *IN VITRO* CULTURES

Cells	F-GαMμ	F-4.22αMδ	MFU 20 F-GαMγ1	F-GαMγ2	Unst*
X16C 8.5	4,675	1,550	595	561	470
K46R	5,001	1,600	362	402	371
BAL 17.7.2	21,395	773	606	554	562
BALB/c spleen	5,521	1,734	1,776	2,234	105
	(56%)†	(48%)	(4%)	(6%)	

*Unst = unstained control cells.
†% positive, MFU 20 for sIg of spleen cells were determined from positive cells for each staining.

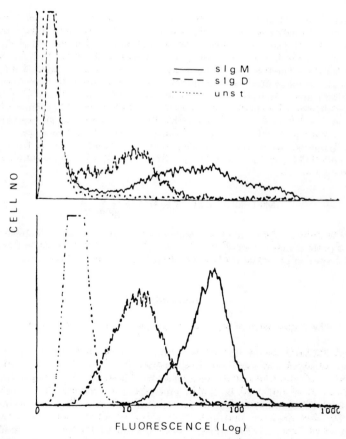

FIGURE 1. The expression of sIgM (—) and sIgD (----) of BALB/c spleen cells (top) and X16C 8.5, BALB/c B lymphoma (bottom). sIgM was stained with F-GαMμ and sIgD was stained with F-4.22αMδ. Unstained control (unst) is shown as dotted line (....). FACS analysis was done on a Log scale.

due to the larger size and greater autofluorescence of tumor cells. Therefore, one should not compare MFU20 of tumor cells directly to those of normal spleen cells even within the same isotype staining. From FMF analysis, we confirmed that X16C 8.5, K46R, and BALENLM 17.7.2. were sIgM$^+$ and sIgD$^+$. BALENLM 17.7.2 expressed much more sIgM but less sIgD, compared to X16C 8.5 and K46R.

FIGURE 1 shows the representative staining profiles of X16C 8.5 and BALB/c spleen cells on a log scale. This figure shows that X16C 8.5 expressed sIgM as well as sIgD. The staining profiles of X16C 8.5 and those of spleen cells with F-GαMγ1, or F-GαM 2 were very close to that of unstained control (data not shown).

In an attempt to induce X16C 8.5 to differentiate further, the effects of LPS on the expression of sIg of X16C 8.5 were examined (FIGURE 2). After stimulation of X16C 8.5 with LPS (10 μg/ml) for two days, the expression of sIgM on X16C 8.5 was increased substantially while that of sIgD was decreased.

The Expression of sIg on A20, In Vitro Cell Lines

A20 cell lines were originally reported as Ig positive, but with unknown heavy chain isotype, by IF staining examined by fluorescence microscopy.[4] A subclone, A20.1.11, was previously reported as IgG2a positive by the incorporation of radio labeled amino acids.[11] However, FMF analysis on several different occasions on different clones, A20, A20.3 and A201.11, failed to reveal the presence of heavy chains even though the presence of kappa chain was readily detectable (TABLE 2). The reasons for the difficulty of typing heavy chain isotypes on these tumor cells were thought to be due to either the low level of expression of the heavy chain or to steric hindrance.

The Effect of In Vivo Growth on the Expression of sIg on A20 Tumor Cells

In order to examine whether the sIg of A20 tumor cells was lost due to mutation or was under an extracellular regulatory mechanism, the effect of *in vivo* passage on the expression of sIg on A20.3 was examined. A20, A20.3 and BALENLM 17.7.2 maintained *in vitro* for one–two years, were injected into BALB/c mice. These tumor cells grew mainly in spleen, mesenteric lymph nodes, or ascites within two–three weeks. The sIg of tumor cells grown *in vivo* was examined (TABLE 3). BALENLM 17.7.2 grown *in vivo* appeared to express bright sIgM and low levels of sIgD, as shown with the tissue culture cell line, but there was also some staining with F-GαMγ2 on BALENLM 17.7.2 grown in mice (day 0 in culture). Further, surprising observations were made with A20 and A20.3. After *in vivo* passage, both A20 and A20.3 stained with F-GαMμ and F-GαMγ2. In addition, A20.3 also stained with F-4.22 αMδ.

It is possible that cytophilic antibodies or antibodies generated against tumor cells would give false positive reactions in detecting sIg on tumor cells.[12] In order to avoid such problems, these tumor cells were retyped after culturing *in vitro* for a short time. A20 grown *in vivo*, which stained with F-GαMμ as well as with F-GαMγ2, continued to express sIgM as well as sIgG2 after incubation for four days *in vitro*. There was a decrease in MFU20 for sIgM, and an increase in sIgG2 after culturing A20 *in vivo* tumor cells. One might argue that the expression of sIgM or sIgG2 could be due to the outgrowth of a subset of A20 *in vivo*. However, it is unlikely because the same result was obtained with A20.3, a subclone of A20; A20.3 tumors passaged *in vivo*, which expressed sIgM, sIgD and sIgG2, continued

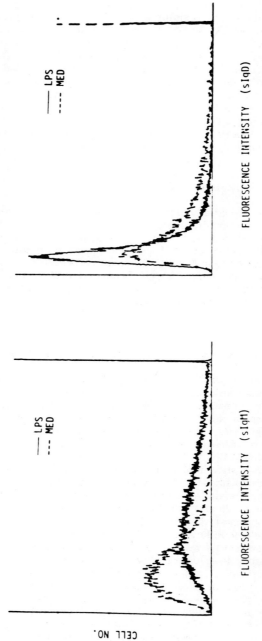

FIGURE 2. FMF analysis of the effect of LPS on the expression of sIgM and sIgD before (----) and after (—) LPS stimulation. Cells (5 × 10⁴ cells/2 ml) were cultured with LPS (10 μg/ml) for two days.

TABLE 2

sIg Expression of A20 in In Vitro Cell Lines

Cells*		F-GαMμ	F-4.22αMδ	MFU 20 F-GαMγ1	F-GαMγ2	F-GαMκ	Unst
A20		398	327	349	523	—	340
A20.3	(1)†	168	323	102	278	1,548	65
	(2)	562	456	393	467	1,929	390
A201.11 (1)		405	416	425	496	—	421
	(2)	130	183	95	184	1,172	70

*A20.3 and A201.11 are subclones of A20.

†( ) = No. of the experiment.

to express these three isotypes after culturing seven days in vitro (TABLE 3, FIGURE 3). However, the level of sIgD decreased significantly while sIgM and sIgG appeared to increase. Therefore, it was concluded that A20.3 tumor cells began to express significant levels of sIgM and sIgG2 after in vivo passage. The expression of sIgD for these tumor cells needs further examination.

Even though there was some difference between the A20.3 in vivo and A20 in vivo tumors, they both appeared to express sIgM and sIgG2 after culturing in vitro for a few days. In contrast to A20.3 and A20, the expression of sIgG2 on BALENLM 17.7.2 in vivo was no longer observed after culturing four days in Click's medium containing FCS, while the bright staining for sIgM and dull staining for sIgD on these cells was continued. Therefore, it was concluded that there was no significant change in sIg expression of BALENLM 17.7.2 by passage in vivo.

DISCUSSION

The present study shows that the A20 maintained in vitro, which did not express any significant levels of heavy chain isotype on the cell membrane, began to express sIgM and sIgG2 after in vivo passage. In contrast to A20, BALENLM 17.7.2 tissue culture lines that express bright sIgM and dull sIgD, were not affected by in vivo passage. Thus, it appears that the expression of sIg of A20 tumors might be subjected to an extracellular regulatory control. Others have shown that T-cell factors may play an important role in the activation of B-cells

TABLE 3

sIg of A20 Tumors after the In Vivo Passage*

Tumors	Source	Days in Culture	F-GαMμ	F-4.22αMδ	MFU 20 F-GαMγ1	F-GαMγ2	F-GαMκ	Unst
A20	AS	0	446	136	95	422	1,579	125
		4	324	200	92	663	—	103
A20	SC	0	262	306	112	390	—	106
		7	327	189	98	540	1,089	96
BAL17.7.2		0	17,965	756	502	692	—	492
		4	15,836	877	433	400	—	469

*Tumor cells obtained from mice were cultured in Click's for four days (5 × 10⁴ cells/well).

using Ig treated spleen cells[13] or BCLI tumor cells.[14] Whether such T-cells factors regulate the expression of sIg on A20 tumors needs further investigation.

It has been postulated that there were different lineages of B-cell development for IgM and IgG plaque forming cells (PFC) as follows: (1) $M^+ \rightarrow M^+D^+ \rightarrow M^+$ PFC. (2) $M^+ \rightarrow M^+G^+ \rightarrow M^+G^+D^+ \rightarrow G^+$ PFC. Thus, K46R and BALENLM 17.7.2 cell lines, which were shown to express sIgM and sIgD, appear to belong to

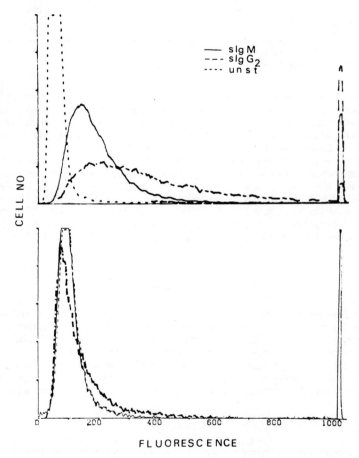

FIGURE 3. The expression of sIgM (—) sIgG2 (----) on A20.3 *in vivo* tumor cells after seven-day culture *in vitro* (top) and those on A20.3 long term cell line (bottom). Unstained controls are shown as dotted lines (....).

the first lineage of B-cell development while A20 belongs to the second lineage. In order to confirm this differentiation scheme, it would be ideal if any B-cell tumor belonging to the first lineage and A20 belonging to the second lineage, could be induced to differentiate further. As an approach, the effect of LPS on the expression of sIgM and sIgD of X16C 8.5 was examined. There was a substantial increase in sIgM but a decrease in sIgD. It has been shown by others[15,16] that LPS stimulation of normal spleen B-cells resulted in a decrease in sIgD expression but no significant change in sIgM. Thus, the effect of LPS on sIgD on X16C 8.5 was similar to that on spleen cells; however, there is a discrepancy in the data obtained for the LPS effects on the expression of sIgM on normal cells and those on X16C 8.5. This difference might be due to the fact that studies with normal cells were done on a heterogenous population while the study with X16C 8.5 was done on a clonal cell population.

It is hoped that A20.3 tumors responding to *in vivo* growth conditions and X16C 8.5 tumors responding to LPS, might be useful tools for the further understanding of B-cell differentiation.

REFERENCES

1. ABNEY, E. R., M. D. COOPER, J. F. KEARNEY, A. R. LAWTON & R. M. E. PARKHOUSE. 1978. Sequential expression of immunoglobulin on developing mouse B lymphocytes: a systematic survey that suggests a model for the generation of immunoglobulin isotype diversity. J. Immunol. **120:** 2041–2049.

2. FRANCUS, T., B. DHARMGRONGARTAMA, R. CAMPBELL, M. D. SCHARFF & B. K. BRISHTEIN. 1978. IgG$_{2a}$-producing variants of an IgG$_{2a}$-producing mouse myeloma cell lines. J. Exp. Med. **147:** 1535–1550.

3. LYNCH, R. G., J. W. RHORER, B. F. ODERMATT, H. M. GEBEL, J. R. AUTRY & R. G. HOOVER. 1979. Immunoregulation of murine myeloma cell growth and differentiation: a monoclonal model of B cell differentiation. Immunol. Rev. **48:** 45–80.

4. KIM, K. J., C. KANELLOPOULOS-LANGEVIN, R. M. MERWIN, D. H. SACHS & R. ASOFSKY. 1979. Establishment and characterization of BALB/c lymphoma lines with B cell properties. J. Immunol. **122:** 549–554.

5. OI, V. T., P. P. JONES, J. W. GODING, L. A. HERZENBERG & L. A. HERZENBERG, 1978. Properties of monoclonal antibodies to mouse Ig allotypes, H-2, and Ia antigens. Curr. Top. Microbiol. Immunol. **81:** 115–129.

6. LOKEN, J. R. & L. A. HERZENBERG. 1977. Analysis of cell populations with a fluorescence activated cell sorter. Ann. N.Y. Acad. Sci. **254:** 163–171.

7. TITUS, J. A., S. O. SHARROW, J. M. CONNOLY & D. M. SEGAL. 1981. Fc (IgG) receptor distributions in homogeneous and heterogenous cell populations by flow microfluorometry. Proc. Natl. Acad. Sci. **78:** 519–523.

8. MCKEEVER, P. E., K. J. KIM, G. B. NERO, R. LASKOV, R. M. MERWIN, W. J. LOGAN & R. ASOFSKY. 1979. Two spontaneous BALB/c lymphomas synthesize IgM; monomers and half molecules are isolated and characterized whereas another molecule resembles IgD. J. Immunol. **122:** 1261–1265.

9. LASKOV, R., J. K. KIM, V. WOODS, P. E. MCKEEVER & R. ASOFSKY. 1981. Membrane immunoglobulins of spontaneous B lymphomas of aged BALB/c mice. Eur. J. Immunol. **11:** 462–468.

10. PARKHOUSE, R. M. E., & M. D. COOPER. 1978. A model for the differentiation of B lymphocytes with implications for the biological role of IgD. Immunol. Rev. **37:** 105–126.

11. WORD, C. J. & W. M. KUEHL. 1982. Expression of surface and secreted IgG$_{2a}$ by a murine B-lymphoma before and after hybridization to myeloma cells. Cell. In press.

12. LOBO, P., F. B. WESTERVELT & P. A. HORWITZ. 1975. Identification of two populations of immunoglobulin-bearing lymphocytes in man. J. Immunol. **114:** 116–119.

13. PARKER, A. C., J. J. FOLLERGILL & D. C. WADWORTH. 1979. B lymphocyte activation by insoluble anti-immunoglobulin: induction of immunoglobulin secretion by a T cell-dependent soluble factor. J. Immunol. **123:** 931–941.

14. ISSAKSON, P. C., E. PURÉ, J. W. UHR & E. S. VITETTA. 1981. Induction of proliferation and differentiation of Neoplastic B-cells by anti-immunoglobulin and I-cell factors. Proc. Nat'l. Acad. Sci. **78:** 2507.

15. BOURGOIS, A., K. KITAJIMA, I. R. HUNTER & B. A. ASKONAS. 1977. Surface immunoglobulins of lipopolysaccharide stimulated spleen cells. The behavior of IgM, IgD and IgG. Eur. J. Immunol. **7:** 151-153.
16. VITETTA, E. S. & J. W. UHR. 1978. IgD and B cell differentiation. Immunol. Rev. **37:** 50-88.

DISCUSSION OF THE PAPER

LEN HERZENBERG: You are probably right in that you have both μ and γ_2 being made by this line after you've got it in culture. However, there was a similar story at Stanford where the same conclusion was reached after LPS stimulation and it was wrong as shown by transfer of the cells into allotype congenic mice. You should be cautious because the γ_2 could be antibody made by contaminating host cells against the tumor.

I. SCHER: In rats infected with *Nippostrongylus* we have seen cells that had IgE, IgM, and IgD on their surface. In trying to test whether the IgE might be cytophilic, cells were treated with enzymes to remove the IgE and it seemed to grow back. Cells were cultured overnight or for longer periods of time and the IgE did not come off. However, if you treated the cells in the cold for one minute at pH4, all the IgE was removed without removing any of the IgD or IgM. I think this reflects how difficult it can be sometimes to show whether an antibody is an anti-cell antibody or a cytophilic antibody. The acid treatment is one that is worth trying.

DEVELOPMENTAL ASPECTS OF RAT IgD EXPRESSION
AND THE CONSEQUENCES OF IgD MODULATION*

Gerrie A. Leslie and Marvin A. Cuchens

Department of Microbiology and Immunology
The Oregon Health Sciences University
Portland, Oregon 97201

and

Department of Microbiology
University of Mississippi Medical Center
Jackson, Mississippi 39216

INTRODUCTION

Despite its discovery over a decade ago[1] the biological function(s) of human IgD remains elusive. Antibody activity within this class has been demonstrated but for the most part only with very sensitive techniques and in special circumstances.[2] Much of the recent interest in IgD has stemmed from the observations that IgD is present on a large percentage of human B-cells and that most of these cells also bear IgM.[2-6] The development of animal models should greatly facilitate our understanding of the role of IgD as an antibody and/or membrane receptor. A murine[2,7-9] and monkey model[2] have been described and most recently, an IgD homologue in rats[2,10] has been demonstrated by antigenic cross reactivity and similar physiochemical properties with human IgD. The initial studies on rat IgD utilized a chicken anti-human IgD (anti-δ) which detected cross-reactive determinants on rat B-lymphocytes. However, primarily because of difficulties with this reagent in fluorescent antibody assays and other limitations imposed with using cross-reactive antibodies, we wished to prepare an antiserum to rat IgD. We report here the preparation of antisera to rat lymphocyte membrane IgD. Using these antisera in fluorescent antibody techniques, the tissue distribution of IgD bearing cells in the rat, the coexpression of IgD and IgM on the same cell, the shared idiotype on membrane IgD and IgM, the ontogeny of membrane IgD and the effects of fetal and neonatal injections of anti-μ and anti-δ are described.

MATERIALS AND METHODS

Immunoadsorbents

Immunoadsorbents (I.A.) were prepared by covalently binding protein to Sepharose 6B (Pharamacia, Uppsala, Sweden) by the CNBr method as described by Wofsy and Burr.[11] I.A. employed in this study were conjugated with normal rabbit IgG, normal chicken IgY, normal rat plasma, normal rat serum, rat IgG, rat IgM or rat IgA.

*This investigation was supported by grants from the National Cancer Institute (7R23 CA28046) and the National Institute of Child Health and Human Development (HD12381).

Antisera

The preparation of goat and sheep anti-rat IgM (anti-μ) and rabbit anti-rat-anti-group A streptococcal carbohydrate antibody (anti-Id-I) have been described.[12,13] The rabbit anti-rat immunoglobulin (Ig) reagent was prepared using an initial subcutaneous footpad injection of 200 μg of rat IgG$_{2a}$ myeloma protein in complete Freund's adjuvant (CFA) followed at regular intervals with 200 μg of normal rat IgG$_{2a}$ in CFA injected subcutaneously. The resulting antiserum demonstrated a strong reactivity with rat L-chains and reacted with each of the rat IgG subclasses, IgM, IgA and myeloma IgE.

Rabbit and sheep anti-rat membrane IgD were prepared in the following manner: twenty-five Sprague-Dawley rats were sacrificed by exsanguination and their spleens, Peyer's patches and submaxillary lymph nodes were excised, trimmed and pooled. Single cell suspensions were prepared and the lymphocytes were isolated from these lymphoid organ cell suspensions and from heparinized blood, using Hypaque-Ficoll centrifugation.[14] The isolated lymphoid cells were then washed three times with phosphate buffered saline (PBS), and lysed with 0.5% (v/v) Nonidet P-40, (Particle Data Laboratories, Ltd., Elmhurst, Ill.) in phosphate-buffered saline (PBS) containing 1mM phenylmethylsulfonyl fluoride at 25° for 10 min. The lysate was centrifuged at 3,000 × g for 30' at 4°C and the supernatant was passed over IA columns containing normal rabbit IgG and normal chicken IgY. The nonadherent material was then passed over an IA column conjugated with specifically purified chicken anti-human δ.[10] Adherent material was eluted with 3M NaSCN, dialyzed against PBS and concentrated to 2.0 ml. The 3M NaSCN elute was centrifuged at 3000 × g for 30' at 4°C and the supernatant (representing 1.7 mg based on an assumed $\epsilon = 14.0$) was emulsified in an equal volume of CFA and used to immunize two New Zealand white rabbits and a sheep subcutaneously. The insoluble material from the above centrifugation procedure was resuspended in 1.0 ml PBS, emulsified in an equal volume of CFA and used to inject one rabbit as above. Animals were boosted with membrane isolates (prepared as described above) after two weeks and subsequently when the activity against human IgD by gel-diffusion was no longer detectable (see below). The antisera were made δ-chain specific by multiple passages over I.A.s. Each antiserum was twice precipitated with 40% saturated (NH$_4$)$_2$SO$_4$ and the dissolved precipitate dialyzed versus PBS or the IgG prepared by ion-exchange chromatography.

A rhodamine-conjugated IgG fraction of rabbit anti-goat IgG and fluorescein labeled goat anti-rabbit IgG were obtained commercially (Miles Labs). Dichlorotrizinylamino-fluorescein and tetramethyl rhodamine isothiocyanate (Research Organics Inc., Cleveland, OH) were conjugated to globulin fractions of anti-Ig and anti-Id-1 antisera using previously described procedures.[15,16] Conjugates with 2 ± 0.2 molar ratios of fluorochrome/protein were used. All sera used in fluorescent antibody assays were ultracentrifuged 60,000 × g for 1.0 hr prior to their use.

Fluorescent Antibody Techniques

Red blood cells were removed from single cell suspensions of fetal livers by lysing with 0.83% NH$_4$Cl. The vaginal plug method was used to accurately time gestational age in order to obtain fetal livers at known periods of development.[17] Lymphocytes from neonatal spleens (and livers at birth) were isolated by

Hypaque-Ficoll centrifugation. All cell suspensions were washed twice with warm (37° C) RPMI-1640 and twice with ice cold PBS containing 1% fetal calf serum (PBS-FCS) prior to staining. One million cells in 0.05 ml were then incubated for 30 minutes on ice with an equal volume of various dilutions of normal or immune serum (fluorescein or rhodamine conjugated serum if directly stained) and washed three times with cold PBS-FCS. For indirect staining the washed cells were resuspended in 0.1 ml of cold, fluorescein or rhodamine-conjugated antiserum, incubated and washed as above. In order to inhibit cap formation NaN$_3$ (0.03M final concentration) was added to the sera and wash solutions. To induce capping the cells were incubated for 60 minutes at 37°C in the absence of NaN$_3$. Cells stained with two contrasting fluorochromes were first examined with a microscope equipped with epi-illumination for the fluorochrome stain localized in a cap (less than half of the cell surface fluorescing). The same cell was then examined for staining with the contrasting fluorochrome (reacted under noncapping conditions). In the case of double staining studies using fluorescein or rhodamine conjugated rabbit anti-Id-1, cells were initially screened for the fluorochrome conjugated to the anti-idiotype. A Zeiss microscope equipped with epi-illumination (barrier, reflector and excitation filters are 520, 510 and 440–490 nm, respectively, for fluorescein and 560, 580 and 510–560, respectively, for rhodamine) was used.

Iodination of Membrane IgD

The material isolated from the chicken anti-human IgD I.A. was radiolabeled with ^{125}I using the method of McConahey and Dixon.[18] ^{125}I-labeled preparations were then reduced and run on SDS-PAGE using previously described techniques.[10]

Statistics

Where statistical analyses were employed, the F test was used for variance analysis, and Student t test was used to determine significances of mean differences.

RESULTS

Specificity of Rabbit and Sheep Anti-Rat Membrane IgD

By immunodiffusion the absorbed anti-rat δ was nonreactive with rat or human IgM, IgG, IgE, pooled normal rat serum or rat saliva. However, the anti-δ formed a single precipitation band of identity with purified human myeloma IgD or normal human serum containing 350 μg/ml of IgD. A band of identity was seen with a Meloy anti-human δ reagent and the various anti-rat δ. Antiserum from each of three rabbits formed a band of identity with human IgD on immunodiffusion. Thus for subsequent work the three antisera were pooled. Adsorption of anti-rat δ with rat thymocytes had no effect on the reactivity of the reagents.

Immunoprecipitation studies of ^{125}I surface labeled splenic lymphocyte lysates with the antisera were carried out to further characterize their specificity. Radioactive profiles of unreduced and reduced immune precipitates, electrophoresed on SDS-polyacrylamide gels, were superimposable on profiles obtained simultaneously with the chicken anti-human δ reagent initially used to characterize rat membrane IgD.[10] The major membrane component recognized ($\sim$187,000 M.W.) was antigenically distinct from rat IgG, IgA, IgE and IgM. Upon reduction of the immune precipitates light chains (23,000) and heavy chains ($\sim$73,000, with the characteristic δ-chain shoulder ($\sim$65,000) and a putative Fc receptor[10] were observed.

Tissue distribution of IgD bearing cells

Using immunofluorescence, the percentage of lymphocytes stained with the anti-δ as well as percentages of μ^+ and total Ig$^+$ lymphocytes in blood, spleen, lymph nodes, Peyer's patches and thymus were determined. The tissue distribution and percentage of δ^+ cells closely correlated with μ^+ and Ig$^+$ staining cells except for Peyer's patch cells where the number of Ig$^+$ cells was approximately two times the number of δ^+ or μ^+ cells (TABLE 1). The highest concentrations of Ig$^+$ cells were detected in the Peyer's patches (79.5%). The thymus had very few positive cells ($<$0.5%). These results were obtained using August strain rats. Similar percentages of δ^+, μ^+ and Ig$^+$ cells also were observed in Fischer (F-344), Copenhagen, Wistar Furth and Sprague Dawley rats.

Preincubation of the anti-δ with rat IgG, IgM, normal rat serum or a cell suspension of pooled thymocytes had no effect on the percentages of δ^+ staining lymphocytes. However, the intensity of staining with anti-δ could be diminished, but not ablated, by preincubation with human myeloma IgD.

Ontogeny of rat membrane IgD

The ontogeny of IgD and IgM on fetal and neonatal rat lymphocyte membranes was studied by immunofluorescence. The percentages of δ^+, μ^+ and Ig$^+$ cells were quantitated in cell suspensions prepared from: 1) fetal livers pooled from individual litters of pregnant rats sacrificed at various gestational ages, 2) neonatal spleens and livers obtained from rats sacrificed immediately after birth (prior to suckling) and 3) spleens obtained at various times after birth. A summary

TABLE 1

TISSUE DISTRIBUTION OF IgD, IgM AND IMMUNOGLOBULIN BEARING LYMPHOCYTES

Source of Cells*	Ig$^+$	δ^+	μ^+
Blood	19.6 (11.7–26.0)†	15.9 (11.0–23.5)	17.7 (11.2–25.7)
Spleen	33.0 (28.6–40.7)	25.4 (21.6–30.2)	28.1 (22.0–36.1)
Lymph Node	39.1 (25.1–54.3)	31.8 (18.1–40.9)	34.0 (19.9–45.0)
Peyer's Patch	79.5 (68.1–92.0)	40.6 (22.5–54.3)	45.8 (29.0–65.3)
Thymus	<0.5	<0.5	<0.5

*Cells from peripheral blood or organ cell suspensions were isolated by Hypaque-Ficoll centrifugation and stained directly for total surface immunoglobulin or indirectly for membrane IgM or IgD.

†Results were compiled from >15 rats (two–three months old), and are presented as the mean of the percent positive with the range in parenthesis. Triplicate determinations per rat, >200 cells examined per determination.

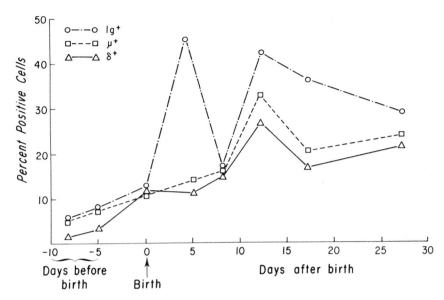

FIGURE 1. Ontogeny of rat membrane immunoglobulins. The number of lymphocytes with membrane immunoglobulin (Ig$^+$), IgM (μ^+) or IgD (δ^+) were quantitated using immunofluorescence. Each point represents a mean value obtained from $\geq$ 6 rats; triplicate determinations per rat; >200 cells examined per determination. Results are expressed as a percent of the total number of cells counted, which demonstrated fluorescence. Prior to birth cells were isolated from fetal livers. After birth spleen cell isolates were examined.

of the results are presented in FIGURE 1. Approximately eight days prior to birth very few (<1%) δ^+ cells were observed. In contrast approximately 5% μ^+ and 5% Ig$^+$ cells were present in fetal livers. Five days prior to birth the percentages of δ^+ and μ^+ cells had increased to approximately 3% and 8%, respectively, and at birth the δ^+, μ^+ and Ig$^+$ percentages were virtually the same (approximately 10%). Percentages of δ^+, μ^+ and Ig$^+$ cells in the newborn spleen and liver were similar.

There was a general increase in the percentage of Ig$^+$ cells in the spleen after birth, with a significant increase occurring by day 12. With the exception of day 5 the percentages of δ^+, μ^+ and Ig$^+$ cells closely paralleled one another. A peak in the number of Ig$^+$ cells was routinely observed on day 5. Since the number of cells expressing IgM and IgD on their surfaces (either independently or coexpressed) could not account for the number of Ig$^+$ cells observed, a transient expression on cell surfaces of other immunoglobulin classes or L chains seems possible. The numbers of δ^+, μ^+ and Ig$^+$ cells of 28-day-old adolescent rats were slightly lower than adult values (see TABLE 1).

Ontogeny of Rat Serum Immunoglobulins

The observation that large numbers (>40%) of rat splenic lymphocytes transiently express isotype(s) other than IgM and IgD (~11%) between 5 and 10 days after birth can be explained in a number of ways. Firstly, during this time a population of B-cells may express one or more IgG subclasses. These cells then could become sequestered in a nonsplenic site or they may cease integrating the IgG into their membranes. In this regard, generally <5% of adult peripheral blood lymphocytes synthesize IgG. Secondly, a transient expression of lambda chains may have occurred. Nothing specific is known about rat lambda chain expression at this time. We are currently investigating this possibility. Thirdly, passively acquired immunoglobulins (maternal) may have interacted with a population of B- and or T-cells during this period.

A review of the literature revealed that no comprehensive study had been made of the ontogeny of rat immunoglobulins. FIGURE 2 gives the results of our investigation. Several points are noteworthy. Virtually no IgM or IgA is transferred across the placenta and detectable quantities are only seen several days after birth. Interestingly, at birth, the rat has very low levels of each of the IgG subclasses, which indicates that the placental transfer of IgG is not particularly efficient. Starting at about four days of age, a dramatic increase in IgG2a, 2b and IgG1 begins and peaks at about 15 days of age. A catabolic decay then occurs and between days 30 and 40 an increase is observed. The exception to these observations is IgG2c. Clearly, placental and milk transfer of IgG2c occurs but not as dramatically as with the other three IgG subclasses.

These results suggest but certainly do not prove, that the high number of Ig-bearing lymphocytes in 5–10 day old rats could be related to the acquisition of maternal immunoglobulins.

Coexpression of IgD and IgM on the Same Cell

Since the tissue distribution and percentage of IgD bearing lymphocytes closely correlated with IgM bearing lymphocytes, double staining techniques were used to determine if IgD and IgM are coexpressed on the same lymphocytes. Direct staining techniques using rhodamine or fluorescein conjugated rabbit anti-δ or goat anti-μ were not sensitive enough to permit accurate quantitation. Therefore indirect staining procedures were used. The procedure used was to react the initial reagent under capping conditions and the subsequent stains under noncapping conditions.

Of the δ^+, μ^+ and Ig$^+$ staining cells 78%, 84% and 80%, respectively formed caps. When anti-δ capped cells were stained with anti-μ or anti-μ capped cells stained with anti-δ, ring staining patterns were observed in 86% and 71% of the capped cells, respectively. Ring staining was not observed when the cells were first capped with anti-Ig. These results indicate that IgD and IgM are coexpressed on a high percentage of the B-lymphocytes in the spleen, can be capped independently by anti-δ or anti-μ and can be cocapped by anti-Ig.

Shared Idiotypic Determinants on Membrane IgD and IgM

An antiserum to a defined idiotype, Id-1, (see MATERIALS AND METHODS) was used to determine if membrane IgD and IgM coexpressed on the same cell share similar idiotypic determinants. The rabbit anti-Id-1 used in these studies was directed towards IgG-anti-group A streptococcal carbohydrate (anti-SACHO) antibodies. The anti-Id-1 reaction to the anti-SACHO has been shown to be hapten (N-acetyl-D-glucosamine) inhibitable.[12,13] Splenic lymphocytes from hyperimmunized rats of a Sprague-Dawley strain (HRP) selectively inbred for their high antibody responsiveness to Group A streptococci[19,20] were isolated by Hypaque-Ficoll centrifugation and used to enhance the detection of idiotype positive cells. Results obtained by double staining immunofluorescence as described above showed that ~0.07–0.08% of the splenic lymphocytes were Id-1$^+$ and represented approximately 2% of the B-cell population. Cells initially

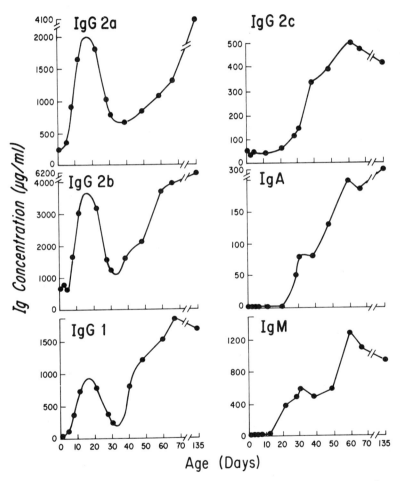

FIGURE 2. The ontogeny of rat serum immunoglobulins. Each point represents the mean concentration for four–six animals, determined by radial immunodiffusion.

capped with anti-δ or anti-μ still demonstrated ring staining with anti-Id-1, whereas anti-Ig capped cells did not. Conversely, ring staining by anti-δ, anti-μ, or anti-Ig was not detected on anti-Id-1 capped cells. Collectively these results indicate that the idiotypic determinants were detected on B-cells, that cells with

TABLE 2

SERUM IMMUNOGLOBULIN ONTOGENY OF COPENHAGEN RATS
INJECTED AT VARIOUS AGES WITH ANTI-μ OR ANTI-δ

Treatments†	n	Day of First Injection‡	% of Control*			
			IgM	IgA	IgG2a	IgG2c
Sheep IgG	4	15 day fetus	100	107	88	95
Sheep IgG	4	18 day fetus	89	100	88	108
Sheep IgG	4	birth	100	100	100	100
Sheep anti-μ	3	15 day fetus	0	0	<1	54
Sheep anti-μ	3	18 day fetus	0	0	<1	60
Sheep anti-μ	3	birth	0	0	1	54
Sheep anti-δ	3	15 day fetus	0	0	13	50
Sheep anti-δ	3	18 day fetus	100	82	51	75
Sheep anti-δ	3	birth	289	230	91	528

*Percentage of uninjected age-matched rats; rats were sacrificed at 15 days of age.
†All reagents were salt precipitated and DEAE-purified.
‡Gestational age based on vaginal-plug method. Additional injections were given one, two, three, five, seven, nine and 11 days after birth.

capped δ or μ determinants still express the idiotype on their surface and that anti-Id-1 cocapped the δ and μ determinants.

Modulation of Rat Serum Immunoglobulin Ontogeny

In 1978 we postulated that an IgD-bearing B-cell was a "pivotal" cell in the developmental pathway of plasma cells.[2] In our original attempt to test this hypothesis we injected rats starting at birth, with anti-δ. The anti-δ treated rats had normal levels of circulating Igs.[22] In view of our recent studies on the ontogeny of IgD-bearing cells (see above) we wished to reevaluate the effect of anti-δ antibody on Ig production and lymphocyte development. Age-matched Copenhagen fetuses and neonates were treated with IgG anti-δ, IgG anti-μ or normal sheep IgG, as indicated in TABLE 2. There were no significant differences between untreated and normal sheep IgG injected rats. In contrast, the anti-μ treated animals totally lacked IgM and IgA, were severely deficient in IgG2a and had depressed IgG2c. Similar results were obtained regardless of the age which the first injection was given (15- and 18-day fetuses or newborn). When rats were given sheep anti-δ starting at birth a marked enhancement of IgM, IgA and IgG2c was seen whereas IgG2a was essentially normal. Anti-δ given first to 18-day fetuses had no effect on IgM, a marginal effect on IgA and IgG2c and caused significant suppression of IgG2a. When anti-δ was given to 15-day fetuses, very pronounced suppression of IgM, IgA, IgG2a and IgG2c occurred. In fact, the results are similar to those obtained with anti-μ. In a separate set of experiments using F-344 rats (Cooper-Willis and Leslie, unpublished) sheep anti-δ given to 17-day fetuses had a marked suppressive effect on IgM, IgG2c, and IgG1 and little or no effect on IgA, IgG2a and IgG2b.

Collectively, these anti-δ data point out the variable effects anti-δ may have depending upon the age at which the animal first receives it. Furthermore, they strongly support the original hypothesis that IgD-bearing B-cells are "pivotal" in the normal developmental pathway of immunoglobulin secreting plasma cells.

Modulation of B-Cell Ontogeny

Fluorescent antibody techniques were used to examine the effects of anti-δ and anti-μ treatments on membrane immunoglobulin-bearing splenic lymphocytes. The results obtained are presented in TABLE 3. There were no detectable μ-bearing cells in the spleen of rats treated with anti-μ during fetal development or at birth. The δ-bearing and total Ig-bearing population were not significantly affected by neonatal anti-μ, but anti-μ when given to 18-day fetuses caused a marked suppression in the number of δ-bearing and Ig-bearing cells. Anti-μ when administered to 15-day old fetuses caused a total depletion of all Ig-bearing cells. In contrast with the anti-μ results, anti-δ when given to neonates as well as 18-day-old fetuses caused significant increases in number of -bearing cells and a concomitant increase in the number of μ-bearing cells. Double staining techniques and the relationship between the total number of Ig-bearing cells and the number of δ-bearing and μ-bearing cells indicate that IgM and IgD are coexpressed on most cells in these anti-δ treated animals. Very different results were obtained when anti-δ was first given to 15-day-old fetuses. Firstly, the anti-δ resulted in animals totally lacking δ-bearing cells. Secondly, the animals had almost a total loss of μ-bearing and Ig-bearing cells (control = 18% vs anti-δ treated = 1%). It is not yet clear if the 1% remaining μ-positive and Ig-positive cells represent immature B-cells that have not yet expressed IgD or if they are a subpopulation of B-cells that do not require IgD expression prior to their development into plasma cells. In this regard, it was noted in TABLE 2 that this group of anti-δ treated rats could synthesize small amounts of IgG2a and IgG2c.

Hypothetical Model of the Role of IgD Plasma-Cell Differentiation

Our original scheme for the development of the plasma-cell line of cells implied that IgM-IgD-dual expressing B-cell was the precursor for most, if not all, plasma cells. We were, however, careful to point out that during the clonal B-cell expansion phase, a cell might be forced into a different differentiation pathway.

TABLE 3

MEMBRANE IMMUNOGLOBULIN-BEARING SPLENIC LYMPHOCYTES OF COPENHAGEN RATS INJECTED AT VARIOUS AGES WITH ANTI-μ OR ANTI-δ*

Treatments	n	Day of First Injection	% of Total†		
			μ^+	δ^+	Ig$^+$
Sheep IgG	4	15 day fetus	18	18	18
Sheep anti-δ	3	15 day fetus	1	0	1
Sheep anti-μ	3	15 day fetus	0	0	0
Sheep IgG	4	18 day fetus	19	18	19
Sheep anti-δ	3	18 day fetus	37	36	37
Sheep anti-μ	3	18 day fetus	0	11	11
Sheep IgG	4	birth	21	21	25
Sheep anti-δ	3	birth	42	41	48
Sheep anti-μ	3	birth	0	19	21

*See legend of TABLE 2 for details.

†Lymphocytes were stained using indirect fluorescent antibody techniques for membrane IgD, IgM and total Ig.

Such may have been the case with 15-day-fetal anti-δ treated rats, which could explain the presence of IgG in these animals. Our current model for the development of the plasma-cell line of cells, which reinforces the possibility of alternative developmental pathways, is given in FIGURE 3.

DISCUSSION

The specificity of the anti-δ reagents used for these experiments is of critical importance. They were made with specifically purified membrane IgD and were used in studies designed to study membrane events. Most previous studies have been done with antisera made against the secreted form of IgD (myeloma) and/or

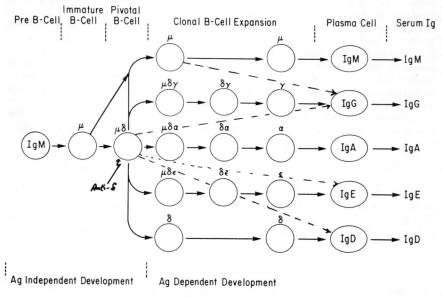

FIGURE 3. A model of B-cell differentiation.

with monoclonal hybridoma anti-δ. Besides the data provided here, rigorous proof of the specificity of our anti-δ, including antigenic cross-reactivity with human and mouse IgD, have been published.[32]

The tissue distribution of IgD bearing lymphocytes reported here is similar to that reported in the mouse,[7,9,24] and in the rat using membrane iodination procedures.[10] With the possible exception of Peyer's patch lymphocytes, the percentages of δ^+ and μ^+ cells when compared with the total Ig$^+$ bearing cells would indicate that a large percentage of the Ig$^+$ cells in the various lymphoid organs coexpress IgM and IgD. Fluorescent antibody double staining of splenocytes and PBL's (results not shown) indicate that this is indeed the case. This conclusion is supported further by previous studies in the human, monkey and mouse[2-9] demonstrating that a high percentage of IgD bearing lymphocytes coexpress IgM. A possible exception is the Peyer's patch cell. The disproportionate percentages of Ig^+ (~80%) cells to μ^+ (~46×) and/or δ^+ (~41%) cells may be explained by an independent expression of IgD and IgM rather than coexpression on this particular lymphoid cell. Thus, the summation of δ^+ and $\mu+$ cells would approximate the percent of Ig^+ cells. However, IgE and IgA bearing cells have been detected in the Peyer's patches of rats (M.A. Cuchens and G.A. Leslie, unpublished observations) and could account for at least some of the discrepancies observed. We are presently examining various lymphoid tissues, especially Peyer's patch cells, for the coexpression of IgA, IgE and IgG with IgM and/or IgD.

With respect to the ontogeny of membrane immunoglobulins, rats are similar to the human and mouse.[2,7,8,9] IgM-bearing lymphocytes appear to be the first predominantly expressed immunoglobulin in the fetal liver, followed shortly thereafter by IgD. The sequence of membrane expression of IgD and IgM determined by immunofluorescence studies confirms an earlier study using ^{125}I-lactoperoxidase labeling procedures.[10] However, IgD was detected much earlier (prenatally as opposed to neonatally) in the present study which is attributed to the greater sensitivity of the immunofluorescence technique employed. The results of these two studies support the contention that there are quantitative differences in the amount of IgD and IgM on fetal and neonatal lymphocytes. A difference between the rat, monkey and human versus the mouse ontogeny data is that rat, monkey and human IgM and IgD are coexpressed at parturition whereas IgD is not detected until several days after birth in the mouse.[2,7,8,9] In this regard one must conclude that the rat is immunologically more mature at birth than the mouse and that in terms of the ontogeny of B-lymphocytes the rat more closely resembles the primates.

Generally there was a gradual increase in the surface immunoglobulin bearing B-cells with the percentages of $Ig^+ > \mu^+ < \delta^+$, although differences (with exception of day 5) were not statistically significant. A peak similar to that observed in the percentages of Ig^+ cells on day 5 has also been reported in neonatal mice after birth.[25] The total number of Ig^+ cells present at day 5 cannot be explained by the independent expression of membrane IgD and IgM. One possible explanation, however, is that some immature lymphocytes are cytophilic for Ig acquired from the mother's colostrum and milk. Following further differentiation, this cytophilic Ig is lost and only de novo synthesized Ig is observed. Alternatively, there may be a period of immunological activity, wherein a differentiation sequence occurs involving cells expressing other surface Ig isotypes or free L-chains while enroute to becoming plasma cells. This point clearly needs to be examined further.

Our observations and those of others that a single cell can express two immunoglobulin isotypes on its membrane surface has led to speculations that the two isotypes may have different functions.[26] An important point regarding the dual functionality hypothesis of IgD and IgM is whether the two isotypes have the same combining site (i.e., the same V-regions). Studies have shown that membrane IgD and IgM on cells from some patients with paraproteins share idiotypic determinants with the paraprotein.[27,28] Others have demonstrated similar antigen binding activity of IgD and IgM on human[29,30] lymphocytes. The present study is the first to examine the similarity of idiotypic determinants on membrane IgD and IgM using a hapten inhibitable anti-idiotype directed towards an antibody with defined specificity. These studies, were restricted due to the low numbers of $Id-1^+$ cells so that the antigen specificity of the $Id-1^+$ cells was not conclusively proven. Our data, however, support the concept that IgD and IgM on the same cell may share similar idiotypic determinants. Further studies on the antigen binding characteristics of IgD and IgM on the same cell are required.

Treatment of fetal and neonatal rats with anti-μ resulted in pronounced hypogammaglobulinemia similar to that reported earlier for neonatally treated rats[22,23] mice[34,35] and chickens.[36,37] Neonatally injected rats had no detectable IgM-bearing cells but IgD-bearing cells were essentially at normal levels. These results differ from those of other workers[33,38] who reported that IgD-bearing cells were also suppressed under these conditions. We do find, however, a total absence of all Ig-bearing cells when the anti-μ is first given to fetuses.

The injection of anti-δ into neonatal rats has yielded variable results. In our original studies[22] there were no changes observed in serum immunoglobulins whereas in the most recent experiments there was a highly significant but selective increase in some classes. Bazin et al.[33] reported that anti-δ strongly suppressed IgD and IgE levels, which we did not measure, had a stimulatory effect on IgG2c and had minimal effects on the other isotypes.

In our studies neonatal anti-δ injection caused a dramatic increase in the number of IgM, IgD and Ig-bearing lymphocytes in the spleen whereas in the Bazin study, anti-δ caused a pronounced decrease in IgM, IgD and Ig-bearing cells in the mesenteric lymph nodes. Layton et al.[39] were the first to show the suppressive effects of anti-δ on IgD and IgM-bearing cells in mice. Recently Tokuhisa et al.[40] reported that injection of anti-paternal mouse IgD allotype antibodies into neonatal (BALB/c × SJL)F1 mice can significantly suppress the appropriate IgM and IgD cells and serum IgG, which would have the paternal allotype. Essentially similar results were reported by Jacobson et al.[41]

There are a number of possible explanations for the apparent differences, stated above, in effects observed with neonatal anti-δ injections. Our experiments, originally used rabbit anti-rat membrane δ and chicken anti-human myeloma δ (cross-reactive with rat-δ) whereas the most recent experiments employed sheep anti-rat membrane δ. In each set of experiments we examined spleen cells whereas Bazin et al. employed mesenteric lymph nodes and used rabbit anti-rat myeloma IgD. In addition, different strains of rats were used. The ontogeny of IgD-bearing cells in rats and mice are totally different. Therefore, the effects of neonatal anti-δ injections should not be expected to be identical. The amount, specificity, affinity, isotype and species of origin of the various anti-δs employed are clearly potential sources of differences.

Rats have significant numbers of IgD-bearing cells at birth. We therefore developed techniques to administer anti-δ to fetuses. The most dramatic results have come from fetuses injected with anti-δ at 15 days of age. These animals have no IgD and ~1% IgM and Ig-bearing lymphocytes and they are markedly hypogammaglobulinemic. Immunologically, their humoral immune system looks very similar to that of animals treated with anti-μ. In spite of the very low number of splenic Ig-bearing cells, even these rats had significant amounts of serum IgG. It would appear therefore that normal humoral immune development requires a pivotal IgD-bearing B-cell but alternative pathways do occur which can be utilized when the IgD-bearing cell population becomes perturbed.

The recent identification of what appears to be IgD in chickens[42] could provide an additional important model for further studies on the role of IgD in humoral immune functions.

SUMMARY

Rat membrane IgD was isolated from lymphocyte lysates utilizing a cross-reactive chicken anti-human IgD immunoadsorbent column. Rabbits and sheep were immunized with the isolated membrane determinants. The resulting antisera were shown to be δ-specific by immunodiffusion, immunoprecipitation studies with ^{125}I-labeled cell lysates and immunofluorescence techniques. The anti-rat membrane IgD (anti-δ) was used to characterize the tissue distribution and ontogeny of IgD-bearing lymphocytes and to determine the effect of prenatal and neonatal anti-δ on subsequent immunoglobulin and B-cell ontogeny in rats. Immunofluorescence studies showed that the percentages of IgD bearing lymphocytes in the various lymphoid organs or peripheral blood usually but not always closely correlated with the percentages of IgM and total immunoglobulin bearing lymphocytes. Less than 1% IgD and approximately 5% IgM-bearing lymphocytes were detectable in the liver of 13-day fetuses. Double staining and capping studies showed that IgD is coexpressed predominately with IgM (~80% of B-cells) and that IgD and IgM cap independently, yet are cocapped by anti-immunoglobulin. Shared idiotypic determinants on IgD and IgM expressed on the same cell were also demonstrated.

Treatment of neonatal or 18 day fetal rats with anti-μ or anti-δ resulted in different manifestations in the ontogeny of the humoral immune system. Anti-μ treatment resulted in hypogammaglobulinemia and the presence of $\mu^-\delta^+$ cells. In contrast, anti-δ treated neonatal or 18-day fetuses had significantly increased numbers of $\mu^+\delta^+$ cells and normal or elevated levels of serum immunoglobulins. The most striking results were obtained when rats were initially injected as 15-day-old embryos with anti-δ or anti-μ. In each case simlar hypogammaglobulinemia occured as well as severe B-cell depletion. The anti-μ treated rats had no detectable B-cells and the anti-δ treated rats had approximately 1% $\mu^+\delta^-$ cells. These results strongly support the important role of IgD-bearing cells in the normal developmental pathway of plasma cells.

ACKNOWLEDGMENTS

We thank Dr. Joan C. Olson for the anti-idiotype reagent, Dr. Herve Bazin for rat myeloma protein containing fluids and our secretarial staffs for their cooperation.

REFERENCES

1. ROWE, D. S. & J. L. FAHEY. 1965. A new class of human immunoglobulins. I. A unique myeloma protein. J. Exp. Med. **121:** 171.
2. LESLIE, G. A. & L. N. MARTIN. 1978. Structure and function of serum and membrane immunoglobulin D (IgD). In Contemporary Topics in Molecular Immunology. I. F. P. Inman and R. A. Reisfeld, Eds.: 1. Plenum Publishing Co. New York, N.Y.
3. ROWE, D. S., K. HUG L. FORNI & B. PERNIS. 1973. Immunoglobulin D as a lymphocyte receptor. J. Exp. Med. **138:** 965.
4. KNAPP, W., R. L. M. BOLHIUS, J. RADL & W. HIJAMANS. 1983. Independent movement of IgD and IgM molecules on the surface of individual lymphocytes. J. Immunol. **111:** 1295.
5. PREUD'HOMME, J. L., J. C. BROUET & M. SELIGMANN. 1977. Membrane-bound IgD on human lymphoid cells, with special reference to immunodeficiency and immunoproliferative disorders. Immunol. Rev. **37:** 127.
6. PERNIS, B. 1977. Lymphocyte membrane IgD. Immunological Rev. **37:** 219.
7. VITETTA, E. S. & J. W. UHR. 1977. IgD and B cell differentiation. Immunological Rev. **37:** 50.

8. PARKHOUSE, R. M. E. & M. D. COOPER. 1977. A model for the differentiation of B lymphocytes with implications for the biological role of IgD. Immunological Rev. **37:** 105.
9. GODING, J. W., D. W. SCOTT & J. E. LAYTON. 1977. Genetics, cellular expression and function of IgD and IgM receptor. Immunol. Rev. **37:** 152.
10. RUDDICK, J. H. & G. A. LESLIE. 1977. Structure and biological function of human IgD. XI. Identification and ontogeny of a rat lymphocyte immunoglobulin having antigenic cross-reactivity with human IgD. J. Immunol. **118:** 1025.
11. WOFSY, L & B. BURR. 1969. The use of affinity chromatography for the specific purification of antibodies and antigens. J. Immunol. **103:** 380.
12. STANKUS, R. P. & G. A. LESLIE. 1974. Cross-idiotypic specificity of rat antibodies to group A streptococcal carbohydrate. J. Immunol. **113:** 1859.
13. STANKUS, R. P. & G. A. LESLIE. 1977. Interspecies and Interantigenic evaluation of a cross-reactive rat idiotype. Immunogen. **4:233.**
14. KERMANI-ARAB. V., G. A. LESLIE, & D. R. BURGER. 1977. Structure and biological function of human IgD. IX. Anti-IgD activation of human lymphocytes. Int. Arch. Allergy Appl. Immunol. **54:** 1.
15. AMANTE, L., A. ANCONA & L. FORNI. 1972. The conjugation of immunoglobulins with tetramethytrodamine isothiocyanate. A comparison between the amorphous and the crystalline fluorochrome. J. Immunol. Methods **1:** 289.
16. BLAKESLEE, D. & M. G. BAINES. 1976. Immunofluorescence using, dichlorotrizinylaminofluorescein (DTAF) I. Preparation and fractionation of labelled IgG. J. Immunol. Methods **13:** 305.
17. BRONSON, F. H., C. P. DAGG & G. D. SNELL. 1966. Reproduction Methods. In Biology of the Laboratory Mouse. E. L. Green, Ed.: 195. McGraw-Hill. New York, N.Y.
18. MCCONAHEY, P. & F. DIXON. 1966. A method of trace iodination of proteins for immunologic studies. Int. Arch. Allergy **29:** 185.
19. STANKUS, R. P. & G. A. LESLIE. 1975. Genetic influences on the immune response of rats to streptococcal A carbohydrate. Immunogen. **2:** 29.
20. STANKUS, R. P. & G. A. LESLIE. 1976. Rat interstrain antibody response and crossidiotypic specificity. Immunogen. **3:** 65.
21. ABNEY, E. R., I. R. HUNTER & R. M. E. PARKHOUSE. 1976. Preparation and characterization of an antiserum to the mouse candidate for immunoglobulin D. Nature **259:** 404.
22. CUCHENS, M. A. & G. A. LESLIE. 1977. B-cell function in rats treated as neonates and adults with anti-IgD and anti-IgM. In Developmental Immunobiology. J. B. Solomon and J. D. Horton Eds.: 197. Elsevier/North Holland Biomedical Press. Amsterdam, the Netherlands.
23. CUCHENS, M. A. & G. A. LESLIE. 1978. The effects of anti-IgD on serum immunoglobulins, antibody production and immunoglobulin bearing cells in adult rats. J. Immunol. **121:** 2257.
24. VITETTA, E. S., U. MELCHER, M. MCWILLIAMS, J. PHILLIPS-QUAGLIATA, M. LAMM & J. W. UHR. 1975. Cell surface immunoglobulin XI. The appearance of an IgD-like molecule on murine lymphoid cells during ontogeny. J. Exp. Med. **141:** 206.
25. BRUYNS, C. G., URBAIN-VANSANTEN, C. PLANARD, C. DE VOS-CLOETENS & J. URBAIN 1976. Ontogeny of mouse B lymphocytes and inactivation   by antigen of early B-lymphocytes. Proc. Natl. Acad. Sci. **73:** 2462.
26. VITETTA, E. S. & J. W. UHR. 1975. Immunoglobulin receptors revisited. Science **189:** 964.
27. SALSANO, F., S. S. FROLAND, J. B. NATVIG & T. E. MICHAELSON. 1974. Same idiotype on B lymphocyte membrane IgD and IgM. Evidence for monoclonality of chronic lymphocytic leukemia cells. Scand. J. Immunol. **3:** 841.
28. FU, S. M., R. J. WINCHESTER, T. FEIZI, P. D. WALZER & H. G. KUNKEL. 1974. Idiotype specificity of surface immunoglobulin and the maturation of leukemic bone marrow derived lymphocytes. Proc. Natl. Acad. Sci. USA. **71:** 4487.
29. PERNIS, B., J. C. BROUET & M. SELIGMANN. 1974. IgD and IgM on the membrane of lymphoid cells in macroglobulinemia. Evidence for identity of membrane IgD and IgM antibody activity in a case with anti-IgG receptors. Eur. J. Immunol. **4:** 776.

30. STERN, C. & I. MC CONNELL. 1976. Immunoglobulins M and D as antigen-binding receptors on the same cells with shared specificity. Eur. J. Immunol. **6:** 225.
31. GODING, J. W. & J. W. LAYTON. 1976. Antigen-induced cocapping of IgM and IgD-like receptors on murine B cells. J. Exp. Med **144:** 852.
32. GOLDING, H., M. A. CUCHENS, G. A. LESLIE & M. B. RITTENBERG. 1979. Cross-reactivity of rat, mouse and human IgD. J. Immunol. **123:** 2751.
33. BAZIN, H., B. PLATTEAU, A. BECKERS. & R. PAUWELS. 1978. Differential effect of neonatal injections of anti-μ or anti-δ antibodies on the synthesis of IgM, IgD, IgE, IgA, IgG1, IgG2a, IgG2b and IgG2c immunoglobulin classes. J. Immunol. **121:** 2083.
34. LAWTON, A. R. & M. D. COOPER. 1974. Modification of B-lymphocyte differentiation by anti-immunoglobulin. Contemp. Top. Immunobiol. **3:** 193.
35. MANNING, D. D. 1975. Heavy chain isotype suppression: a review of the immunosuppressive effects of heterologous anti-Ig heavy chain antisera. J. Ret. Soc. **18:** 63.
36. KINCADE, P. W., A. R. LAWTON, D. E. BOCKMAN & M. D. COOPER. 1970. Suppression of immunoglobulin G synthesis as a result of antibody mediated suppression of immunoglobulin M synthesis in chickens. Proc. Natl. Acad. Sci. U.S.A. **67:** 1918.
37. LESLIE, G. A. & L. N. MARTIN. 1973. Modulation of immunoglobulin ontogeny in the chicken. Effect of purified antibody specific for μ-chain on IgM, IgY and IgA production. J. Immunol. **110:** 959.
38. COOPER, M. D., J. F. KEARNEY, P. M. LYDYARD, C. E. CROSS & A. R. LAWTON. 1976. Studies of generation of B-cell diversity in mouse, man and chicken. Cold Spring Harbor Symposia on Quantitative Biol. **41:** 139.
39. LAYTON, J. E., G. R. JOHNSON, D. W. SCOTT & G. J. V. Nossal. 1978. The anti-δ suppressed mouse. Eur. J. Immunol. **8:** 325.
40. TOKUHISA, T., F. T. GADUS, L. A. HERZENBERG & L. A. HERZENBERG. 1981. Monoclonal antibody to an IgD allotype induces a new type of allotype suppression in the mouse. J. Exp. Med. **154:** 921.

41. JACOBSON, E. B., Y. BAINE, Y.-W. CHEN, T. FLOTTE, M. J. O'NEIL, B. PERNIS, G. W. SISKIND, G. J. THORBECKE & P. TONDA. 1981. Physiology of IgD. I. Compensatory phenomena in B lymphocyte activation in mice treated with anti-IgD antibodies. J. Exp. Med. **154:** 318.
42. LESLIE G. A. 1980. Idiotypy and IgD isotypy of chicken immunoglobulins. *In* Phylogeny of Immunological Memory. M. J. Manning, Ed.: 253 Elsevier/North-Holland Biomedical Press. Amsterdam, the Netherlands.

DISCUSSION OF THIS PAPER BEGINS ON PAGE 154.

EXPRESSION OF IgD AS A FUNCTION OF B-CELL DIFFERENTIATION*

Max D. Cooper, Taro Kuritani, Chen-lo Chen, Joyce E. Lehmeyer, and William E. Gathings

Cellular Immunobiology Unit of the Tumor Institute
Departments of Pediatrics and Microbiology
and
Comprehensive Cancer Center
University of Alabama in Birmingham
Birmingham, Alabama 35294

INTRODUCTION

The role of IgD has remained an enigma since its discovery in 1965.[1] It was the last immunoglobulin isotype to be identified because of the relative rarity of IgD myelomas and the low frequency of normal plasma cells which produce IgD. Later it was discovered that IgD is present on the majority of B-lymphocytes.[2,3] Thus, IgD is though to play its primary role as an antigen receptor through which B-cells can be activated.[4] Although there is considerable evidence indicating that B-cell behavior can be influenced via cross linkage of surface IgD receptors, there is still no convincing evidence for a unique influence of IgD antibody receptors.

We have sought insight into the role of surface IgD by examining its phylogenetic representation, expression relative to other immunoglobulin isotypes during development, and persistence during later phases of B-cell differentiation.

SEARCH FOR AN IgD ANALOGUE IN CHICKENS

If IgD is indeed an important receptor molecule for regulation of the immune response, it would be expected to be a highly conserved molecule widely represented among vertebrates. So far, IgD expression has been identified with certainty only on B-cells from mammals, i.e., humans, monkeys, mice, rats and rabbits.[2,5-10]

Several investigators have mentioned suggestive immunofluorescence evidence of an IgD analogue in chickens[11,12] (J. R. Pink, cited in reference 13), but a clear delineation of this issue has not been forthcoming. A significant obstacle has been the paucity of well-defined isotype specific antibodies. After a long and frustrating search for a chicken IgD analogue using heterologous antibodies to heavy and light chain determinants, we prepared monoclonal antibodies to chicken μ-, γ-, α- and light chains for this purpose. Using these in indirect immunofluorescence assays, we noted that the majority of chicken B-lymphocytes bore surface IgM. The frequency of μ-, γ- and α- B-cells in blood was 20%, 2% and 0.2%, respectively. After μ determinants were capped, monoclonal antibodies to a light chain determinant were still reactive with determinants distributed over the entire surface of IgM B-cells. We then proceeded with an

*This work was supported by Grants CA 16673, CA 13148, awarded by the National Cancer Institute; 5M01-RR32, awarded by National Institutes of Health; and 1-608 awarded by March of Dimes Birth Defects Foundation.

0077-8923/82/0399-0146 $01.75/0 © 1982, NYAS

immunochemical analysis of surface immunoglobulins on chicken lymphocytes. Surface proteins were radiolabeled by the lactoperoxidase method, solubilized, selectively precipitated with monoclonal anti-immunoglobulin antibodies, and analyzed under reducing conditions by gel electrophoresis. FIGURE 1 illustrates experimental results which suggest the existence of an IgD analogue on chicken splenocytes. After precipitating from the supernatant all of the surface μ-, γ- and α- chains reactive with the monoclonal antibodies, heavy chains of 81,000 daltons were still precipitated with monoclonal anti-light chain antibody. The same basic

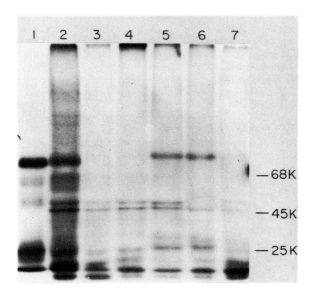

FIGURE 1. Analysis of immunoglobulin molecules on chicken B-cells. Purified splenic lymphocytes were surface-radiolabeled with ^{125}I-NaI by the lactoperoxidase-catalyzed method.[14] The cells were lysed with 0.5% NP-40 containing protease inhibitors. Immune complexes were precipitated with heat-killed Cowan's *Staphylococcus aureus*,[15] reduced, and analyzed by SDS-PAGE[16] using a 5–12% polyacrylamide gradient gel. Lane 1, I[125]-labeled chicken serum IgM molecular weight marker. Lane 2, band precipitated with monoclonal anti-chicken μ antibody (M-3). Lane 3, bands precipitated subsequently with monoclonal anti-μ, anti-γ, and anti-α. Lysate was divided in half, and in lane 4, one-half was precipitated again with M-3. In lane 5, the other half was precipitated with monoclonal anti-light chain. Lane 6, the supernatant from lane 4 was precipitated with goat anti-chicken μ. Lane 7, the supernatant from lane 5 was precipitated with goat anti-chicken light chain.

result was obtained after removal of μ-chains by precipitation with an alloanti-chicken IgM antiserum. It is noteworthy that the putative IgD analogue was also precipitated by the affinity-purified goat antibodies to chicken μ-chains.

We conclude from these studies that chicken B-cells may express surface immunoglobulin molecules of a fourth isotype (non-μ, -γ, -α), and that this candidate IgD analogue shares at least one antigenic determinant with chicken IgM. The latter feature may be responsible for much of the previous difficulty in identifying a chicken IgD analogue.

ONTOGENY OF IgD EXPRESSION IN MICE

Although expressed by most IgM B-cells in adults, membrane IgD is acquired significantly later than IgM during B-cell ontogeny.[6,7,17] Earlier, we examined the ontogeny of IgD expression in relation to the other immunoglobulin isotypes.[17] We confirmed the fact that few of the IgM B-cells present at birth had IgD on their surface. A gradual acquisition of surface IgD was then noted over the first nine days of life. Our most interesting findings concerned B-cells undergoing immunoglobulin isotype switches. As B-cells expressing IgG1, IgG2a, IgG2b, IgG3 or IgA emerged, they continued for a time to express surface IgM. The surprising finding was that IgD was not seen on most B-cells with IgG and IgA isotypes in three-day-old mice, whereas by day nine virtually all IgG and IgA B cells appeared to express both IgM and IgD as well. With further maturation most IgG and IgA B-cells appeared to cease expression of IgM and IgD, as most of these cells were "singles" in adult mice. A similar ontogenetic pattern has been noted in developing humans.[18] One possible interpretation of these observations was given in the model of B-cell differentiation shown in FIGURE 2. Subsequently the order of the immunoglobulin constant region genes was shown to be μ, δ, γ_3, γ_1, γ_{2b}, γ_{2a}, and α on chromosome 12 in mice.[19,20] The continued expression of IgM and IgD by B-cells switching to the expression of another isotype could be explained simply by the persistence of long-lived μ and δ messages after deletion of the μ and δ genes.[21] More difficult to explain would be an expression sequence of $\mu \rightarrow \mu\gamma \rightarrow \mu\gamma\delta$, for example.

With this in mind, we have reexamined the ontogeny of immunoglobulin isotype expression in mice. Affinity purified heterologous antibodies specific for each isotype were conjugated with either rhodamine or fluorescein and used in two-color immunofluorescence assays. The anti-δ antibodies were a gift from Dr. Fred Finkelman, the other isotype specific antibodies were made in our laboratory. The results, shown in FIGURE 3, essentially confirm our previous results using a

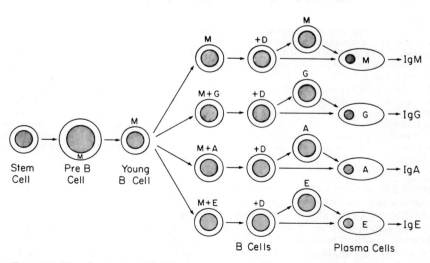

FIGURE 2. Hypothetical model of the generation of isotype diversity in a B-cell clone.

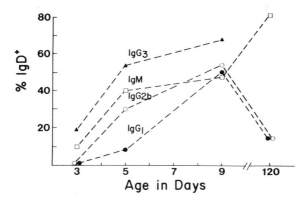

FIGURE 3. Ontogeny of IgD expression on mouse B-cells.

different set of antibodies. The proportion of IgG and IgA B-cells with detectable IgD was very low at three days, and gradually increased over the next few days. Not shown in the figure is the fact that virtually all B-cells expressing IgG and IgA isotypes over the first nine days of life were also stained for surface IgM.

The explanation for this interesting pattern of isotype diversification during B-cell differentiation is not immediately clear. One possibility would be a complex splicing or translational control of long-lived δ messages. Another might be the existence of multiple pathways of isotype switching, e.g., (i) $\mu \rightarrow \mu\gamma \rightarrow \gamma$ and (ii) $\mu \rightarrow \mu\delta \rightarrow \mu\delta\gamma \rightarrow \gamma$. In other words, it seems possible that some B-cells may switch directly from expression of IgM to the expression of other isotypes without expressing IgD. If so, our results suggest that most of the B-cells which undergo isotype switches in the first few days of life follow this pattern.

EXPRESSION OF THE SURFACE IgD AS A FUNCTION OF HUMAN B-CELL DIFFERENTIATION

As in mice, IgD expression occurs relatively late during B-cell ontogeny in humans.[18] While IgM⁺ B cells are present by the ninth week of fetal life, IgD⁺ B-cells are not seen before the twelfth week. By the time of birth IgD is seen on the surface of almost all IgM B-cells and, together with IgM, on the great majority of the IgG and IgA B-cells. The pattern of isotype expression changes again after birth, probably as a result of exposure to environmental antigens and T-cell influences. The adult pattern includes IgD expression by more than 80% of IgM B-cells, but no more than 30% of IgG and 10% of IgA B-cells bear IgD and/or IgM.

We have used pokeweed mitogen (PWM) to induce polyclonal B-cell proliferation and differentiation as a model system to study expression of the various immunoglobulin isotypes at different stages in the B-cell pathway. PWM induces a subpopulation of B-cells that is gradually expanded during infancy.[22] The activation of PWM responsive precursors of IgM, IgG and IgA plasma cells requires T-cell help, via non-MHC restricted factors.[23,24] The PWM responsive B-cells have a relatively low buoyant density,[25] lack receptors for mouse erythrocytes,[26] and are easily and selectively inhibited by isotype specific antibodies.[27,28]

Monoclonal antibodies specific for μ, γ, α and α_1 subclass were used to examine the immunoglobulin isotypes expressed by the B-lymphocyte precursors of plasma cells producing IgM, IgG, IgA, or IgA_2. All of the monoclonal antibodies inhibited PWM induced differentiation of B-cells, but each in a different way. Anti-μ antibody suppressed differentiation not only of IgM plasma cells but also of IgG and IgA plasma cells in a dose-related fashion. The concentration of anti-μ antibody required to suppress development of IgG and IgA plasma cells was approximately 100 times higher than that needed for suppression of IgM plasma cell precursors. Selective depletion of IgM^+ B-cells, before culture of blood mononuclear cells (MNC) with PWM, diminished the number of IgM plasma cells induced by >90% and of IgG and IgA plasma cells by approximately 50%.

The addition of monoclonal anti-γ or anti-α antibody to PWM treated cultures of blood MNC selectively inhibited the development of IgG and IgA plasma cells, respectively, and did not affect differentiation of plasma cells producing other isotypes. The concentrations of anti-γ and anti-α antibodies required for selective suppression of IgG and IgA plasma cell precursors were very low (≤ 0.1 $\mu g/ml$), and the degree of suppression achieved with the highest concentrations (≥ 100 $\mu g/ml$) of anti-γ and anti-α was greater than with the same concentrations of anti-μ antibody. Removal of IgG^+ or IGA^+ B-cells before culture of blood MNC was as effective in reducing IgG or IgA plasma cell differentiation as was incubation with anti-γ or anti-α antibodies throughout the seven-day culture interval. Removal of IgG B-cells selectively impaired IgG plasma cell differentiation, and depletion of IgA B-cells likewise inhibited only the development of IgA plasma cells. Similarly anti-α_1 antibodies affected only the PWM induced differentiation of IgA_1 plasma cell precursors; IgA_2 plasma cell differentiation was unaffected.

Thus, several subpopulations of PWM inducible B-cell precursors of plasma cells were defined in these experiments (FIGURE 4): (i) $sIgM^+$ precursors of IgM plasma cells that do not express IgG or IgA isotypes, (ii) $sIgG^+$ precursors of IgG plasma cells that may or may not express residual sIgM, but do not express IgA, and (iii) $sIgA^+$ precursors of IgA plasma cells that do not express IgG, but approximately half of which express functional IgM receptors. The IgA B-cell subpopulation is further divisible into two separate sublines of IgA_1 and IgA_2 B-cells, as suggested from earlier studies of their ontogeny.[29] These results further suggest that normal human B-cells can switch from μ directly to each of the other heavy chain isotypes, and these represent the main switch pathways. A similar

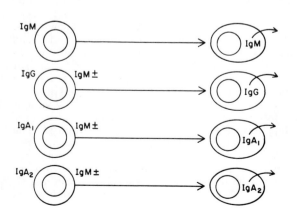

FIGURE 4. Pokeweed mitogen responsive subpopulations of B-cells.

FIGURE 5. Hypothetical scheme in which PWM responsive B-cells represent a relatively mature IgD⁻ subpopulation.

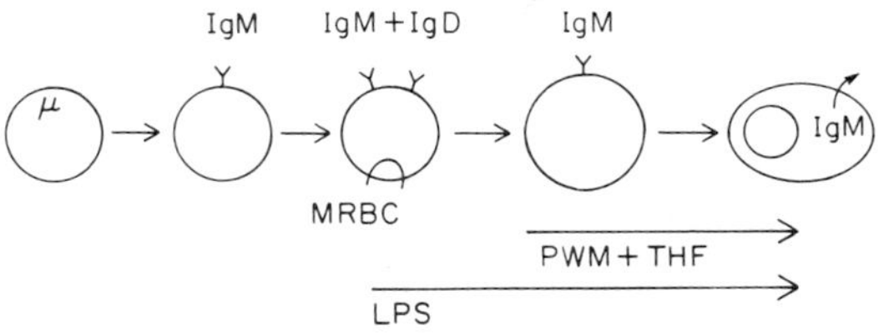

model for immunoglobulin isotype switching has been proposed on the basis of studies in mice.[17,30]

In contrast to the suppressive effects of anti-μ, -γ and -α antibodies, we noted that monoclonal anti-δ antibodies did not suppress PWM-induced plasma cell differentiation. Variable effects of anti-δ antisera on PWM-induced differentiation had been noted by others.[31,32] In order to examine further the expression of IgD on the PWM inducible subpopulations of B-cells, we used monoclonal anti-δ antibodies to selectively remove IgD⁺ B-cells from blood MNC preparations before culture with PWM. Although the great majority of B-cells were removed, the numbers of IgM-, IgG- and IgA- plasma cells induced by PWM were unaffected. This was a reproducible result in experiments employing either a "panning" procedure or a fluorescence activated cell sorter for sIgD⁺ B-cell depletion. The PWM-responsive, IgD⁻ B-cells were further shown to be relatively large, have a relatively low buoyant density, and lack surface receptors for mouse erythrocytes.

The non-PWM responsive B-cells were primarily small IgM⁺ IgD⁺ lymphocytes with surface receptors for mouse erythrocytes. In another series of experiments we found that pretreatment of these IgD⁺ B-cells with anti-δ antibodies moved some of them into the PWM responsive compartment. Small IgD⁺ B-cells were also found to be inducible by LPS stimulation. FIGURE 5 incorporates these results into a hypothetical model of B-cell differentiation.

CONCLUSIONS

We have presented evidence suggesting that B-cells in the chicken, as a representative avian species, may express a surface immunoglobulin analogue of mammalian IgD. This implies that IgD is a highly conserved molecule as would be expected if it serves an important role as an immunoregulatory receptor molecule.

We have confirmed the relatively late appearance of IgD during B-cell ontogeny. Our data indicate that IgD may be expressed together with IgM for an undefined, but presumably brief, period of time after some of the members of B-cell clones switch to the expression of an IgG or IgA isotype. More surprisingly, some of the first B-cells that undergo such isotype switches bear IgM but lack detectable surface IgD. This finding could reflect an unusual switch pattern of a primitive B-cell subpopulation or an unpredictably complex pattern of usage of long-lived δ mRNA.

Our studies of the various immunoglobulin isotypes expressed at different stages during human B-cell differentiation are consistent with a model of B-cell differentiation that has similarities with the stages in mouse B-cell differentiation described by Melchers and colleagues.[33] They found that a population of small resting B-cells are triggered by antigen and Ia-complementary specific helper T-cells, by LPS or by anti-Ig antibodies and transformed into large activated B-cells. The latter exhibit responsiveness, in a non-MHC restricted fashion, to T-cell factors which induce polyclonal B-cell replication and maturation. We would also suggest that the large "pre-progenitor" B-cell described by Shortman and Howard[34] is analogous to the large PWM-responsive, IgD⁻ B-cell in our model and to the large, pre-activated B-cell in the model of the Basel group. One reason for drawing this conclusion is the recent demonstration that the mouse "pre-progenitor" cells are largely IgD⁻.[35]

One feature emphasized in this model is that IgD expression is missing both early and late during B-cell differentiation. Earlier studies have established that anti-μ or antigen induced cross-linkage of IgM receptors on immature B-cells aborts further differentiation (Reviewed in references 36, 37]. Our present studies indicate that cross-linkage of IgM receptors also imparts a negative signal to the preactivated IgD⁻ precursor so as to block terminal plasma cell differentiation. In contrast, our data suggest that anti-δ antibody can induce IgM⁺IgD⁺ B-cells to become responsive to PWM induction. Others have shown that both anti-μ and anti-δ antibodies can induce B-cell proliferation and increased Ia expression.[38,39] We would, therefore, offer a very simple hypothesis for the special role of IgD as a B-cell surface receptor. A basic assumption is that both IgM and IgD transmit similar signals to the B-cell. IgM is expressed on immature cells and preactivated mature B-cells, both of which may receive negative signals from surface immunoglobulin cross-linkage. However, IgD is only expressed by the B-cell during an intermediate stage in differentiation during which the B-cell responds positively to cross-linkage of surface antibodies regardless of the isotype. The main virtue of IgD would be that it is not expressed on the cell surface during stages in differentiation when the B-cell responds negatively to cross-linkage of antibody receptors. Thus, we view the complex regulation of IgD expression as a sophisticated mechanism for fine tuning of B-cell responses.

ACKNOWLEDGMENTS

We thank Dr. John F. Kearney for helpful discussions and monoclonal antibodies, Mrs. Ann Brookshire for typing the manuscript, and Mrs. Maxine Aycock for help with illustrations.

REFERENCES

1. ROWE, D. S. & J. L. FAHEY. 1965. A new class of human immunoglobulins. I. A unique myeloma protein. J. Exp. Med. **121:** 171.
2. ROWE, D. S., K. HUG & L. FORNI. 1973. Immunoglobulin D as a lymphocyte receptor. J. Exp. Med. **138:** 965.
3. KNAPP, W., R. L. M. BOLHUIS, J. RADL & W. HIJMANS. 1973. Independent movement of IgD and IgM molecules on the surface of individual lymphocytes. J. Immunol. **111:** 1295.
4. VITETTA, E. S. & J. W. UHR. 1975. Immunoglobulin receptors revisited. Science **189:** 964.
5. MARTIN, L. N. & G. A. LESLIE. 1977. Lymphocyte surface IgD and IgM in Macaca monkeys: ontogeny, tissue distribution and occurrence on individual lymphocytes. Immunol. **33:** 865.

6.   ABNEY, E. R. & R. M. E. PARKHOUSE. 1974. Candidate for immunoglobulin D present on murine B lymphocytes. Nature (Lond.) **252**: 600.
7.   MELCHER, U., E. S. VIETETTA, M. MCWILLIAMS, M. E. LAMM, J. M. PHILLIPS-QUAGLIATA & J. W. UHR. 1974. Cell surface immunoglobulin X. Identification of an IgD-like molecule on the surface of murine splenocytes. J. Exp. Med **140**: 1427.
8.   RUDDICK, J. H. & G. A. LESLIE. 1977. Structure and biologic function of human IgD. XI. Identification and ontogeny of a rat lymphocyte immunoglobulin having antigenic cross-reactivity with human IgD. J. Immunol. **118**: 1025.
9.   ESKINAZI, D. P., B. A. BESSINGER, J. M. MCNICHOLAS, A. L. LEARY, & K. L. KNIGHT. 1979. Expression of an unidentified immunoglobulin isotype on rabbit Ig-bearing lymphocytes. J. Immunol. **122**: 469.
10. WILDER, R. L., C. Y. YUEN, S. A. COYLE & R. G. MAGE. 1979. Demonstration of a rabbit cell surface Ig that bears light chain and V_H, but lacks μ- α-, and γ-allotypes-rabbit IgD? J. Immunol. **122**: 464.
11. LESLIE, G. A. & L. N. MARTIN. 1978. Structure and function of serum and membrane immunoglobulin D (IgD). Contemp. Top. Mol. Immunol. **7**: 1.
12. PARKHOUSE, R. M. E. & M. D. COOPER. 1977. A model for the differentiation of B lymphocytes with implications for the biological role of IgD. Immunol. Rev. **37**: 105.
13. LERMAN, S. P., M. D. GREBENAU, D. S. CHI, M. A. PALLADINO, J. GALTON & G. J. THORBECKE. 1980. Transfer of agammaglobulinemia in the chicken. II. Characterization of the target of suppression. Cell. Immunol. **51**: 109.
14. GODING, J. W. 1980. Structural studies of murine lymphocyte surface IgD. J. Immunol. **124**: 2082.
15. KESSLER, S. W. 1975. Rapid isolation of antigens from cells with a staphylococcal protein A-antibody adsorbent: parameters of the interaction of antibody-antigen complexes with protein A. J. Immunol. **115**: 1617.
16. Laemmli, U. K. 1970. Cleavage of structural proteins during the assembly of the head of bacteriophage T4. Nature **227**: 680.
17. ABNEY, E. R., M. D. COOPER. J. F. KEARNEY, A. R. LAWTON & R. M. E. PARKHOUSE. 1978. Sequential expression of immunoglobulin on developing mouse B lymphocytes. A systematic survey which suggests a model for the generation of immunoglobulin isotype diversity. J. Immunol. **120**: 2041.
18. GATHINGS, W. E., A. R. LAWTON & M. D. COOPER. 1977. Immunofluorescent studies of the development of pre-B cells, B lymphocytes and immunoglobulin isotype diversity in humans. Eur. J. Immunol. **7**: 804.
19. Liu, C. P., P. W. TUCKER, J. J. MUSHINSKI & F. R. BLATTNER. 1980. Mapping of heavy chain genes for mouse immunoglobulins M and D. Science (Wash., D.C.) **209**: 1348.
20. SHIMIZU, A., N. TAKAHASHI, Y. YAMAWAKI-KATAOKA, Y. NISHIDA. T. KATAOKA & J. HONJO. 1981. Ordering of mouse immunoglobulin heavy chain genes of molecular cloning. Nature (Lond.) **289**: 149.
21. GATHINGS, W. E., H. KUBAGAWA & M. D. COOPER. 1981. A distinctive pattern of B cell immaturity in perinatal humans. Immunol. Rev. **57**: 107.
22. WU, L. Y. F., A. BLANCO, M. D. COOPER & A. R. LAWTON. 1976. Ontogeny of B-lymphocyte differentiation induced by pokeweed mitogen. Clin. Immunol. Immunopathol. **5**: 208.
23. JANOSSY, G. & M. GREAVES. 1975. Functional analysis of murine and human B-lymphocyte subsets. Transplant. Rev. **24**: 177.
24. KEIGHTLEY, R. G., M. D. COOPER & A. R. LAWTON. 1976. The T cell dependence of B cell differentiation induced by pokeweed mitogen. J. Immunol. **117**: 1538.
25. DAGG, M. K. & D. LEVITT. 1981. Human B lymphocyte subpopulations. I. Differentiation of density-separated B lymphocytes. Clin. Immunol. Immunopathol. **21**: 39.
26. LUCIVERO, G., A. R. LAWTON & M. D. COOPER. 1981. Rosette formation with mouse erythrocytes defines a population of human B lymphocytes unresponsive to pokeweed mitogen. Clin. Exp. Immunol. **41**: 185.
27. LUCIVERO, G., A. R. LAWTON & M. D. COOPER. 1981. Pokeweed mitogen-induced differentiation of human peripheral blood B lymphocytes. II. Suppression of plasma cell differentiation by heavy chain specific antibodies and development of immunoglobulin class restriction. Hum. Lymph. Diff. **1**: 27.

28. KURITANI, T. & M. D. COOPER. 1982. Human B cell differentiation. I. Analysis of immunoglobulin heavy chain switching using monoclonal anti-immunoglobulin M, G, and A antibodies and pokeweed mitogen-induced plasma cell differentiation. J. Exp. Med. In press.

29. CONLEY, M. E., J. F. KEARNEY, A. R. LAWTON & M. D. COOPER. 1980. Differentiation of human B cells expressing the IgA subclasses as demonstrated by monoclonal hybridoma antibodies. J. Immunol. **125:** 2311.

30. Manning, D. D. 1975. Heavy chain isotype suppression. A review of the immunosuppressive effects of heterologous anti-Ig heavy chain antisera. J. Reticuloendothelial Soc. **18:** 63.

31. FINKELMAN, F. D. & P. E. LIPSKY. 1978. Immunoglobulin secretion by human splenic lymphocytes *in vitro:* The effects of antibodies to IgM and IgD. J. Immunol. **120:** 1465.

32. CHIORAZZI, N., S. M. FU & H. G. KUNKEL. 1980. Stimulation of human B lymphocytes by antibodies to IgM and IgG: Functional evidence for the expression of IgG on B-lymphocyte surface membrane. Clin. Immunol. Immunopathol. **15:** 301.

33. MELCHERS, F., J. ANDERSON, W. LERNHARDT & M. H. SCHREIER. 1980. Roles of surface-bound immunoglobulin molecules in regulating the replication and maturation to immunoglobulin secretion of B lymphocytes. Immunol. Rev. **52:** 89.

34. HOWARD, M. C., J. M. FIDLER, J. HAMILTON & K. SHORTMAN. 1978. Antigen-initiated B lymphocyte differentiation. XII. Nonspecific effects of antigenic stimulation on the physical properties of AFC-progenitors. J. Immunol. **120:** 911.

35. LAYTON, J. E., J. BAKER, P. E. BARTLETT & K. SHORTMAN. 1981. Antigen-initiated B lymphocyte differentiation. XVIII. Pre-progenitor B cells that give primary adoptive responses are s-IgM⁺IgD⁻Ia⁺. J. Immunol. **126:** 1227.

36. COOPER, M. D., J. F. KEARNEY, W. E. GATHINGS & A. R. LAWTON. 1980. Effects of anti-Ig antibodies on the development and differentiation of B cells. Immunol. Rev. **52:** 29.

37. KLINMAN, N. R., D. E. WYLIE & J. M. TEALE. 1981. B-cell development. Immunol. Today **2:** 212.

38. SIECKMANN, D. G. 1980. The use of anti-immunoglobulins to induce a signal for cell division in B lymphocytes via their membrane IgM and IgD. Immunol. Rev. **52:** 181.

39. MOND, J. J., E. SEGHAL, J. KING & F. D. FINKELMAN. 1981. Increased expression of I-region-associated antigen (Ia) on B cells after cross-linkage of surface immunoglobulin. J. Immunol. **127:** 881.

DISCUSSION OF THE TWO PRECEDING PAPERS

J. C. CAMBIER: Max, do you think the anti-α and anti-γ suppression that you see in that system is affecting or working through a mechanism acting on the second stage with the progenitor, or the large cell, or the first, the $\mu\delta$ cell?

M. D. COOPER: Well, since we're only looking at the large responsive cells we think we're looking in pokeweed driven assay at a more mature cell.

CAMBIER: Do you assume they've already lost α and γ?

COOPER: No, I didn't put γ and α in that last slide just for simplicity reasons. But it would be hard to go back over that reason. They actually don't have γ and α on their surface because we couldn't pull them out by anti-γ and anti-α antibodies, but we are studying a committed mature subpopulation.

I. SCHER: When you sorted for δ^- cells you showed very few μ positive cells in that population and had excellent stimulation with pokeweed mitogen. How is that data compatible with your hypothesis and couldn't it also be that the pokeweed mitogen is, in fact, stimulating a cell that doesn't express any immuno-globulin on the surface?

COOPER: It could be, but numerically one wouldn't think so because if you pulled those cells out to start with that express M, G, or A, it eliminates almost all the cells that are triggerable to those classes of plasma cells.

J. W. GODING: I have a question for Dr. Leslie. It concerns the protein that you call Fc receptor. It would seem to me that this sort of observation has been made over many years. Is this protein actin, which becomes labeled in the cytoplasm of dead cells?

G. A. LESLIE: That could be because we haven't proven it to be Fc receptor in any way. All that I know is that irrelevant antigen antibody complexes will bring it down, but we have not characterized it.

GODING: My experience is that as you improve the conditions of the cells before iodination that peak gradually goes away. These days we don't see it anymore at all.

LESLIE: The only thing I can say is that in some of the experiments the cell viability was better than 95% and we still saw this peak.

E. S. VITETTA: As you know, in the human and in the rat, cells from maternal breast milk can be transferred to the neonate. Considering the low numbers of gamma positive cells you see in the first three days after birth, I wonder whether it wouldn't be worthwhile to use parents of two different γ allotypes and then to look at the allotype of the γ bearing cells in the neonate to see if they are in fact maternal B-cells?

COOPER: Yes, part of the reason we haven't considered this is because we thought most people who have tried to produce that entry of maternal breast milk cells by the gut hadn't been able to do so.

VITETTA: I think the question is what the numbers are rather than whether it can be done or not, but your numbers are certainly low enough so that they could be consistent with a few maternal cells trafficking across. The allotype should tell you that very easily.

F. R. BLATTNER: Do you know whether IgD crosses the placenta?

LESLIE: In only 1 of the 98 newborns in which we found IgD in cord blood could we prove that there had been a leaky placenta that could be responsible. In at least 94 of the others there appeared to be prenatal synthesis. I think the general feeling is that there is very little that crosses the placenta.

BLATTNER: Does δ serve as an antibody? Now you showed a lot of proteins in various disease states that bind antigens, but is there any case where somebody has immunized with something and gotten a response in the IgD class?

LESLIE: As far as I know there's been no intentional immunization with the possible exception of Rajewsky's anti-DNP hydridomas.

BLATTNER: But the point isn't whether it's possible for this molecule, which we know has a V region, to bind to something.

LESLIE: Well, let me approach that another way. In diabetics who get insulin over a long period of time, a significant number will have IgD anti-insulin antibodies.

F. R. BLATTNER: In most humans we're probably not doing the kind of immunizations that lead to making IgD antibodies.

PARTICIPANT: It seems as though, as is true in the mouse and the human, you find IgM positive cells before you do find IgD positive cells in the rat. Yet, if you inject anti-delta on day 15 after fertilization you seem to block the appearance of IgM positive cells.

LESLIE: Yes, we block down to roughly 1% as opposed to 10 or 15% if we start later. It's as though the anti-delta were blocking the differentiation of the B-cells. It may well be that there's just that very small population of cells that will always be a μ only cell.

M. KLEIN: It's a point that seems to be different in the mouse studies, as you know. About four years ago Peter Lipsky and I published some fairly similar data with combinations of anti-μ or anti-δ plus pokeweed *in vitro*. One thing that was a bit different is that we found that we could block about 80 or 90% of the IgG response stimulated with pokeweed with either anti-μ or anti-δ. Most of our work was done with spleen rather than peripheral blood.

We found different effects on IgM production with different doses of both anti-μ and anti-δ. When we optimized culture conditions and used a low quantity of either anti-μ or anti-δ we could stimulate the amount of IgM that was being secreted. If we used large quantities of anti-μ or anti-δ we could suppress IgM production in most cases again with either anti-isotype antibody. Yet, if we tried to compare what given doses of anti-μ would do versus the same dose of anti-δ, anti-μ always seemed to be less stimulatory or more suppressive, and we concluded that both anti-μ and anti-δ could exert stimulatory or suppressive effects on B-cells and that the sum total of these counter balancing effects was more suppressive for anti-μ and more stimulatory for anti-δ.

COOPER: We have had similar results as far as inhibition with heterologous purified anti-μ and anti-γ, but we haven't used anti-δ except the monoclonal.

DISTINCT δ^+ AND δ^- B-LYMPHOCYTE LINEAGES
IN THE RAT*

H. Bazin,† D. Gray,‡ B, Platteau,† and I. C. M. MacLennan‡

†Experimental Immunology Unit
University of Louvain UCL 3056
30 Clos Chapelle aux Champs
1200 Brussels, Belgium

‡Department of Immunology
The Medical School
University of Birmingham
Birmingham B15 2TJ, United Kingdom

INTRODUCTION

In general, the expression of IgD on the surface of B-lymphocytes has become associated with distinct stages of B-cell development. Hence μ^+ δ^- populations are well recognized as a feature of the earliest stages of B-cell differentiation[1-4] as well as comprising a subset of memory cells appearing after antigenic stimulation.[5,6] However, the existence of a distinct δ^- B-cell lineage separating from cells which transiently or permanently express δ in differentiation has been supported by relatively little evidence. In this paper we present data which indicate that many of the mature δ^- B-cells found in the spleen of rats have developed without ever expressing δ. The experimental approach has been to treat rats from birth with rabbit-anti-rat-δ^7 in order to eliminate δ expressing B-cells as they appear. It is shown that these rats acquire δ^- B-cells in secondary lymphoid organs which are not obviously different from those δ^- B-cells found in control animals. The range of immunoglobulin isotypes which are produced in these rats has been assessed. This suggests that the profile of antibody synthesized by this δ^- population does not totally overlap that produced by B-cells that have expressed δ during their development.

MATERIALS AND METHODS

Rats

(Lou × DA) F_1 hybrid rats were used in the study of the distribution of surface immunoglobulin isotypes in secondary lymphoid organs of healthy adult (10–14 weeks of age) rats.

IgD suppression experiments were performed in outbred rats having the rnu mutation. Groups of rnu/rnu athymic rats and rnu/$^+$ rats with a thymus were used.

*This research was carried out, in part, under contract No. BIO-c-358-B, radiation protection program of the Commission of the European Communities. Contribution No. 1840 of the radiation protection program.

157

Antisera

Rabbit anti-rat immunoglobulin isotype sera were prepared as described in reference 7.

Immunohistology

Spleens and other lymphoid tissue were snap frozen in liquid nitrogen and stored at −70°C. Staining for surface membrane immunoglobulin on lymphocytes was carried out using the peroxidase-anti-peroxidase technique.[8] Frozen sections were cut at 5µm, mounted on formol-gelatin-coated slides, thoroughly dried at room temperature and fixed in acetone at 4°C for 20 minutes. These were then washed in 0.05 M tris HCl-buffered saline pH 7.6. A 1 in 20 dilution of normal swine serum in the same buffer was then laid onto the sections for 15 minutes. (All dilutions of antisera were made in this solution). Next the first layer rabbit anti-rat immunoglobulin isotype was added to the sections followed sequentially by swine anti-rabbit immunoglobulin (Dakopatts) and peroxidase rabbit anti-peroxidase complex (Dakopatts) with intermediate washing stages. Peroxidase activity was revealed with 3'3'-diamin obenzidene (Sigma). The sections were then counterstained lightly in haemotoxylin to demonstrate nuclei.

Fluorescein and Rhodamine Labelling of Ox Red Blood Cells (RBC)

Ox RBC were washed three times in saline and made up to a 10% suspension in 0.15M sodium bicarbonate. Four mg of fluorescein isothiocyanate (BDH Chemicals) was dissolved in 5 ml of 0.15M sodium bicarbonate. This solution is added to 6 ml of the 10% ox RBC suspension. A substituted rhodamine isothiocyanate (Research Organics Inc., Cleveland, Ohio, U.S.A.) was used, 3 mg being dissolved by grinding in a small mortar in 6 ml of 0.15M of sodium bicarbonate. This suspension was spun before being added to 6 ml of 10% ox RBC suspension. These mixtures are placed at 4°C for 2 hr and inverted occasionally. The labelled cells were washed six times in sterile saline and were then ready for coating with antibodies. This labelling method is based on that of Dhaliwal et al.[9]

Coating of Ox RBC with Antibody

The chromic chloride method was used to coat 0.1 mg of protein onto RBC as described by Ling et al.[10] Fluorescein labelled ox RBC were coated with anti-IgM antibodies, while the rhodamine labelled RBC were coated with anti-IgD antibodies. Instead of Hepes buffered RPMI 1640 the coated cells were resuspended in Gey's tissue culture medium containing 0.1% BSA. Neither phenol red nor nystatin were added as these interfere with the fluorescence. As lysis of fluorescent labelled cells occurs more rapidly than unlabelled cells preparations were used within two weeks of coating.

Lymphocyte Preparations

Spleen and lymph node cell suspensions were prepared in exactly the same way. A lymph node or weighed portion of spleen was first chopped into fine pieces in a petri dish using crossed scalpel blades and then dispersed further by pressing between artery forceps. Tissue culture medium (RPMI 1640) was then added and the suspension taken up through a 21G needle. Cells were then washed twice before use. Blood lymphocytes were separated on 9% Ficoll-Triosil. Blood was diluted 1 in 2 with RPMI, layered onto 9% Ficoll-Triosil and spun at 500g for 20 mins. The mononuclear cells at the interface were taken off and washed twice.

Double Rosette Assay

A technique based on that of Dhaliwal et al.[9] was used: $30\mu l$ of anti-IgM-coated fluorescein labelled cells and $30\mu l$ of anti-IgD-coated rhodamine-labelled cells were added to small plastic tubes containing 150 μl of Gey's solution plus 0.1% BSA. After mixing, $60\mu l$ of a $2 \times 10^6/ml$ lymphocyte suspension was added.

The contents were mixed and left on the bench for 10 minutes before being spun at 150g for 2 min. The tubes were left for 30 minutes at 4°C, after which the cells were resuspensed by gentle inversion. Rosette chambers were prepared by sticking two coverslips to a microscope slide, approximately half a coverslip width apart. A coverslip placed on top made a chamber of 0.2mm approximate depth. Rosette suspensions were placed into these chambers using a pipette with widened bore. Acridine orange was added to suspensions to make the lympho-cyte nuclei fluoresce. The proportion of lymphocytes rosetting was first deter-mined and then each rosette assessed as mixed or single. The rosettes were viewed using a Leitz Dialux microscope fitted with a Ploemopak 2.3 fluorescence illuminator and comprising two interchangeable filter systems, filter system 12 for FITC and filter system N2 for TRITC. A triple rosette assay was attempted; however, the results indicated that the number of rosettes of certain isotypes were less when two other isotypes were being detected at the same time. The reason for the discrepancy is probably competition of the coated RBC for sites on the lymphocyte surface. Comparison of single and double rosette (μ and δ) results showed that there was no competition in the double rosette system, i.e., the total number of rosettes formed with either anti-μ or anti-δ-coated ox red cells when assessed singly was not significantly different from that when both were assessed together. This control was performed in all experiments using double rosettes.

Anti-δ Treatment

Rats were injected every other day, from birth (day 0) until day 10 with rabbit anti-rat-δ antibody. From day 10 to day 55 the animals were injected three times a week. Control animals were injected with normal rabbit serum. This suppression protocol is described in Bazin et al.[7]

Measurement of Serum Immunoglobulin Isotype Levels

The serum IgM, IgA, IgG1, IgG2a, IgG2b and IgG2c concentrations were measured using single radial immunodiffusion. IgD and IgE levels were determined by a radioimmunoassay, as described in Bazin *et al.*[11]

RESULTS

Distribution of δ^+ and δ^- B-Cells in Secondary Lymphoid Organs in the Adult Rats

Serial frozen sections were taken from lymph node, spleen and Peyer's patch of healthy adult rats. These were processed as described in the methods to demonstrate surface membrane immunoglobulin of different isotypes. The most obvious δ^- population of B-cells is seen in the spleen (FIGURE 1; a, b, c, d). Here a substantial $\mu^+\delta^-$ population is resident in the marginal zones. This area is clearly identified in the rat as it is separated from the follicles and periarteriolar lymphocytic sheath by a distinct marginal sinus. While very few marginal zone cells express δ (FIGURE 1b), there is a substantial number of α^+ cells in this compartment (FIGURE 1c) and rather fewer cells expressing γ2c. γ1 γ2a and γ2b bearing cells were not demonstrated in the marginal zone. The main δ^+ population is located in the follicles although there are collections of δ^+ cells: deep to the marginal sinus; in marginal zone bridging channels and on the outer edge of the marginal zone. In addition there are substantial numbers of isolated δ^+ cells seen throughout the red pulp. No predominantly $\mu^+ \delta^-$ area analogous to the marginal zone is seen in lymph nodes (FIGURE 2 a,b,c,d), or Peyer's patch (FIGURE 3 a,b). The isotype expression, appearance and distribution of B-cells in adult rnu/rnu rats was found to be qualitatively similar.

The Numbers of μ and δ Expressing B-Cells in Dissociated Secondary Lymphoid Organs and in Peripheral Blood of Adult Rats

Double marker studies were performed on these lymphocyte preparations to determine the numbers of: (1) $\mu^+ \delta^-$, (2) $\mu^+ \delta^+$ and (3) $\mu^- \delta^+$ B-cells. The results are shown in TABLE 1. These assays show that $\mu^+ \delta^-$ B-cells comprise a third of spleen B-cells, 17 percent of lymph node B-cells and 18 percent of blood B-cells. These data indicate that although there is no anatomical site dominant in $\mu^+ \delta^-$ cells in lymph nodes, the lymph node follicles do contain a substantial minority of these cells. The proportion of $\mu^- \delta^+$ B-cells in the spleen is surprisingly low when one simply compares follicular with marginal zone B-cell numbers. This result suggests that the scattered δ^+ cells outside the follicles in the spleen are numerically as important as those in the follicles.

The Effect of Neonatal and Continued Rabbit anti-δ Treatment on the Isotype Expression and Distribution of B-Cells

Rats treated for eight weeks with rabbit-anti rat-δ serum were sacrificed three days after the last serum injection. Their secondary lymphoid organs were

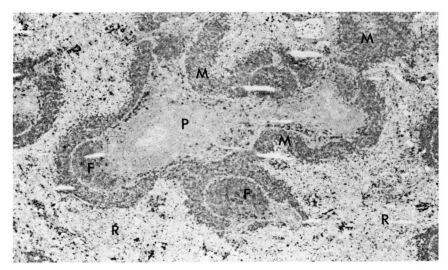

FIGURE 1A. Normal adult, rat spleen serial section. Stained for surface μ showing both follicular (F) and marginal zone (M), B-cells are positive. The marginal sinus is clearly seen separating the marginal zone from the periarteriolar lymphocytic sheath (P) and the follicles. R = red pulp, × 140.

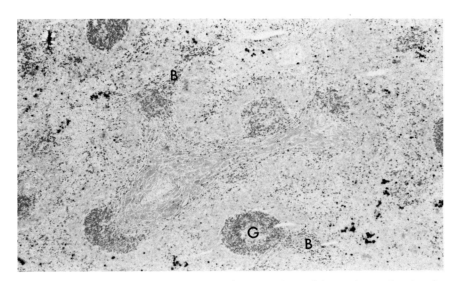

FIGURE 1B. Normal adult, rat spleen serial section. Stained for surface δ showing the majority of follicular B-cell express IgD. The marginal zone contains very few δ^+ cells. There are substantial large numbers of isolated δ^+ B-cells in the red pulp, on the inner and outer aspects of the marginal zone and in marginal zone bridging channels (B). The follicle marked G contains a germinal center, × 140.

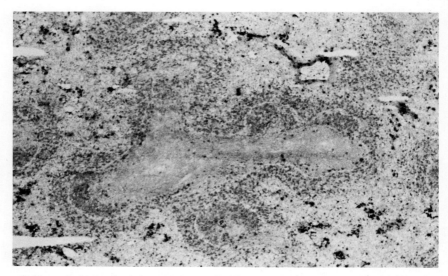

FIGURE 1C. Normal adult, rat spleen serial section. Stained for surface α show large numbers of follicular and marginal zone B-cells express surface α, × 140.

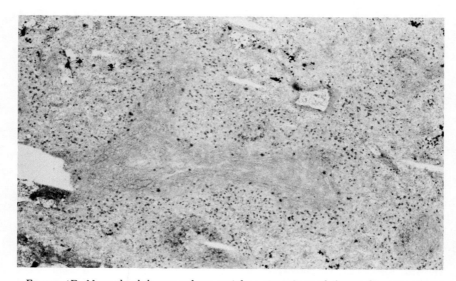

FIGURE 1D. Normal adult, rat spleen serial section. Stained for surface $\gamma2c$ shows approximately 20% of marginal zone cells are positive while rather fewer follicular B-cells are stained, × 140.

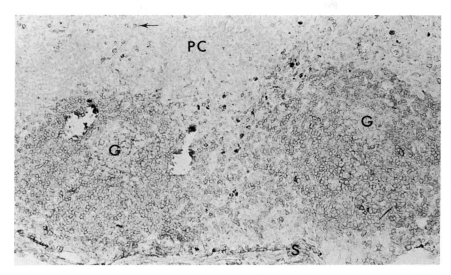

FIGURE 2A. Serial frozen section of normal rat axillary lymph node showing two follicles, × 350. Stained for μ the edge of two germinal centers are cut where μ-containing immune complex is demonstrated on follicular dendritic cells. Occasional μ^+ cells are seen in the cortex, presumably in transit to or from follicles. The edge of the capsular sinus is seen, (S) × 350.

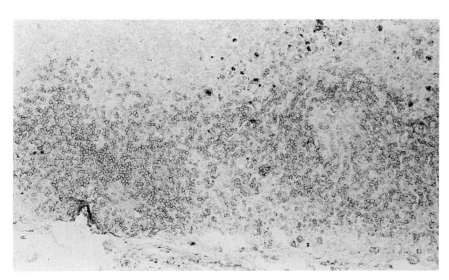

FIGURE 2B. Serial frozen section of normal rat axillary lymph node showing two follicles stained for δ, immune complexes are not picked up in the germinal centers. Otherwise the δ^+ cells are distributed as in the section stained with anti-μ, × 350.

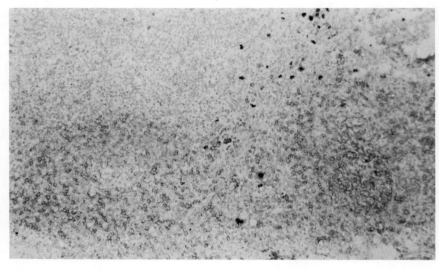

FIGURE 2C. Serial frozen section of normal rat axillary lymph node showing two follicles stained for α, α-positive cells are scattered throughout both follicles, α-containing immune complex is seen on follicular dendritic cells in the right hand follicle, $\times$ 350.

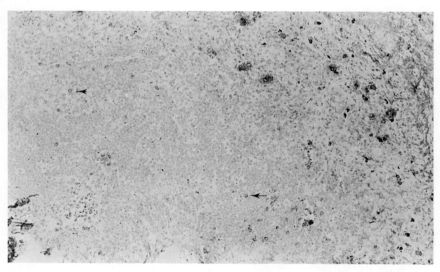

FIGURE 2D. Serial frozen section of normal rat axillary lymph node showing two follicles stained for γ2c, only very occasional positive cells seen, $\times$ 350.

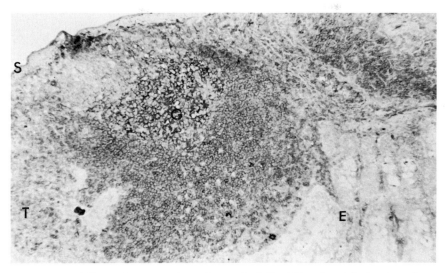

FIGURE 3A. Adjacent frozen sections of normal adult rat Peyer's patch showing a large secondary follicle. Stained for μ, immune complex on follicular dendritic cells is clearly seen surrounded by μ^+ small lymphocytes. G = germinal center, E = epithelium, S = serosal surface, and T = T-cell zone, $\times$ 350.

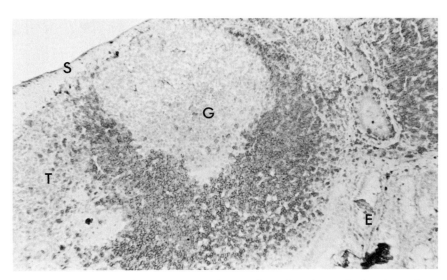

FIGURE 3B. Adjacent frozen sections of normal rat Peyer's patch showing a large secondary follicle. Stained for δ, small δ^+ B-lymphocytes show the same distribution as that of μ^+ B-cells, $\times$ 350.

TABLE 1

SURFACE μ AND δ EXPRESSION IN NORMAL ADULT RAT SPLEEN,
LYMPH NODE AND BLOOD

	Spleen	*Lymph Node	Blood
Total lymphocyte count $\times 10^6$	160 ± 13	2.3 ± 0.6	4.4 ± 0.3
Total rosetting cells $(\mu + \delta + \mu\delta$ cells) % of total count	41.1 ± 1.6	30.3 ± 0.3	28.3 ± 0.7
Surface immunoglobulin phenotype as % of total rosetting cells			
% $\mu^+ \delta^-$ lymphocytes	33.7 ± 0.7	17.5 ± 0.6	18.4 ± 1.1
% $\mu^+ \delta^+$ lymphocytes	60.1 ± 0.7	64.9 ± 0.4	63.8 ± 1.1
% $\mu^- \delta^+$ lymphocytes	6.2 ± 0.2	17.6 ± 0.7	17.9 ± 0.7

*Axillary lymph node; mean values ± standard error; groups comprised eight rats.

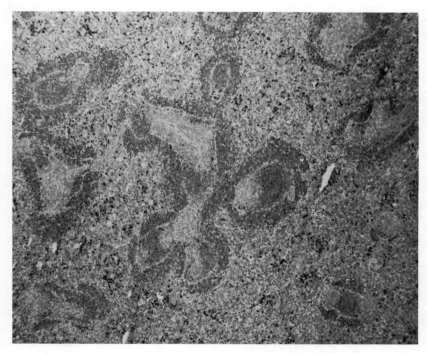

FIGURE 4A. Adjacent frozen section of spleen from a 55-day-old rnu/$^+$ rat given neonatal and continued treatment with anti-δ antibody. Stained for μ, marginal zones and some follicles are seen. Follicular formation in this section is unusually prominent for an anti-δ treated rat, × 90.

examined immunohistologically. In most rats no δ^+ B-cells were demonstrated, however, in 3 rats occasional isolated δ^+ cells were clearly seen in follicular areas. These rats served to demonstrate that there was no technical problem in demonstrating δ^+ in this group of rats. In the spleen the marginal zones contained substantial numbers of $\mu^+ \delta^-$ cells (FIGURE 4 a,b). α and γ2c positive cells were also seen in this area (FIGURE 4 c,d). Surprisingly a substantial $\mu^+ \delta^-$ population was also seen in splenic follicles. However, lymph node follicles contained relatively few B-cells in these rats. These data appear to indicate that a substantial $\mu^+ \delta^-$ population of the spleen can develop from precursors which have never expressed δ. On the other hand, lymph node and Peyer's patch B-cell development is severely curtailed if δ^+ B-cells are eliminated. These results, therefore,

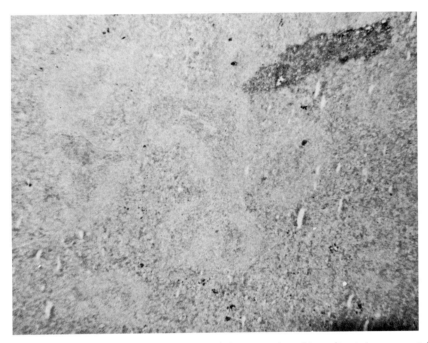

FIGURE 4B. Adjacent frozen section of spleen from a 55-day-old rnu/$^+$ rat given neonatal and continual treatment with anti-δ antibody. Stained with anti-δ, there is a total absence of δ^+ cells even in the follicles. The only positive cells are occasional red pulp macrophages showing endogenous peroxidase activity, $\times$ 90.

imply that a $\mu^+ \delta^-$ spleen seeking B-cell population develops as an independent lineage from the majority of lymph node B-cells.

Immunoglobulin Isotypes in the Blood of Rats Treated from Birth with anti-δ antibody

Groups of rnu/rnu athymic rats and rnu/$^+$ rats were suppressed from birth with rabbit anti-δ antibody. Serum immunoglobulin levels were assessed at 35

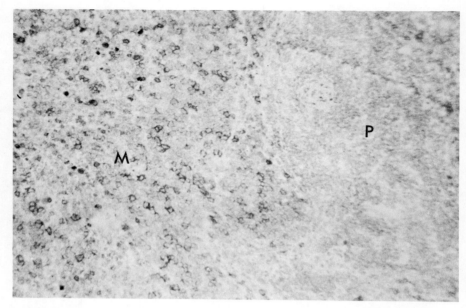

FIGURE 4C. High power of spleen from the same rat as in FIGURES 4A and 4B that show a portion of marginal zone (M) and periarteriolar lymphocytic sheath (P). Stained for α, frequent α positive B-cells can be noted in the marginal zone, × 640.

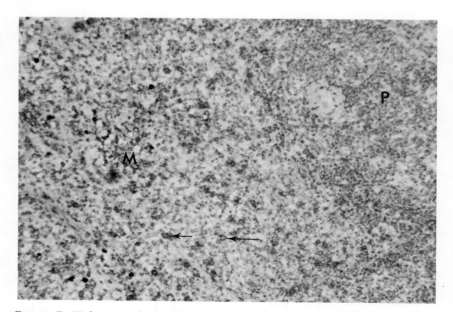

FIGURE 4D. High power of spleen from the same rat as in Figures 4A and 4B that show a portion of marginal zone (M) and periarteriolar lymphocytic sheath (P). Stained for $\gamma 2c$, some $\gamma 2c$-positive B-cells can be noted in the marginal zone, × 640.

and 55 days of age. Comparisons were made with groups of control rats injected with normal rabbit serum only. The results are shown in TABLE 2a and b and FIGURE 5a and b. γ2a and γ1 was present in athymic rats at 35 days but its maternal origin is made clear as these isotypes were no longer detectable at 55 days. Similarly IgE was not detected in the serum of athymic controls. The effect of anti-δ treatment is illustrated in FIGURES 4a and b. In rnu/$^{+}$ rats the main effects were gross depression of δ and γ2a with some potentiation of α and γ2c. By comparison the effect of γ1 γ2b and μ was essentially neutral. In the athymic rats the results were similar although there was no potentiation of γ2c levels.

DISCUSSION

We have previously shown that B-cells of the marginal zone in rats have properties which distinguish them from the majority of splenic and lymph node follicular cells.[12,13] These differences include: (1) larger average size with less condensed chromatin, (2) failure to recirculate, (3) strong complement receptors, and (4) the μ^{+} δ^{-} surface membrane immunoglobulin phenotype. The marginal zones acquire normal numbers of lymphocytes in athymic rnu/rnu rats[12] and develop in rats bred and maintained in germ free conditions.[14,15] Reconstitution experiments in rats depleted of marginal zone cells by high dose cyclophosphamide or X-irradiation indicate that marginal zone B-cells originate from recirculating precursors.[16] These studies also show that there is a maturation period of some three weeks between the pre B-cell stage and a cell becoming resident in the marginal zone. In more recent experiments we have shown that depletion of circulating B-lymphocytes results in marked and selective loss of δ^{+} follicular B-cells with relative sparing of the μ^{+} δ^{-} population.[13] The current studies suggest that a substantial component of the marginal zone B-cell compartment can develop from B-cells which have never expressed δ. These findings suggest that in the case of this population, there is divergence from δ^{+} B-cells at an early stage in differentiation. This is not to say, however, that other B-cells may only express surface membrane δ at certain times during their differentiation. Such a pattern has been strongly suggested by both Black et al.[5] and Zan-Bar et al.,[6] who have studied isotype expression in successive cell transfer experiments. They separated cells to be transferred by isotype using the fluorescence-activated cell sorter. In the experiments by both these groups they show switching on and off of δ expression. However, these workers have confined their interest to T-dependent antigens which evoke strong γ1 γ2a responses.[17] In our current experiments we have shown that the animals deprived of δ^{+} B-cells fail to produce γ2a levels detectable in the serum. Der-Balian et al. have emphasized that γ isotype production is strongly linked to inducing antigen in both the mouse and rat.[18] They have classified antigens into those inducing predominantly γ2c, those including γ2c and γ2b and those inducing γ1 and γ2a responses. DNP-albumin and DNP-KLH, which have been used in the successive transfer experiments mentioned above,[5,6] fall into the γ1 γ2a inducing antigen class. In our current studies the thymus dependency of the γ1 γ2a and to a lesser extent γ2b production in the rat is emphasized. γ2c levels on the other hand are maintained or even increased in athymic rats compared to controls. However, it is interesting to note that anti-δ treatment of rats with normal T-cells causes augmentation of γ2c responses. In nude rats, on the other hand, where control levels of γ2c are higher than those of their heterozygous counterparts further augmentation is not seen on anti-δ treatment.

TABLE 2

LOG MEDIAN: SERUM IMMUNOGLOBULIN LEVELS IN CONTROL AND δ-SUPPRESSED RATS

	IgE ng/ml	IgD ng/ml	IgA µg/ml	IgM mg/ml	IgG1 mg/ml	IgG2a mg/ml	IgG2b mg/ml	IgG2c mg/ml
35 days								
rnu/+NRS*	0	3.13	1.53	0.049	−0.357	−0.483	0.154	0.358
rnu/+anti-δ†	0	−1.0	1.672	0.283	−0.268	−0.441	0.357	0.959
rnu/rnu NRS	0	1.964	0.954	−0.276	−2.222	−0.754	−0.485	0.496
rnu/rnu anti-δ	0	0.079	1.279	−0.222	−2.301	−1.387	−0.807	0.512
55 days								
rnu/+NRS	1.80	2.944	1.568	0.053	−0.341	−0.315	0.452	0.336
rnu/+anti-δ	0	0.544	1.653	0.079	−0.351	0	0.435	1.084
rnu/rnu NRS	0	1.857	1.114	0.0086	0	0	−0.004	0.797
rnu/rnu anti-δ	0	0.47	1.312	0.025	0	0	−0.49	0.516

*Animals injected with normal rabbit serum.
†Animals injected with anti-δ antibody; groups comprized eight rats.

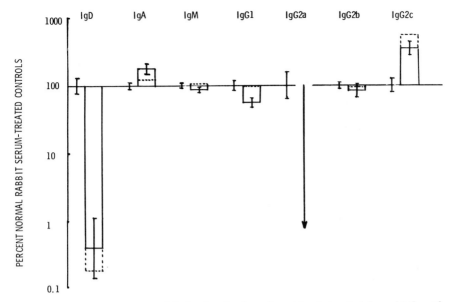

FIGURE 5A. Serum immunoglobulin levels of 55-day-old rats treated from birth with rabbit anti-rat δ. The results are expressed as percent deviation from the log mean of a control group of rats treated with normal rabbit serum. Standard errors of the groups of eight animals are shown. Dotted lines indicate the percent deviation of the medians of the groups. Here are the data from groups of rnu/$^+$ rats. The arrow falling from IgG2a indicates that no IgG2a was detected in the serum of the anti-δ treated group.

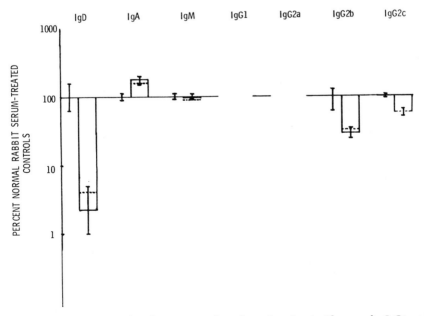

FIGURE 5B. Here are the data from groups of rnu/rnu athymic rats. The gaps for IgG1 and IgG2 indicate that no antibody of these classes was detected in these groups.

SUMMARY

Analysis of surface membrane immunoglobulin isotype expression in rats indicates that there is a major $\mu^+ \delta^-$ population in the spleen. This population is mainly confined to the marginal zones of the white pulp and differs from the major follicular B-cell population of the spleen, lymph nodes and gut associated lymphoid tissue. These latter express μ and δ on their surfaces. These $\mu^+ \delta^+$ cells are selectively reduced when recirculating lymphocytes are depleted, while the $\mu^+ \delta^-$ population of the spleen is retained. Deletion of δ^+ B-cells *in vivo* has been achieved using neonatal and continued treatment with rabbit anti-rat δ antibody. In these animals lymph node and Peyer's patch B-lymphocytes are substantially reduced while they are less markedly reduced in the spleen, which selectively retains its marginal zone population. However, some follicular cells of $\mu^+ \delta^-$ phenotype are seen in the spleen of these animals. The expression of α and $\gamma 2c$ by a proportion of marginal zone cells is apparent in both normal and nude rats treated from birth with anti-δ antibody. Serum immunoglobulin measurements in δ-depleted rats show selective loss of IgE, IgD and IgG2a with conservation of IgM IgG1 and IgG2b and augmentation of IgG2c and IgA. It is concluded that, while there is substantial overlap between the products of δ^+ and δ^- B-cells this overlap is not complete.

In conclusion, we deduce that the static population of splenic marginal zone B-cells contains a substantial component of cells which has never expressed δ. These cells are capable of producing all isotypes of immunoglobulin except $\gamma 2a$ but they appear to have a particular contribution in the maintenance of serum IgA and IgG2c. The overlap in isotype production may well explain functional similarities between δ^+ and δ^- populations.[19] However, our current data suggest that this overlap is complemented with substantial independent function, which may be more apparent if studies are made with an extensive range of antigens.

REFERENCES

1. KEARNEY, J. F., M. D. COOPER, J. KLEIN, E. R. ABNEY R. M. E. PARKHOUSE & A. R. LAWTON. 1977. Ontogeny of Ia and IgD on IgM-bearing B lymphocytes in mice. J. Exp. Med. **146:** 297.
2. COFFMAN, R. L. & M. COHN. 1977. The class of surface membrane immunoglobulin on virgin and memory B-lymphocytes. J. Immunol. **118:** 1806.
3. RAFF, M. C. 1977. Development and modulation of B lymphocytes: studies of newly formed B cells and their putative precursors in the haemopoietic tissues of mice. Cold Springs Harbor Symp. Quart. Biol. **41:** 159.
4. LAYTON, J. E., J. BAKER, P. F. BARTLETT & K. SHORTMAN. 1981. Antigen-initiated B lymphocyte differentiation XVIII. Preprogenitor cells B cells that give primary adoptive responses are S-IgM+ IgD−Ia+. J. Immunol. **126:** 1227.
5. BLACK, S. J., T. TOKUHISA, L. A. HERZENBERG & L. A. HERZENBERG. 1980. Memory B cells at successive stages of differentiation: expression of surface IgD and capacity for self renewal. Eur. J. Immunol. **10:** 846.
6. ZAN-BAR, I., S. STROBER & E. S. VITETTA. 1979. The relationship between surface immunoglobulin isotype and immune function of murine B lymphocytes. IV. Role of IgD bearing cells in the propagation of immunologic memory. J. Immunol. **123:** 925.
7. BAZIN, H., B. PLATTEAU, A. BECKERS & R. PAUWELS. 1978. Differential effect of neonatal injections of anti-μ or anti-δ antibodies in the synthesis of IgM, IgD, IgE, IgA, IgG1, IgG2a, IgG2b and IgG2c immunoglobulin classes. J. Immunol. **121:** 2083.
8. HOFFMAN-FREZER, G., H. RODT, H. EALITZ & S. THIERFELDER. 1976. Immunohistochemi-

cal identification of T- and B-lymphocyte delineated by the unlabelled antibody enzyme method. I. Anatomical distribution of theta positive and Ig positive cells in lymphoid organs of mice. J. Immunol. Methods **13**: 261.

9. DHALIWAL, H. S., N. R. LING, S. BISHOP, & H. CHAPEL. 1978. Expression of immunoglobulin G on blood lymphocytes in chronic lymphocytic leukaemia. Clin. Exp. Immunol. **31**: 226.

10. LING, N. R., S. BISHOP, & R. JEFFERIS. 1977. Use of antibody-coated red cells for the sensitive detection of antigen and in rosette tests for cells bearing surface immunoglobulins. J. Immunol. Methods **15**: 279.

11. BAZIN, H., A. BECKERS, G. URBAIN-VANSANTEN, R. PAUWELS, C. BRUYNS, A. F. TILKIN, B. PLATTEAU & J. URBAIN. 1978. Transplantable IgD immunoglobulin-secreting tumors in rats. J. Immunol. **121**: 2077.

12. KUMARARATNE, D. S., H. BAZIN, & I. C. M. MACLENNAN. 1981. Marginal zones: the major B cell compartment of rat spleens. Eur. J. Immunol. **11**: 858–864.

13. KUMARARATNE, D. S. I. C. M. MACLENNAN, H. BAZIN & D. GRAY. 1981. Marginal zones: The largest B cell compartment of the rat spleen. Proceedings of the 7th International Conference on Lymphatic Tissues and Germinal Centers in Immune Reactions. M. G. Hanna, P. Nieuwenhuis & Van den Broek, Eds. Plenum Press. In press.

14. COTTIER, H., N. ODARTCHENKO, R. SCHINDLER & C. C. CONGDON, Eds. 1967. Germinal Centers in Immune Responses: 343. Springer Verlag. Berlin, German Federal Republic.

15. IIJIMA, S. & G. YAMANE. 1968. *In* Advances in Germfree Research and Gnotobiology. M. Miyakawa & T.D. Luckey, Eds. Iliffe Books Ltd. London, England.

16. KUMARARATNE, D. S. & I. C. M. MACLENNAN. 1981. Cells of the marginal zone of the spleen are lymphocytes derived from recirculating precursors. Eur. J. Immunol. **11**: 865–869.

17. SLACK, J., G. P. DER-BALIAN, M. NAHM, & J. M. DAVIE. 1980. Subclass restriction of murine antibodies. II. The IgG plaque-forming cell response to thymus-independent type 1 and type 2 antigens in normal mice and mice expressing an X-linked immunodeficiency. J. Exp. Med. **151**: 853.

18. DER-BALIAN, G. P., J. SLACK, B. L. CLEVINGER, H. BAZIN, & J. M. DAVIE. 1981. Subclass restriction of murine antibodies. III. Antigens that stimulate IgG3 in mice stimulate IgG2c in rats. J. Exp. Med. **152**: 209.

19. LAYTON, J. E., B. L. PIKE, F. L. BATTYE & G. J. V. NOSSAL. 1979. Cloning of B cells positive or negative for surface IgD. I. Triggering and Tolerance in T-independent systems. J. Immunol. **123**: 702.

DISCUSSION OF THE PAPER

R. M. E. PARKHOUSE: Just to remind you that four years ago John Kear published that fetal liver cells and newborn spleen cells which, just as in the mouse system, contain no δ positive cells, can in fact, be stimulated under the influence of LPS to produce plasma cells making all the common Ig classes.

D. E. MOSIER (*Institute For Cancer Research, Philadelphia, Pa.*): Sixty percent of all B-cells you recover express both μ and δ. The total volume of cells contained in the marginal zones must be in excess of the total volume of cells contained in primary and secondary folicules in normal rat spleen. So I'm confused by the finding that the marginal zone seems to contain only μ positive cells. That doesn't seem to me in accord with the data you get when you make a spleen cell suspension.

H. BAZIN: We found that among the cells in the marginal zone there are some

IgD positive cells, but much less than in the follicle and there could be at least partially circulating cells.

BAZIN: In the germinal centers, we only detected μ and α, but no δ-containing immune complex on follicular dendritic cells. It is possible that other Ig isotypes can also be demonstrated.

G. J. THORBECKE: In mice suppressed with anti-δ from birth we find good immune responses of both 19S and 7S antibody in spleen, but extremely poor responses in lymph nodes. Because of these findings, Drs. Skelly, Baine, Ahmed and I did a detailed analysis of the μ only cells in spleen and lymph nodes. While the normal mouse spleen has approximately 5% such cells, anti-δ treated mice show a doubling of that population, but the lymph node has 1-2% in both normal and in anti-δ suppressed mice. If you immunize in such a way that you primarily reach the spleen, the defect in B-cells created by anti-δ treatment is not noticeable, while immunization via intraperitoneal or subcutaneous administration of antigen brings out a large difference. It, therefore, depends entirely on how the antigen reaches the immune system what effect of anti-δ treatment you will see. These results suggest, however, that the percentage of μ^+, δ^- cells in the mouse is much lower than in the rat, particularly in lymph nodes.

MEMBRANE IgD EXPRESSION AND DYNAMICS IN CLONES OF HUMAN B-LYMPHOBLASTOID CELLS*

Philip Roth, Paolo Tonda and Benvenuto Pernis

Departments of Microbiology and Medicine
Cancer Center/Institute of Cancer Research
College of Physicians & Surgeons
Columbia University
New York, New York 10032

Introduction

Immunoglobulin D (IgD) was initially described as a human serum immunoglobulin present in very low concentrations relative to other immunoglobulin (Ig) classes.[1] In marked contrast, the proportion of B-cells with membrane IgD is very high. In fact, the majority of antigen reactive B-lymphocytes in peripheral lymphoid organs express two classes of membrane immunoglobulins (mIg), IgM and IgD,[2,3] which share immunoglobulin light chain types,[2] idiotypes,[4,5] and specificity for antigen.[6-8] These two isotypes have been similarly demonstrated on the membranes of human B-lymphoblastoid cell lines (B-LCL),[9] which, in addition to mIg, display many B-cell markers[10] and functions.[11] Prior evidence suggesting that mIgM and mIgD are simultaneously synthesized by the cells bearing them[12,13] has been supported by recent data on the organization of Ig genes showing a uniquely short distance (2.3 kilobases) between the $C\mu$ and $C\delta$ gene segments when compared to other C-region genes.[14] This close proximity would be conducive to production of primary transcripts containing μ and δ sequences. It is therefore important that analyses of mIg physiology take into account this simultaneous synthesis of two isotypes with apparently identical receptors. We have attempted to address this question by studying the relative expression of mIgM and mIgD on clones of human B-lymphoblasts as well as mouse and human small B-lymphocytes and the differences in dynamics between these two classes of receptor.

Human B-Lymphoblastoid Cells

Human B-LCL MW derived from Epstein-Barr virus-transformed normal peripheral blood lymphocytes was received from Dr. S. Litwin (Cornell University, New York), and clone BL derived from a human lymphoma has been previously described.[12] Cell line MW was cloned in soft agarose by the method of Coffino and Scharff.[15] All cells were maintained as suspension cultures in RPMI-1640 supplemented with 16.7% fetal calf serum, 2 mM glutamine, 100 μg/ml penicillin, 100 μg/ml streptomycin and 0.25 μg/ml Fungizone (GIBCO, Grand Island, New York). The phenotypes, which were highly stable, of the clones that were studied and of the MW parental line are shown in Table 1.

*This work was supported by a research grant from the National Institutes of Health, U.S.P.H.S., AI ROI 14398 and by Grant IM-191 from the American Cancer Society.

175

0077-8923/82/0399-0175$01.75/0 © 1982, NYAS

Relative Expression of mIgM and mIgD by Lymphoblastoid Clones

The presence of mIg of different classes on B-lymphoblasts was demonstrated by immunofluorescence using tetramethyl rhodamine isothiocyanate (TRITC) and fluorescein isothiocyanate (FITC)-conjugated rabbit antibodies to human IgM and IgD, as previously described.[16] The density of mIgM or mIgD on single cells was determined by measuring fluorescence intensities of single cells with a Leitz MPV microscope photometer (Leitz, Wetzler, Germany) attached to a Leitz dialux microscope with Ploemopak vertical illuminator. Cells stained with both TRITC anti-μ and FITC anti-δ antibodies were applied in straight lines with a quill on microscope slides, fixed for 15 minutes in ice cold ethanol, washed with phosphate-buffered saline and then mounted with elvanol. Measurements were then carried out as follows: The diameter of the fluorescence intensity measuring field was adjusted to accommodate single cells and then kept constant for all measurements. Fluoresence intensities for both fluorescein and rhodamine were corrected for background fluorescence by taking multiple readings in fields containing no cells and subtracting the average values of rhodamine and fluorescein backgrounds from the respective readings. A "dot plot" of the mIgM and IgD densities on BL cells is shown in FIGURE 1. Within this single clone there is a wide range of μ/δ ratios ranging from predominance of IgM to predominance of IgD. This heterogeneity is entirely consistent with earlier observations made with both normal and malignant B-cell populations.[6,12,17] Furthermore, re-cloning of lymphoblast populations yielded subclones which resembled each other as well as their respective parental clone with respect to expression of IgM and IgD and the heterogeneity in the ratio of these two receptors. Taken together, these observations argue strongly against the occurrence of an irreversible shift in the μ/δ ratio secondary to a μ to δ or δ to μ switch in these cells, but rather favor the possibility that the cells oscillate between expression of different ratios of mIgM and mIgD, both of which they are capable of simultaneously synthesizing.

Unlike their *in vivo* B-cell counterparts, the B-lymphoblast clones do not seem to show any clustering of subpopulations around discrete μ/δ ratios (Herzenberg *et al.*, this volume, references 18, 19) but rather show a continuum of values between the two extremes. It is possible that the presence of subpopulations with particular μ/δ ratios *in vivo* may result from immunoregulatory or selective processes, while B-lymphoblast clones display the full potential range of ratios in the unperturbed, i.e., unregulated state.

TABLE 1

Ig PHENOTYPES OF PARENTAL AND CLONED CELLS

Cell population	Membrane Ig†			Cytoplasmic Ig‡
	% μ^+	% $\mu^+\delta^+$	% δ^+	% μ^+
MW	7.2	12.9	21.5	19.2
MW-E*	2.4	12.7	24.1	18.8
BL*	24.2	70.6	0.6	0.0

*Lymphoblastoid cell clones

†Data determined by immunofluorescence using a TRITC-conjugated rabbit anti-μ antibody and an FITC-conjugated rabbit anti-δ antibody.

‡Data determined by immunofluorescent staining of cytocentrifuge slides with TRITC-conjugated rabbit anti-μ antibody.

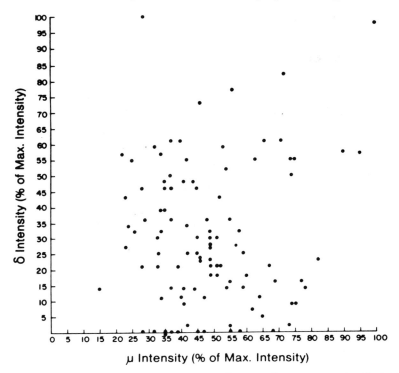

FIGURE 1. mIgM and mIgD densities on BL cells. BL cells were stained with TRITC-anti-μ and FITC-anti-δ antibodies, fixed and mounted, followed by measurement of fluorescence intensities as described in the text. Each point represents the μ and δ intensity of a single cell relative to the maximum μ and δ intensities, respectively, of the cell population.

Effect of Cross-linking of mIgM and mIgD in B-Lymphoblasts

Cells were exposed *in vitro* to class specific anti-immunoglobulin antibodies to determine if there were any differences in the fate of cross-linked mIgM and mIgD. Anti-immunoglobulin antibodies were prepared, purified and conjugated to fluorochromes as described elsewhere.[16] In order to distinguish between membrane immunoglobulin molecules that had been internalized from those that had remained on the membrane, the following approach was employed: First, cells were treated with FITC-conjugated anti-Ig antibodies (Ab#2) and washed, all at 4°C. Following incubation for two–six hours at either 0°C or 37°C, the cells were restained in suspension with TRITC-conjugated antibodies (Ab#w) directed at the first immunofluorescent reagent, Ab#1, which was either a rabbit or goat antibody. Membrane Ig molecules which remained on the membrane throughout all treatments would be stained with both fluorochromes, while those which were internalized would be inaccessible to staining by Ab#2 and thus would be positive for fluorescein only. MW-E cells treated with rabbit anti-μ antibodies at 37°C displayed IgM-containing cytoplasmic vacuoles, whereas cells treated with rabbit anti-δ antibodies contained IgD vacuoles in only a minimal proportion of cells and these latter vacuoles were smaller and present in smaller numbers per cell than their μ counterpart. Furthermore, intracytoplasmic vacuoles, when present, also stained positively for rabbit Ig, as well as kappa light chains. The data of several experiments with MW-E exposed to anti-Ig antibodies for 24 hours are shown in TABLE 2.

These results suggest that mIgD is generally not endocytosed after cross-linking in B-lymphoblasts unless cross-linked to mIgM as by anti-total Ig antibodies. On the other hand, mIgM-anti-μ complexes are internalized via repeated rounds of endocytosis and re-expression of mIgM as suggested previously by the work of Kearney et al.[20] Similar experiments with BL demonstrated μ vacuoles in nearly 100% of cells following anti-μ treatment in marked contrast to the 1–2% of cells containing δ vacuoles following anti-δ treatment.

Membrane IgM and IgD also differed in that the former could be still demonstrated indirectly following anti-μ exposure by positive immunofluorescent staining for rabbit Ig on the membranes of the B-lymphoblasts, while this was not the case for the latter isotype following anti-δ treatment (TABLE 3).

TABLE 2

APPEARANCE OF Ig-CONTAINING VACUOLES AFTER TREATMENT WITH
ANTI-IMMUNOGLOBULIN ANTIBODIES

24 hr culture* in the presence of:	% μ^+ vacuoles	% δ^+ vacuoles
PBS	0.0 ± 0.0	0.0 ± 0.0
RIgG	0.0 ± 0.0	0.0 ± 0.0
Anti-μ	29.4 ± 3.7	0.0 ± 0.0
Anti-δ	0.0 ± 0.0	1.7 ± 1.2
Anti-total Ig	42.8 ± 5.6	19.0 ± 3.0
Anti-μ + anti-δ	38.7 ± 0.0	0.0 ± 0.0

*Cell at a density of 4×10^5/ml were cultured for 24 hours in medium containing normal rabbit IgG (500 μg/ml), specific rabbit IgG antibodies (500 μg/ml) or an equivalent volume of PBS.

In order to exclude the possibility that mIgD was actually endocytosed but was so rapidly degraded intracellularly as to avoid detection by immunofluorescence, the following ^{125}I-antibody consumption experiments were performed. Briefly, cells were incubated for 20 hours in a 37°C, 5% CO_2 humidified atmosphere or at 0°C with affinity-purified anti-μ and anti-δ antibodies, respectively, that had been radioiodinated by the chloramine-T method[21] to specific activities of 2–5 μCi/μg, in concentrations that were determined to be well in excess of the amount needed to saturate all mIgM and mIgD. Cell-free medium incubated with ^{125}I-antibodies served as controls. If continuous endocytosis of mIg antibody complexes with subsequent intracellular degradation of ^{125}I-antibodies followed by mIg replacement were taking place, then consumption of ^{125}I-antibody would be detected.[22] This was assayed by incubating 20 μl of supernatant from control or experimental samples at 37°C for 30 minutes with shaking with an excess of either Sepharose 4B-coupled IgM for the ^{125}I-anti-μ samples or Sepharose 4B-coupled IgD for the ^{125}I-anti-δ samples. Corrections for nonspecific binding were made by performing the assay in the presence or absence of soluble IgM or IgD at 200 μg/ml, a

TABLE 3

PRESENCE OF RABBIT ANTIBODIES ON BL CELLS TREATED
WITH ANTI-IMMUNOGLOBULIN ANTIBODIES

24 hour culture in the presence of:	% RIg*
PBS	0.0 ± 0.0
RIgG	0.3 ± 0.3
Anti-μ	45.1 ± 4.9
Anti-δ	1.5 ± 1.0
Anti-total Ig	26.0 ± 1.2
Anti-μ + anti-δ	20.4 ± 7.4

*Cells were treated as described in TABLE 2. After 24 hours, cells were stained with fluorochrome-conjugated sheep-anti-rabbit Ig antibodies.

concentration sufficient to give maximal inhibition of binding, and subtracting the bound counts per minute of those aliquots inhibited with excess soluble IgM or IgD from those assayed in the absence of soluble Ig.

The Sepharose pellets were then washed three times with PBS + 1% fetal calf serum and counted in a Searle gamma counter. The specific cellular consumption of ^{125}I-antibody could then be determined by comparison of antibody counts recovered specifically from supernatants of cell-containing samples with those from samples containing medium alone. Representative experiments with clone MW-E are shown in TABLE 4. During incubation with ^{125}I-labelled anti-μ antibodies, the cells consumed approximately 32% of the specific IgM-binding radioactivity found in medium controls (Experiments A and B). In marked contrast, the cells consumed none of the ^{125}I-labelled anti-δ antibodies (Experi-

TABLE 4

CONSUMPTION OF ^{125}I-LABELLED ANTIBODIES BY MW-E

Expt.	Cells* or medium	Temp.	^{125}I-antibody	Metabolic† inhibitor	% ^{125}I-antibody consumed
A	medium	37°C	anti-μ	—	0.0
	MW-E	37°C	anti-μ	—	+31.6
	medium	37°C	anti-δ	—	0.0
	MW-E	37°C	anti-δ	—	−0.3
B	medium	37°C	anti-μ	—	0.0
	MW-E	37°C	anti-μ	—	+32.0
	MW-E	37°C	anti-μ	cycloheximide 50 μg/ml	+18.9
C	medium	0°C	anti-μ	—	0.0
	MW-E	10°C	anti-μ	—	−1.5

*MW-E (6.4 × 10^5 cells/ml) or culture medium were incubated in the presence of ^{125}I-anti-μ or anti-δ for 20 hours at either 37°C or 0°C.

†Cycloheximide, where indicated, was added at the initiation of cultures to a final concentration of 50 μg/ml.

‡Radioactivity associated with nonconsumed antibody in 20 μl of each supernatant was determined by measuring the amount of specific binding to Sepharose-coupled IgM or IgD. % Antibody consumption was calculated by the following formula:

$$\% \text{ Consumption} = \frac{\text{(Cell-free control supt) cpm bound} - \text{(MW-E supt) cpm bound}}{\text{(Cell free control supt) cpm bound}} \times 100$$

ment A) during 20 hours of culture. The possibility that consumption of labelled anti-μ was due to nonspecific factors released by the cells into the culture supernatants was eliminated when incubation of ^{125}I-antibody with spent culture supernatant from this clone did not result in any decrease of specific IgM-binding radioactivity (data not shown). In addition, the existence of proteolytic factors which selectively degrade anti-μ and not anti-δ antibodies is unlikely. If, in fact, the consumption of ^{125}I-anti-μ was the outcome of multiple rounds of endocytosis and intracellular degradation of mIgM-anti IgM complexes, and new synthesis of IgM with subsequent insertion into the membrane, then metabolic inhibitors which block these processes should totally or partially block the consumption of ^{125}I anti-μ. When cells were treated with cycloheximide, an inhibitor of protein synthesis, anti-μ consumption was reduced from 32% to approximately 19% (Experiment B). In addition, if the experiments were carried out at 0°C, a condition known to greatly decrease membrane fluidity and inhibit capping, MW-E consumed no anti-μ antibody at all when compared to controls (Experiment C). The "consumption" of ^{125}I-anti-μ by MW-E was the result of endocytosis, and intracellular degradation and not simple competition for ^{125}I-anti-μ combining sites between secreted IgM and Sepharose 4B-coupled IgM in the assay. If only simple competition were occurring, then in the presence of the large excess of labelled anti-μ antibodies added to the cultures and the low levels of secreted IgM in MW-E, soluble complexes would have formed. Thus, no labelled anti-IgM would have been removed from the solution, become unable to bind in our assay, and consequently been measured as "consumed."

In marked contrast to anti-μ, anti-δ antibodies were not consumed, confirming that mIgD was not endocytosed. However, shedding of mIgD with replacement at a rate of insertion that is normal or subnormal is likely when considering this experiment together with the immunofluorescence data described above. Since shedding would contribute only small amounts of IgD to the culture fluid already containing excess anti-IgD, soluble complexes would form and no antibody consumption would be detected in our assay.

Thus, in B-lymphoblasts, cross-linking of mIgM results in internalization, while cross-linking of mIgD results in shedding. Furthermore, these results were not a property of the antibodies used since multiple preparations from different rabbits as well as goats yielded the same basic results.

Dynamics of Cross-linked mIgM and mIgD in Mouse and Human Small B-Lymphocytes

Similar cross-linking experiments were performed with mouse splenocytes and human peripheral blood lymphocytes. Exposure of mouse spleen cells to rabbit anti-mouse μ antibodies resulted in internalization of mIgM in virtually 100% of B-cells. On the other hand, the same cells treated with rabbit anti-mouse δ antibodies (kindly provided by Dr. F. Finkelman) showed internalization of mIgD but only in approximately two-thirds of B-lymphocytes with very small and few IgD-containing vacuoles in some of these cells. Thus, despite equivalent if not greater expression of MIgD when compared to mIgM on murine splenic B-cells,[19,23] there is still more extensive internalization of mIgM. Internalization of mIgD, however, is clearly in contrast to results with human B-lymphoblasts (see below).

The identical experiments were performed with human peripheral blood lymphocytes using the same rabbit anti-μ and anti-δ preparations used in the experiments with B-lymphoblasts. Results with human peripheral B-lymphocytes were very similar to those with mouse splenocytes in that virtually all the cells showed internalization of mIgM with a large subpopulation also showing concurrent internalization of mIgD.

CONCLUSIONS

The outcome of cross-linking of mIgD by ligands does not seem to be a uniform property of all B-lymphoid cells. The difference in behavior observed between the B-lymphoblasts and the small B-lymphocytes may stem from different dynamic interactions of cross-linked mIg with underlying elements of the membranes of these cells. Whether these underlying dynamics are a property of cell type, i.e., lymphoblasts vs. lymphocytes or of particular clones with particular properties is unknown. Clearly, either point of view may be invoked to explain our data on *clones* of B-lympho*blasts* and *polyclonal* populations of B-lympho*cytes*. Furthermore, in light of current data demonstrating multiple δ membrane mRNA species in B-lymphocytes (Mushinski *et al.*, this volume), it is possible that these transcripts are translated in different cell types or clones into different δ membrane molecules capable of contacting different components of the B-lymphocyte membrane and displaying different properties and consequently functions.

REFERENCES

1. ROWE, D. S. & J. L. FAHEY. 1965. A new class of human immunoglobulins. II. Normal serum IgD. J. Exp. Med. **121**: 185–199.
2. ROWE, D. W., K. HUG, L. FORNI & B. PERNIS. 1973. Immunoglobulin D as a lymphocyte receptor. J. Exp. Med. **138**: 965–972.
3. MELCHER, U., E. S. VITETTA, M. MCWILLIAMS, M. E. LAMM, J. M. PHILLIPS-QUAGLIATA & J. W. UHR. 1974. Cell surface immunoglobulin. X. Identification of an IgD-like molecule on the surface of murine splenocytes. J. Exp. Med. **140**: 1427–1431.
4. SALSANO, F., S. S. FROLAND, J. B. NATVIG & T. E. MICHAELSEN. 1974. Same idiotype of B-lymphocyte membrane IgD and IgM. Formal evidence for monoclonality of chronic lymphocytic leukemia cells. Scand. J. Immunol. **3**: 841–846.
5. FU, S. M., R. WINCHESTER, T. FEIZI, P. D. WALZER & H. G. KUNKEL. 1974. Idiotypic specificity of surface immunoglobulin and the maturation of bone marrow derived lymphocytes. Proc. Natl. Acad. Sci. USA **71**: 4487–4490.
6. PERNIS, B., J. C. BROUET & M. SELIGMANN. 1974. IgD and IgM on the membrane of lymphoid cells in macroglobulinemia: Evidence for identity of membrane IgD and IgM antibody activity in a case with anti-IgG receptors. Eur. J. Immunol. **4**: 776–778.
7. STERN, C. & I. MCCONNELL. 1976. Immunoglobulins M and D as antigen-binding receptors on the same cell, with shared specificity. Eur. J. Immunol. **6**: 225–227.
8. GODING, J. W. & J. E. LAYTON. 1976. Antigen-induced co-capping of IgM and IgD-like receptors on murine B cells. J. Exp. Med. **144**: 852–857.
9. VAN BOXEL, J. A. & D. N. BUELL. 1974. IgD on cell membranes of human lymphoid cell lines with multiple immunoglobulin classes. Nature (London) **251**: 443–444.
10. WINCHESTER, R. J., S. M. FU, P. WERNET, H. G. KUNKEL, G. DUPONT and C. JERSILD. 1975. Recognition by pregnancy serums of non-HL-A alloantigens selectively expressed on B lymphocytes. J. Exp. Med. **141**: 924–929.
11. KOSBOR, D., M. STEINITZ, G. KLEIN, S. KOSKIMIES & O. MÄKELÄ. 1979. Establishment of

anti-TNP antibody producing human lymphoid lines by preselection for hapten binding followed by EBV transformation. Scand. J. Immunol. **10:** 187–194.

12. PERNIS, B., L. FORNI & A. LUZZATI. 1977. Synthesis of multiple immunoglobulin classes by single lymphocytes. Cold Spring Harbor Symp. Quant. Biol. **41:** 175–183.

13. HURLEY, J. N., S. M. FU, H. G. KUNKEL, G. MCKENNA & M. D. SCHARFF. 1978. Lymphoblastoid cell lines from patients with chronic lymphocytic luekemia: Identification of tumor origin by idiotypic analysis. Proc. Natl. Acad. Sci. USA **75:** 5706–5710.

14. LIU, C-P., P. W. TUCKER, J. F. MUSHINSKI & F. R. BLATTNER. 1980. Mapping of heavy chain genes for mouse immunoglobulins M and D. Science **209:** 1348–1353.

15. COFFINO, P. & M. D. SCHARFF. 1971. Rate of somatic mutation in immunoglobulin production by mouse myeloma cells. Proc. Natl. Acad. Sci. USA **68:** 219–223.

16. FERRARINI, M., G. VIALE, A. RISSO & B. PERNIS. 1976. A study of the immunoglobulin classes present on the membrane and in the cytoplasm of human tonsil plasma cells. Eur. J. Immunol. **6:** 562–565.

17. PERNIS, B. 1977. Lymphocyte membrane IgD. Immunological Reviews **37:** 210–218.

18. VITETTA, E. S., M. MCWILLIAMS, J. M. PHILLIPS-QUAGLIATA, M. E. LAMM & J. W. UHR. 1975. Cell surface immunoglobulin. XIV. Synthesis, surface expression and secretion of immunoglobulin by Peyer's patch cells in the mouse. J. Immunol. **115:** 603–605.

19. VITETTA, E. S., U. MELCHER, M. MCWILLIAMS, M. LAMM, J. M. PHILLIPS-QUAGLIATA & J. W. UHR. 1975. Cell surface immunoglobulin. XI. The appearance of an IgD-like molecule on murine lymphoid cells during ontogeny. J. Exp. Med. **141:** 206–215.

20. KEARNEY, J. F., J. KLEIN, D. E. BOCKMAN, M. D. COOPER & A. R. LAWTON. 1978. B cell differentiation induced by lipopolysaccharide. V. Suppression of plasma cell maturation by anti-μ: mode of action and characteristics of suppressed cells. J. Immunol. **120:** 158–166.

21. GREENWOOD, F. C., W. M. HUNTER & J. S. GLOVER. 1963. The preparation of ^{131}I-labelled human growth hormone of high specific radioactivity. Biochem. J. **89:** 114–123.

22. KNOPF, P. M., A. DESTREE & R. HYMAN. 1973. Antibody-induced changes in expression of an immunoglobulin surface antigen. Eur. J. Immunol. **3:** 251–259.

23. SCHER, I., S. SHARROW, R. WISTAR, R. ASOFSKY & W. E. PAUL. 1976. B lymphocyte heterogeneity: Ontogenetic development and organ distribution of B lymphocyte populations defined by their intensity of surface immunoglobulins. J. Exp. Med. **144:** 494–506.

DISCUSSION OF THE PAPER

R. WHITE: There was a paper last year by Satir's group which showed that μ chains may interact with actin, I believe it was a lymphoblastoid line. Is that kind of information available for the interaction of δ in any system with actin? If it isn't could that be a possible lesion in your system, i.e., δ in this BL line does not interact with actin when it's cross linked by itself but maybe when it's cross linked with μ now can interact with coded pits?

B. G. PERNIS: Yes, that is the next step.

D. JARTA: My question follows on this one and has to do with the coated pits. Is there any evidence that either IgM or IgD are internalized through special organelles, such as coated pit, or do they just enter at any place on the cell surface?

PERNIS: I asked myself the same question. I couldn't see any obvious evidence of that but clearly this has to be repeated with new preparations and new staining.

E. S. VITETTA: Do the lymphoblastoid lines have a S2L2 or are they SL? I'm curious if there could be any correlation with the form of the membrane IgD and the fact that it will or will not be internalized?

PERNIS: We have not investigated this point.

SURFACE IgD PHENOTYPE OF ELECTROPHORETICALLY FRACTIONATED MOUSE LYMPHOID CELLS

Francis Dumont,* Robert C. Habbersett, and Aftab Ahmed

Department of Immunology
Merck, Sharp and Dohme Research Laboratories
Rahway, New Jersey 07065

INTRODUCTION

Preparative electrophoresis[1] enables one to physically fractionate cell suspensions on the basis of differences in electrophoretic mobility (EPM), a parameter that reflects the net cell-surface charge arising from the overall biochemical composition of the plasma membrane.[2] This technique has been efficiently used to separate mouse B- and T-lymphocytes, the former having on average a lower EPM than the latter.[3-5] Evidence indicating that the B-lymphocyte compartment is itself electrophoretically heterogeneous has also been obtained. Thus, the electrophoretic separation of different types of progenitors for antibody-forming cells has been reported.[6,7] Also, ontogenetic studies have revealed developmental changes in the electrokinetic properties of B-cells[8] suggesting that subsets representing stages in the B-cell differentiation pathway can be enriched by electrophoresis.

This report summarizes a series of studies initiated in order to evaluate further the electrophoretic separability of mouse B-cell subsets as defined by their surface phenotype with special reference to sIgD expression. We used single- and dual-parameter flow cytofluorometry (FCF) analyses[9] to quantitate the cell surface binding of fluorochrome-conjugated antibodies to IgD and to total Ig, IgM and Ia antigen on electrophoretically fractionated cells from mouse spleen and Peyer's patches. By this approach, we could delineate several electrophoretically distinct B-cell subsets differing in their sIgD phenotype and in their organ distribution. The influence of the CBA/N xid mutation[10] on these subsets in the spleen was also investigated.

MATERIALS AND METHODS

Mice

CBA/J and NZB/BINJ mice were obtained from the Jackson Laboratories (Bar Harbor, Me). CBA/N × DBA/2 (CND2) and DBA/2 × CBA/N (D2CN) males were obtained from Dominion Laboratories (Dublin, Va). NZB XY and NZB xid Y (9th to 11th backcross generations) mice were a gift from Dr. Eric Gershwin (Davis University, Ca).

*On leave of absence from the Unit of Experimental Cancerology, INSERM U95, Vandoeuvre les Nancy, France.

0077-8923/82/0399-0184 $01.75/0 © 1982, NYAS

Preparation of Cell Suspensions

Mice were killed by cervical dislocation. Spleens or Peyer's patches were gently teased in ice-cold RPMI 1640 medium (GIBCO, Grand Island, N.Y.) supplemented with 5% heat inactivated foetal calf serum (RS medium). Cell suspensions were passed through nylon mesh and washed in RS medium.

Cell Separation with Free-Flow Electrophoresis

Cell suspensions were gradually transfered into low ionic strength electrophoresis buffer and filtered through cotton wool. Cells were fractionated in a Hannig's free-flow electrophoresis apparatus model FF48 (Desaga, Heidelberg, Germany) as described elswhere.[11]

Fluorescent Staining of the Cells

Rabbit anti-mouse IgD antiserum and rabbit anti-mouse IgM antiserum were obtained from Dr. Fred Finkelman. Monoclonal antibodies against mouse Ig5a (clone 10-4-22) and IaK (clone 11-5-2) were purchased from Becton-Dickinson (Mountain View, Ca). Polyvalent rabbit anti-mouse Ig antiserum was obtained from Polysciences (Warrington, Pa). The monoclonal antibody 14G8 was a gift from Dr. John Kung (NIH, Bethesda). These antibodies were either fluorescein (Fl)-conjugated or biotin-conjugated. In the latter case, Fl-, Rhodamine (Rh)- or Texas red (TxR)-avidin (Becton Dickinson) were used as second-step reagents. All these reagents were ultracentrifuged (100,000 g, 10 min.) immediately before use.

For single-color staining, 10^6 cells in 100 μl of RS medium containing 0.1% NaN$_3$ were incubated on ice for 30 minutes in the presence of saturating amounts of antibody. Cells were washed, and when required, were further incubated for 30 minutes with Fl-avidin. Cells were again extensively washed, and were resuspended in phenol red-free Hanks medium (GIBCO) containing 5% foetal calf serum and 0.1% NaN$_3$. For two-color analysis, cells were stained with a first biotinylated antibody as described above, using Rh- or TxR-avidin, and then were incubated with a second Fl-conjugated antibody.

Flow Cytofluorometry (FCF) Analysis

Quantitative fluorescence measurements were performed on a FACS IV (Becton Dickinson, FACS Systems, Mountain View, Ca) equipped with two lasers (Models 164-05 and 164-01, Spectra-Physics). Single-parameter or dual-parameter (Fluorescence vs. light scatter) analysis of cells stained with Fl-conjugated reagents was carried out with the Argon-ion laser operated at 300 mW. For single-color analysis, 20,000 viable cells, as identified by forward light scatter signals, were scored in each sample. The date were collected in 256 channel linear distributions, stored and processed in a PDP 11 computer (Digital Equipment, Maynard, Ma). The Krypton-ion laser, exciting at 568 nm and 120 mW was utilized in the two-color fluorescence analyses. Green and red fluorescence intensities were measured simultaneously on 100,000 individual cells. Correlated two parameter data were collected and stored in the computer as cell number in a

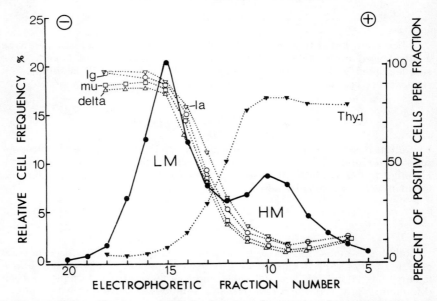

FIGURE 1. Electrophoregram of CBA/J splenocytes showing the relative frequency of all cells in the various fractions as a function of the relative EPM of these fractions (●). The cells migrated in the electric field from the cathode (left) to the anode (right). LM: low mobility cells, HM: high-mobility cells. The frequency distributions of cells positive for various surface markers as evaluated by FACS analysis in each electrophoretic fraction are also represented: Thy-1 (▼), sIg (O), sIa (∇), sIgD (△), sIgM (□).

64 × 64 matrix of green fluorescence (X axis) and light scatter or red fluorescence (Y axis) and displayed as contour plots.[12]

RESULTS AND DISCUSSION

Electrophoretic Fractionation and FCF Analysis of CBA/J Splenocytes

Following separation by preparative electrophoresis, the splenocytes from two to three month-old CBA/J mice were distributed in a distinctly bimodal pattern (FIGURE 1). The predominant peak, accounting for 55–60% of the whole profile was arbitrarily designated as the low-mobility (LM) population, the other peak, with a more anodic velocity, was called the high-mobility (HM) population. The various cell fractions thus collected were analyzed for the expression of several surface antigens using single-color FCF. As shown in FIGURE 1, the frequency of cells bearing the T-lymphocyte marker Thy-1 was low in the LM region but rapidly rose to 80–85% in the fractions of increasing EPM. In contrast, the cells stained with a polyvalent anti-mouse Ig antiserum were considerably enriched in the LM fractions and depleted in the HM fractions. Therefore, the LM population of splenocytes represents mostly B-cells and the HM population mostly T-cells.[3-5]

Accordingly, cells bearing sIgD were found to segregate in the LM region of the electrophoretic profile. The distribution of these sIgD[+] cells paralleled that of sIg[+] cells detected with the polyvalent anti-Ig antiserum but in all fractions there was always 5–10% less of the former than of the latter cell type. The electrophoretic distribution of the other Ig isotype known to be expressed on most B-cells,[13] i.e. IgM, was also almost identical to that of sIgD. The surface expression of Ia antigen, another B cell marker,[14] was also investigated by FCF analysis. The distribution of sIa[+] cells was close to that of sIg[+] cells although the frequency of sIa[+] cells slightly exceeded that of sIg[+] cells, especially in those fractions intermediate between the LM and HM peaks.

Examples of series of fluorescence staining profiles for the four B-cell markers above mentioned as obtained with the various electrophoretic fractions of CBA/J splenocytes are presented in FIGURES 2 and 3. In the cases of sIg and sIa, the shapes of the profiles indicated no major shift in the intensity of staining as a function of EPM. This was more accurately quantitated by calculating the median fluorescence intensity for each individual profile. For sIg and sIa this value varied slightly although no consistent trend was observed (FIGURE 2). In contrast,

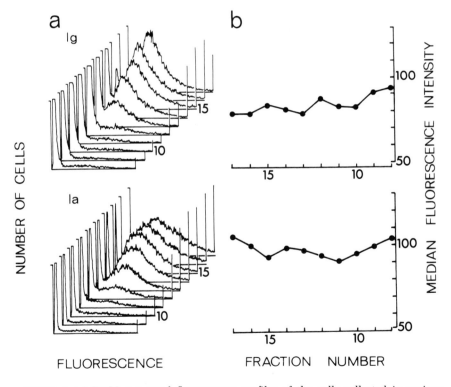

FIGURE 2. (a) FACS-generated fluorescence profiles of the cells collected in various electrophoretic fractions of CBA/J splenocytes and stained for sIg or sIa. (b) Median fluorescence intensity of the marker-positive population as a function of the fraction number.

there was a marked shift in the intensity of staining for sIgD as a function of EPM (FIGURE 3). Thus, the sIgD-bearing cells with lowest EPM (fractions 15–17) were brighter than those with higher EPM (fractions 12–14). Pronounced differences in the median fluorescence intensity of staining for sIgM were also observed depending on the EPM of the fractions. However, this trend for sIgM was the opposite of that seen for sIgD staining (FIGURE 3). Thus, the fractions that were stained dimly for sIgD were relatively bright for sIgM and conversely, those which were stained brightly for sIgD were dull for sIgM.

These observations indicate that existence of at least two types of sIgD-bearing splenocytes differing in the amount of sIgD exposed on their surface and possessing distinct electrokinetic properties. Correlated FCF analysis of light scatter vs. sIgD staining intensity of the various electrophoretic fractions of CBA/J splenocytes revealed that these two sIgD-bearing cell subsets also slightly differ in their light scattering properties (FIGURE 4). Since the degree of light scattering by cells is mainly related to cell size,[9] these data suggest that the dull sIgD$^+$ cells are slightly larger than the bright sIgD$^+$ cells.

Two-color FCF analysis was used to define more precisely the correlation between the expression of IgD and other B-cell markers on the surface of electrophoretically fractionated CBA/J splenocytes. Typical contour maps resulting from such experiments are depicted in FIGURE 5. The analysis of cells

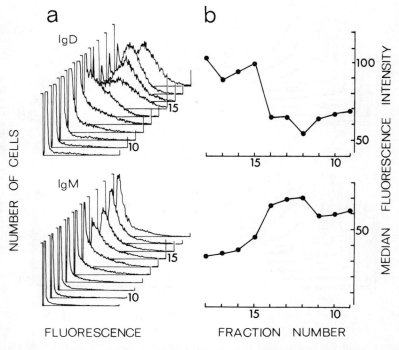

FIGURE 3. (a) FACS-generated fluorescence profiles of the cells collected in various electrophoretic fractions of CBA/J splenocytes and stained for sIgD or sIgM. (b) Median fluorescence intensity of the marker-positive population as a function of the fraction number.

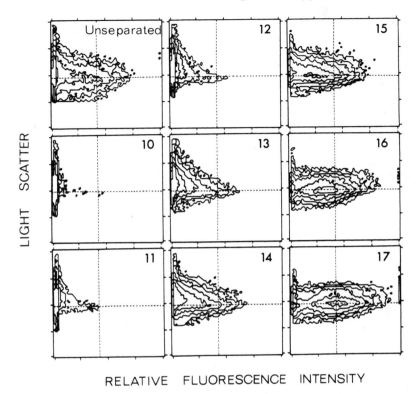

LIGHT SCATTER

RELATIVE FLUORESCENCE INTENSITY

FIGURE 4. Contour plots of correlated light scatter vs. fluorescence FCF analysis of unseparated or electrophoretically separated CBA/J splenocytes stained with Fl-anti-IgD (Ig5a) antibody. The fraction number is indicated on each plot. Each contour represents increasing numbers of cells (levels: 1 = 10, 2 = 20, 3 = 40, 4 = 80, 5 = 160, 6 = 320). The dashed lines are centered on the modal fluorescence intensity and modal light scatter intensity of the bright sIgD⁺ subset in fraction 17.

simultaneously stained for sIa and sIg demonstrated a positive correlation between the expression of these two determinants (FIGURE 5a). In agreement with the single-color FCF data, in the anodic LM fractions (e.g. fraction 13) there was a small proportion (8–12%) of sIa⁺ cells possessing low amounts or devoid of sIg while in the LM fractions of the cathodic side of the profile (e.g. fraction 16), all the cells which were sIa⁺ were also sIg⁺. As shown in FIGURE 5b, staining of splenocytes with biotinylated-anti-IgD (Ig5a) antibody followed by Rh-avidin and by Fl-anti-IgM antibody revealed that most of the B-cells express both Ig isotypes on their surface. However, the cells that were bright for sIgD were dull for sIgM and vice versa. In fraction 13, there was an enrichment for dull sIgD⁺ bright sIgM⁺ cells whereas in fraction 16, most of the cells were bright sIgD⁺ and dull sIgM⁺. The patterns of sIgD vs. sIa staining (FIGURE 5c) demonstrated that bright and dull sIgD⁺ splenocytes have very similar amounts of sIa antigen.

These observations demonstrate that in CBA/J mice, at least two phenotypically distinct subsets of sIgD-bearing splenocytes can be partially separated on the basis of surface-charge differences. The first of these subsets, characterized as $sIgD^+$ $sIgM^{++}$ sIa^+ was enriched in the anodic part of the LM peak which also contained up to 25% T-cells. To obtain this B-cell subset in a more purified form, it will be useful to combine preparative electrophoresis with a procedure to remove T-cells. The other B-cell subset, defined as $sIgD^{++}$ $sIgM^+$ sIa^+ was enriched in the cathodic part of the HM peak.

The monoclonal antibody used in these studies (10-4-22) has been shown to recognize an allotypic determinant (43) located in the Fc region of the lymphocyte $sIgD$.[15,16] It is conceivable that depending on the cell type, this part of the IgD molecule might be more or less buried into the cell membrane and thus might be more or less accessible to the 10-4-22 antibody. If so, the changes in intensity of $sIgD$-staining observed here might reflect a change in accessibility of the 43 determinant rather than changes in the total number of $sIgD$ molecules exposed

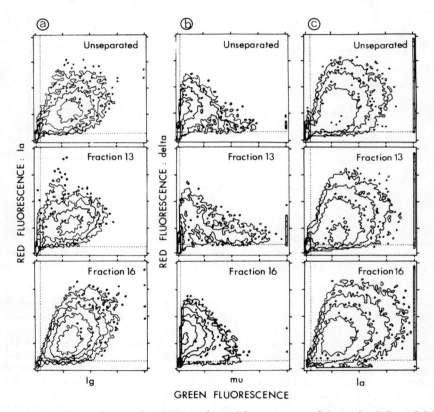

FIGURE 5. Two-color correlated FCF analysis of the expression of sIa vs. sIg, sIgD vs. sIgM and sIgD vs. sIa on the surface of unseparated or of electrophoretically separated CBA/J splenocytes. The staining patterns of two representative LM fractions are shown: fast LM fraction (13), slow LM fraction (16). Each contour represents increasing number of cells (levels: 1 = 10, 2 = 20, 3 = 40, 4 = 80, 5 = 160, 6 = 320). The background fluorescence intensities of control samples, stained with only one of the two fluorochrome labelled antibodies, are delimited by the dotted lines.

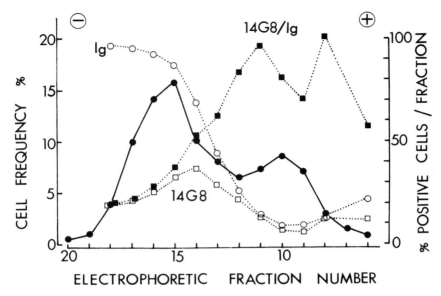

FIGURE 6. Electrophoregram of CBA/J splenocytes (●) and frequency distribution of sIg⁺ (○) or 14G8 (□) cells in the various fractions. The ratio of 14G8⁺/sIg⁺ cells (■) in these fractions is also shown.

on the cell surface. However, in preliminary experiments, using a rabbit anti-mouse IgD antiserum known to react with a common determinant present on the Fab fragment of IgD,[15] we found similar differences in sIgD-staining of slow and fast LM splenocytes as those reported here, which suggests that the hypothesis just mentioned is unlikely and that the differences observed do reflect changes in the amount of sIgD.

The distribution on electrophoretically fractionated CBA/J splenocytes of another B-cell surface antigen, recently described by Dr. John Kung, was also studied. This determinant is recognized by a monoclonal antibody (14G8) and has been shown to be present on Lyb-5⁻Ig⁺ cells (John Kung, personal communications). As demonstrated in FIGURE 6, 14G8⁺ cells were found to display an electrophoretic distribution pattern clearly different from that of sIg⁺ cells. The highest frequency of these 14G8⁺ cells was encountered in fraction 14.

Moreover, consideration of the ratio of 14G8⁺ cells/sIg⁺ cells indicated that 60–90% of sIg⁺ cells present in the HM region bear the 14G8 antigen as compared to only 20–30% in the fractions with lowest EPM. This suggests that while most sIgD⁺ sIgM⁺⁺ sIa⁺ B-cells are 14G8⁺ (Lyb-5⁻), the majority of sIgD⁺⁺ sIgM⁺ sIa⁺ B-cells are 14G8⁻ (Lyb-5⁺).

Electrophoretic Fractionation and FCF Analysis of NZB Splenocytes

Spleen cells from two to three month-old NZB mice exhibited a bimodal electrophoretic distribution but the proportion of LM cells was consistently found to be lower than in CBA/J mice. FCF analysis of sIg and Thy-1 expression demonstrated that in NZB, like in CBA/J mice, the LM population corresponds predominantly to B-cells and the HM population to T-cells (FIGURE 7a). sIgD-bearing cells could be detected using the 10-4-22 monoclonal antibody.[16] As shown in FIGURE 7b, their frequency did not exceed 10–15% in the HM fractions, but reached 80–85% in the LM fractions. Also, the distribution of these sIgD-bearing cells closely paralleled that of sIgM-bearing cells.

Two-color correlated FCF analysis was also carried out to determine the relationship between the surface expressions of IgD and IgM on electrophoreti-cally fractionated NZB splenocytes. The results of this study, presented in FIGURE 8, are essentially similar to those above described for CBA/J mice. Thus, the cells recovered in the very low EMP fractions made up a cluster of bright sIgD+, dull sIgM+ cells (fractions 17–15). In contrast, those sIgD-bearing cells present in the fractions with higher EPM were predominantly dull for sIgD and bright for sIgM.

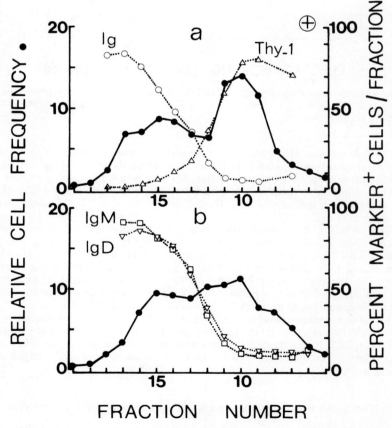

FIGURE 7. (a) Electrophoregram of splenocytes from three month-old NZB mice (●) showing the frequency distribution of sIg+ (O) and Thy-1+ (△) cells in the various fractions. (b) Electrophoregram of NZB splenocytes (●) and frequency distribution of sIgD+ (▽) and sIgM+ (□) cells. LM = low-mobility cells, HM = high-mobility cells.

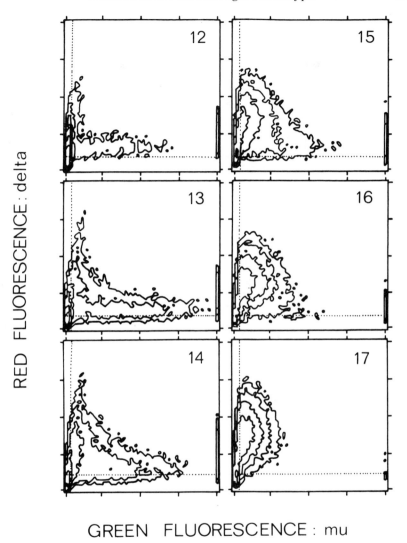

FIGURE 8. Two-color correlated FCF analysis of sIgD vs. sIgM expression on electrophoretically fractionated splenocytes from three month-old NZB mice.

Therefore, the two electrophoretically and phenotypically distinct sIgD-bearing cell subsets: sIgD$^+$ sIgM^{++} and sIgD^{++} sIgM$^+$ recognizable in immunologically normal mice are also present in the autoimmunity-prone NZB mice. However, in agreement with other studies[17] we found that during aging in NZB mice, but not in CBA/J or BALB/c mice, there is an expansion of the sIgD$^+$ sIgM^{++} cell subset in the spleen resulting in a progressive masking of the sIgD^{++} sIgM$^+$ cells (data not shown). Such a phenomenon probably reflects the hyperac-

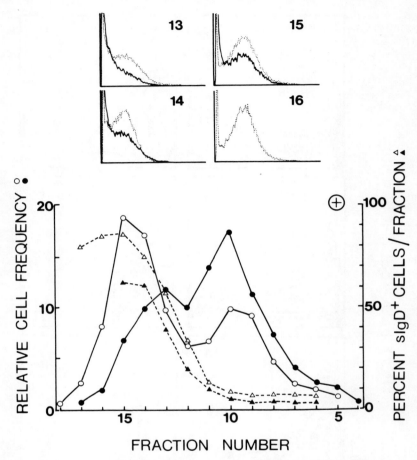

FIGURE 9. Electrophoregrams of splenocytes from D2CN (normal, ○) and CND2 (xid-bearing, ●) male mice. The frequency distribution of sIgD-bearing cells in the various splenocyte fractions of D2CN (△) and CND2 (▲) mice are represented. The inset on top of this figure shows the FACS-generated sIgD-staining profiles of four LM fractions in D2CN (·····) and CND2 (—) mice. Note that in CND2 mice, fraction 16 did not contain enough cells to permit FCF analysis.

tivation of the B-cell compartment which is a characteristic of autoimmune strains.[18]

Influence of the xid Mutation on the Electrophoretic Subsets of sIgD-Bearing Splenocytes

The sex-linked xid mutation which occurred in the CBA/N mouse strain results in an immune deficiency manifested by a number of phenotypic and

functional abnormalities of B-cells.[10] In many respects, the B-lymphocyte compartment of adult mice carrying this mutation behaves like that of neonatal
normal mice. Thus, xid mice lack a unique subpopulation of B-cells appearing
late during ontogeny in normal mice and characterized by large amounts of sIgD
and low amounts of sIgM.[19]

In view of the above-mentioned findings indicating a relationship between
the EPM of B-cells and their sIgD phenotype, it seemed of interest to investigate
the electrokinetic properties of splenocytes from such xid mice. In a first series of
experiments, we compared the electrophoretic distribution of splenocytes from
xid-bearing CND2 males with that of splenocytes from normal D2CN males.
FIGURE 9 demonstrates that while LM cells prevailed (63%) in the spleen of D2CN
males, these LM cells accounted for less than 40% of CND2 male splenocytes.
Such a decreased frequency of LM cells in CND2 is consistent with the known
numerical B-cell deficiency of these mice.[10] Moreover, although in both types of
hybrids the HM population (T-cells) appeared electrophoretically similar, in
CND2 mice, the LM population was usually shifted by two fractions towards a
higher EPM (peak fraction: 13) as compared to D2CN mice (peak fraction: 15). The
evaluation of sIgD-bearing cells by FCF analysis revealed a distribution of these
cells in D2CN mice comparable to that observed in CBA/J mice. However, the
frequency of these cells in the LM fractions was much lower in CND2 mice than
in D2CN mice. Most interestingly, the fractions which were depleted in the xid
mice correspond to those containing the bright sIgD$^+$ cells, whereas the fractions
with proportionally higher cell numbers in CND2 mice than in D2CN mice
correspond to those enriched for dull sIgD$^+$ cells.

We also studied the electrokinetic properties of splenocytes from NZB mice
carrying the xid mutation and produced by Dr. Eric Guershwin.[20] Their spleen
cells were shown to exhibit the same phenotypic features as those of other xid
mice with different genetic backgrounds. The fluorescence profiles depicted in
FIGURE 10 show that compared to normal NZB mice, these NZB xid presented a
relative decrease of sIgD^{++} splenocytes and a relative increase of sIgM^{++}
splenocytes. The distribution patterns observed after electrophoretic fractiona-

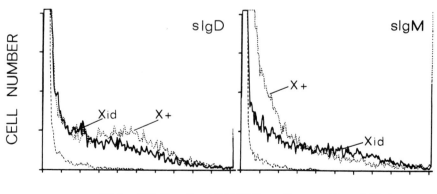

FIGURE 10. FACS-generated fluorescence profiles of unseparated splenocytes from three
month-old NZB XY (·····) and NZB xid Y (—) mice stained with Fl-anti-IgD (Ig5a) or
Fl-anti-IgM antibodies.

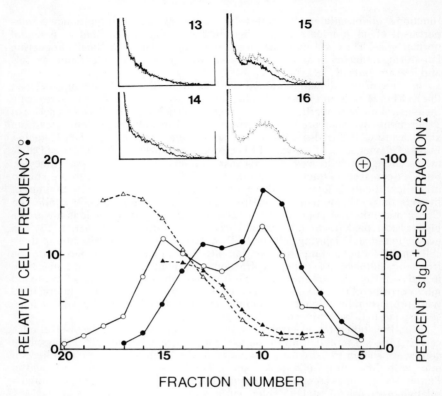

FIGURE 11. Electrophoregrams of splenocytes from NZB XY (O) and NZB xid Y (●) mice. The frequency distributions of sIgD-bearing cells in the various splenocyte fractions of NZB XY (△) and NZB xid Y (▲) mice are represented. The inset on top of this figure shows the FACS-generated sIgD-staining profiles of four LM fractions in NZB XY (·····) and NZB xid Y (—) mice.

tion of these splenocytes were essentially bimodal (FIGURE 11). However, the majority of LM cells in NZB xid mice possessed a higher EPM than LM cells in NZB X$^+$ mice. The FACS profiles presented in FIGURE 11 confirmed that the LM cells depleted in NZB xid mice are sIgD.$^{++}$

These studies on xid mice further support the notion that sIgD$^+$ and sIgD^{++} splenocytes are endowed with distinctive EPM. Since the immune defect of xid mice is believed to involve an arrest in the development and/or maturation of the B-cell population,[10] the fact that splenic B-cells with very low EPM are depleted in these mice is in accord with our earlier finding that in normal mice the mean EPM of the B-cell population tends to decrease in the course of ontogeny.[8] Thus, the B-cells with very low EPM (sIgD^{++}) may be more mature than those with high EPM (sIgD$^+$). However, such an interpretation is speculative since sIgD^{++} mature B-cells have been found to lose their sIgD[21] and increase their EPM upon mitogenic stimulation.[22] Then, it is possible that the sIgD$^+$ cells recovered in the anodic part of the LM population may represent both activated B-cells and less mature B-cells.

Electrophoretic Fractionation and FCF Analysis of Peyer's Patch Cells from CBA/J Mice

Peyer's patches (PP) are known to contain a large proportion of mature B-cells.[23] Since these B-cells have been reported to differ phenotypically and functionally from splenic B-cells,[23-25] in the context of the present work it appeared of interest to investigate their electrokinetic properties and sIgD staining properties.

In FIGURE 12 are superimposed the electrophoretic distribution profiles of splenocytes and PP cells as obtained in experiments run under identical conditions. The frequency of LM cells in PP was close to that of LM cells in the spleen, and in both tissues, these LM cells peaked at fraction 15. In PP, like in spleen, sIgD-bearing cells were confined to the LM fractions.

Although the percentages of sIgD-bearing cells in the various fractions of PP cells were always lower than for the spleen, the electrophoretic distribution curves of these cells in the two tissues were parallel, which suggests that overall, sIgD-bearing cells in PP possess a surface-charge close to that of splenic sIgD-bearing cells.

Contrarily to what was observed for splenocytes, there was no major change in the magnitude of sIgD staining in the various electrophoretic fractions of PP cells (FIGURE 13). Moreover, as shown in FIGURE 14, the subset of sIgD$^+$ sIgM^{++} cells that was clearly visible in the spleen was undetectable in PP. Indeed, the sIgD-bearing cells present in the unseparated PP cell population appeared

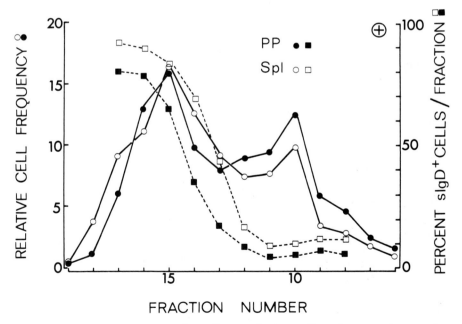

FIGURE 12. Electrophoregrams of PP cells (●) and spleen cells (○) from CBA/J mice. The frequency distributions of sIgD-bearing cells as determined by FCF analysis in the various fractions of PP cells (■) or spleen cells (□) are also shown.

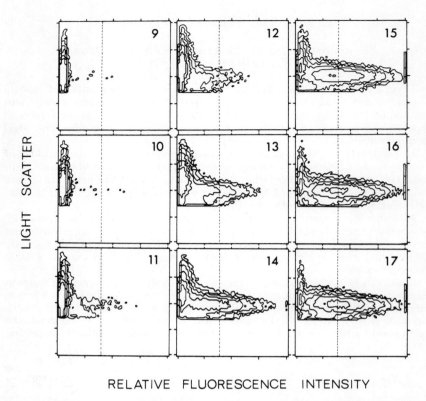

LIGHT SCATTER

RELATIVE FLUORESCENCE INTENSITY

FIGURE 13. Contour plots of correlated light scatter vs. fluorescence FCF analysis of electrophoretically separated CBA/J PP cells stained with Fl-anti-IgD (Ig5a) antibody.

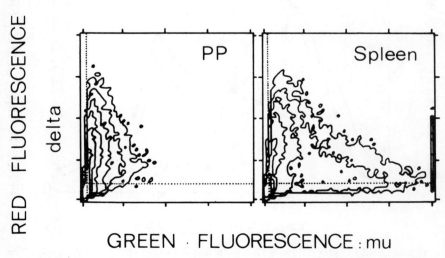

RED FLUORESCENCE

delta

GREEN · FLUORESCENCE : mu

FIGURE 14. Two-color correlated FCF analysis of sIgD vs. sIgM expression on unseparated PP cells and spleen cells from CBA/J mice.

uniformly dull for sIgM. Also, the sIgM-bearing cells recovered in the various electrophoretic fractions of PP cells were in majority dimly fluorescent without any consistent shift in the intensity of staining as a function of EPM, (data not shown). Therefore, the electrophoretic heterogeneity of sIgD-bearing cells from PP cannot apparently be related to variations in their sIg phenotype. In both the anodic part and the cathodic part of the LM population, these cells can be defined as $sIgD^{++} sIgM^+$.

Recent studies have demonstrated that PP cells express higher amounts of sIa than splenocytes.[25] This was confirmed here by two-color FCF analysis of cells stained for both sIa and sIgD. The contour maps presented in the top part of FIGURE 15 indicate that in PP, sIgD-bearing cells are much brighter for sIa than in the spleen. Interestingly, although there was no direct correlation between the intensities of sIgD and sIa staining of PP cells, a subpopulation of $sIgD^- sIa^+$ cells, accounting for about 10% of PP cells, was clearly distinguishable. The determination of the sIgD vs. sIa staining patterns of the electrophoretic fractions of PP cells revealed that despite the absence of variation in the brightness of sIgD staining, there was a definite increase in the intensity of sIa staining with decreasing EPM of the fractions. Although this shift in sIa staining as a function of EPM was progressive, it seems appropriate to distinguish at least two types of sIgD-bearing cells in PP: the fast LM cells which are sIa^+ and the slow LM cells which are sIa^{++}.

FIGURE 15 also shows that $sIgD^- sIa^+$ cells were somewhat more abundant in the anodic LM fractions (e.g. fraction 12: 20%) than in the cathodic LM fractions (e.g. fraction 17: 8%). The nature of these $sIgD^- sIa^+$ PP cells was investigated by two-color FCF analysis. A large proportion of these cells was found to be devoid of T-cell markers (Thy-1, Lyt-1 and Lyt-2) but to carry surface receptor(s) for peanut agglutinin (PNA) (data not shown). The patterns presented in FIGURE 16 indicate that such $sIa^+ PNA^+$ cells were enriched in the anodic LM fractions of PP cells. Recent histological studies have identified the PNA^+ cells from mouse PP as germinal center cells.[26]

CONCLUDING REMARKS

The present studies demonstrate that electrophoretic fractionation combined with FCF analysis provides a powerful tool for the delineation of lymphocyte subsets with distinct surface phenotypes. This approach allowed us to identify two subsets of sIgD-bearing cells in the spleen of CBA/J and NZB mice. The first subset, with relatively high EPM, was characterized as $sIgD^+ sIgM^{++}$ and was present in mice carrying the CBA/N xid defect. The other subset possessed a very low EPM, was $sIgD^{++} sIgM^+$ and was relatively depleted in xid mice. This apparent relationship between the amount of sIgD exposed on the cell surface and cell EPM might be interpreted as the indication that sIgD influences the ionization of the cell surface. However, preliminary experiments of removal of sIgD from the cell surface by capping, suggest that the contribution of sIgD to the cell surface-charge is only marginal. Instead, the electrophoretic disparity observed between these two sIgD-bearing splenocyte subsets probably arise from the expression of other surface molecules which may be quantitatively different on these two subsets.[14] The notion that the amount of sIgD is not per se a major factor determining the electrophoretic heterogeneity of B-cells is indeed sup-

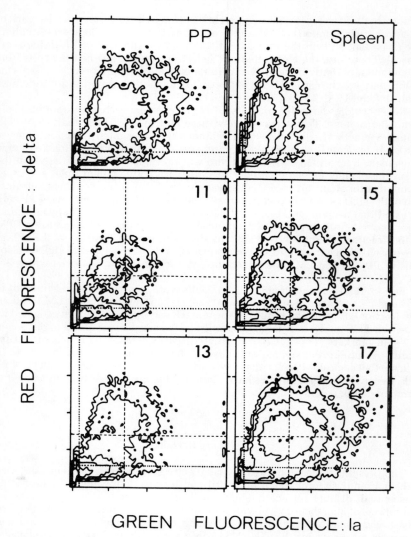

FIGURE 15. Two-color correlated FCF analysis of sIgD vs. sIa expression on unseparated PP cells and spleen cells from CBA/J mice (top) and on electrophoretically fractionated PP cells. The dashed lines are centered on the modal fluorescence intensities of sIgD and sIa stainings. The dotted lines indicate the background fluorescence thresholds.

ported by the finding that in PP, B-cells with different EPM have the same sIgD phenotype. In this case, at least two subsets of sIgD-bearing cells could nevertheless be distinguished on the basis of differences in sIa expression. Thus, the fast LM fractions of PP cells included sIgD^{++} sIgM$^+$ sIa$^+$ cells while the slow LM fractions contained mainly sIgD^{++}sIgM$^+$sIa^{++} cells. Additionally, a significant proportion of PP cells appeared sIgD⁻ sIa⁺. The developmental relationship between these various subsets of splenic and PP sIgD-bearing cells described here remains to be established. The potential of obtaining enriched sIgD-bearing cell subsets by preparative electrophoresis will prove useful for functional studies aimed at the characterization of the biological significance of these subsets.

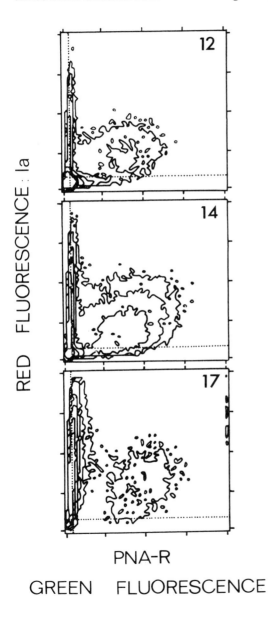

PNA-R

GREEN   FLUORESCENCE

FIGURE 16. Two-color correlated FCF analysis of sIa vs. PNA-R expression on electrophoretically separated PP cells from CBA/J mice.

ACKNOWLEDGMENTS

We wish to thank Dr. Alan Rosenthal for scientific support, Dr. Regina Skelly for administrative help and critical reading of the manuscript and Miss Eileen Frees for typing this manuscript.

REFERENCES

1. HANNIG, K. 1971. Free-flow electrophoresis. In Methods of Microbiology. J. R. NORRIS & D. W. RIBBONS, Eds.: 5B: 513. Academic Press. London, England.
2. MEHRISHI, J. N. 1972. Molecular aspects of the mammalian cell surface. In Progress in Biophysics and Molecular Biology. J. A. BUTLER & D. NOBLE, Eds.: 25: 1. Pergamon Press. Oxford, England.
3. WIOLAND, M., D. SABOLOVIC & C. BURG. 1972. Nature New Biol. 237: 274.
4. ANDERSSON, L. C., S. NORDLING & P. HAYRY. 1973. Cell. Immunol. 8: 235.
5. BOEHMER, H. VON, K. SHORTMAN & G. J. V. NOSSAL. 1974. J. Cell. Physiol. 83: 231.
6. SCHLEGEL, R. A., H. VON BOEHMER & K. SHORTMAN. 1975. Cell. Immunol. 16: 203.
7. ZEILLER, K., G. PASCHER & K. HANNIG. 1976. Immunology 31: 863.
8. DUMONT, F. & P. BISCHOFF. 1977. Ann. Immunol. 128C: 771.
9. HERZENBERG, L. A. & L. A. HERZENBERG. 1979. Analysis and separation using the fluorescence-activated cell sorter (FACS). In Handbook of Experimental Immunology. D. M. WEIR, Ed. 22: 1. Blackwell Scientific Publications. Oxford, England.
10. SCHER, I. 1981. B. lymphocyte development and heterogeneity. Analysis with the immune-defective CBA/N mouse strain. In Immunologic Defects in Laboratory Animals. M. E. GERSHWIN and B. MERCANT, Eds. Vol. 1: 163. Plenum Press, New York, N.Y.
11. DUMONT, F. Combination of two physical parameters for the identification and the separation of lymphocyte subsets. In Methods of Cell Analysis. N. CATSIMPOOLAS, Ed.: 1 Plenum Press, New York, N.Y. In press.
12. MILLER, M. H., J. I. POWELL, S. O. SHARROW & A. R. SCHULTZ. 1978. Rev. Sci. Instrum. 49: 1137.
13. GODING, J. W. & J. E. LAYTON. 1976. J. Exp. Med. 144: 852.
14. AHMED, A. & A. H. SMITH. CRC Rev. Immunol. In press.
15. KESSLER, S. W., V. L. WOODS, F. D. FINKELMAN & I. SCHER. 1979. J. Immunol. 123: 2772.
16. WOODS, V. J., S. W. KESSLER, F. D. FINKELMAN, A. LIEBERMAN, I. SCHER & W. E. PAUL. 1980. J. Immunol. 125: 2699.
17. COHEN, P. L., F. S. LIGLER, M. ZIFF & E. S. VITETTA. 1978. Arthritis Rheum. 21: 551.
18. IZUI, S., P. J. MCCONAHEY & F. J. DIXON. 1978. J. Immunol. 121: 2213.
19. SCHER, I., A. K. BERNING, S. KESSLER & F. D. FINKELMAN. 1980. J. Immunol. 125: 1686.
20. OHSUGI, Y., M. E. GERSHWIN & A. AHMED. 1981. J. Immunogenetics 8.
21. BOURGOIS, A., K. KITAJIMA, I. R. HUNTER & B. A. ASKONAS. 1977. Eur. J. Immunol. 7: 151.
22. DUMONT, F. 1975. Ann. Immunol. 126C: 453.
23. KRCO, C. J., S. J. CHALLACOMBE, W. P. LAFUSE, C. S. DAVID & T. B. TOMASI. 1981. Cell Immunol. 57: 420.
24. MATTINGLY, J. A. & B. H. WAKSMAN. 1978. J. Immunol. 121: 1878.
25. MOND, J. J., S. KESSLER, F. D. FINKELMAN, W. E. PAUL & I. SCHER. 1980. J. Immunol. 124: 1675.
26. ROSE, M. & F. MALCHOIDI. 1981. Immunology 42: 583.

DISCUSSION OF THE PAPER

P. W. KINCADE: Herima Genucchi in my lab, using NZB mice, has found that there is a very rapid decline in B-cell precursors in the bone marrow. By the time the mice are about 15 weeks old they have virtually no cells in their bone marrow that are identifiable as precursors of B-cells, which might suggest that they aren't making a lot of B-cells after that time. This is also true for CB and normal mice but these mice need to be over two years old. My question to you and perhaps also to Dr. Vitetta relates to the IgD expression in NZB mice. It seemed to me there was some difference with 12-week-old spleens, between your results and those that she reported earlier regarding the $\mu = \delta$ expression in these mice. Did you look at NZB Peyer's patches?

F. DUMONT: Not yet.

KINCADE: Has anybody looked at very old normal mice?

DUMONT: In NZB mice as they age, a shift in the pattern of sIgD versus sIgM staining appears. The sIgD bright cells tend to disappear or to be flooded by a large number of sIgD dull cells. Also, in these NZB mice there is actually a lower frequency of B-cells than in other mouse strains. They have about 10 to 15% less B-cells than CBA or DBA2 mice.

KINCADE: And you haven't looked at very old normal mice?

DUMONT: In very old normal mice there is no significant change in the pattern when the mice are healthy.

I. SCHER: This looks like a very powerful multi-technique for separating out B-cells and I was just wondering if you had an opportunity to look at the function of these cells separated by this technique in terms of their responses to antigens or their MLS reactivity?

DUMONT: We have preliminary experiments in collaboration with Dr. R. Skelly regarding the response to TNP *ficoll* and TNP-LPS. The responses appear to correlate with what is known of the response of the B-cells subset to these antigens. That's all we have done so far.

F. FINKELMAN: You seem to get a good degree of separation of the spleen cell populations but there is still considerable overlap. If you subject a population that has gone through electrophoresis once to a repeat electrophoresis do you get further separation or do you really have overlap between the μ - δ ratios in different populations?

DUMONT: You cannot get higher resolution. What should be done is associate this with other physical techniques. There is a limitation in the resolution of the separation with the presently available equipment..

FINKELMAN: Can you say anything about the surface μ δ phenotype of the PNA positive cells from spleen or Peyer's patches?

DUMONT: In the spleen the frequency of these PNA positive cells is very low, on the order of 5%. In the Peyer's patches it varies between 15 and 25% and there these cells, at least when examined in the FACS on linear amplification, appear completely negative for sIgD, negative for sIgM and very dull for total sIg and it's possible that they are positive for sIgA, but very dull. And the other markers are Ia and FC receptor.

THE DISTRIBUTION OF SURFACE IgD ON B-LYMPHOCYTES OF MICE: TWO PARAMETER CORRELATION WITH SURFACE IgM AND Ia*

I. Scher, J. A. Titus, S. O. Sharrow,
J. J. Mond, and F. D. Finkelman

Naval Medical Research Institute
and
Department of Medicine
Uniformed Services University of the Health Sciences
and
Immunology Branch, National Cancer Institute
National Institutes of Health
Bethesda, Maryland 20205

INTRODUCTION

B-cells are distinguished from other lymphoid cells by the presence of easily detected immunoglobulin (Ig) on their surfaces.[1,2] This surface Ig (sIg) serves as an antigen specific receptor for these cells and marks different B-cell populations. These subpopulations have been distinguished by studies using developing immunologically normal and immune-defective CBA/N mice.[3] Early studies on this topic using immunoprecipitation and sodium-dodecylsulfate-polyacryl-amide-gel-electrophoresis, demonstrated IgM on the surface membranes of B-cells from neonatal mice. This sIgM persisted during maturation and was supplemented with sIgD during the second and third weeks of life.[4] More recent analysis of the sIg of B-cells using single parameter flow microfluorometric techniques with the Fluorescence Activated Cell Sorter (FACS), confirmed that sIgD appeared after sIgM during development, and demonstrated that immature murine splenic B-cells have a high density of sIgM and had no, or low densities of sIgD.[5,6] As mice matured, the relative density of their B-cell sIgM decreased, coincident with an increase in their B-cell sIgD. It was also shown that the density of B-cell surface Ia encoded antigens (sIa) also distinguished different B-cell subpopulations, since B-cells of immature mice had higher densities of sIa than B-cells of adult mice.[7] These data were limited, because the sIgM, sIgD and sIa characteristics of individual B-cells could only be inferred on the basis of these findings. Thus, although the relative mean density of the sIgM and sIa on B-cells of adult mice was low, and that of sIgD was high when compared to the relative mean density of these surface membrane markers on the B-cells of adult mice, the surface membrane phenotype of individual cells could not be determined.

*This work was supported in part by the Naval Medical Research and Development Command Research Task No. M0095-PN.001.1030; in part by the Uniformed Services University of the Health Sciences Research Protocol No. C08310 and in part by the National Naval Medical Center Clinical Investigation No. 3-06-132. The opinions and assertions contained herein are the private ones of the author and are not to be construed as official or reflecting the views of the Navy Department or the naval service at large. The experiments reported herein were conducted according to the principles set forth in the current edition of the *Guide for the Care and Use of Laboratory Animals,* Institute of Laboratory Animals Resources, National Research Council.

0077-8923/82/0399-0204/0 $01.75 © 1982, NYAS

Therefore, it was possible that subpopulations of B-cells existed that had densities of sIgM, sIgD or sIa that were distinct from the mean densities of these constituents, as determined by single parameter analysis.

In this study we have utilized a dual laser, dual parameter FACS to characterize the density of two surface markers, sIgD and sIgM, or sIgD and sIa on individual B-cells derived from the lymphoid organs of normal and immune defective CBA/N mice. Two major subpopulations of B-cells have been defined after analysis with anti-μ and anti-δ antibodies. These groups appear at different times during development and represent varying frequencies of the total sIg$^+$ cells in the spleen and bone marrow of mice during development. The data obtained when using anti-δ and anti-Ia antibodies confirm that the sIa density of B-cells decreases during development; however, cells labeled with these reagents do not segregate into two distinct subpopulations when analyzed with the dual parameter FACS.

MATERIALS AND METHODS

Source of Animals, Preparation and Staining of Lymphoid Cells

The C3H/HeN and (CBA/N × DBA/2)F$_1$ mice used in this study were obtained from the Small Animal Section, Division of Research Services, National Institutes of Health, Bethesda, Maryland and Flow Laboratories, Rockville, Maryland, respectively. The techniques used to prepare single cell suspensions of lymphoid cells derived from mice sacrificed by cervical dislocation have been previously described.[5,6] These cells were labeled by incubating 1×10^6 cells in 50 μl of RPMI-1640, with 10% fetal calf serum and 1% sodium azide, using optimum amounts of one each of the following fluorescence conjugated (Fl) or biotinylated antibodies (B); 1) Fl rabbit anti-mouse δ (RaMδ), 2) Fl RaMμ, 3) Fl RaFerritin (RaFer), 4) the mouse anti-mouse Ia^k hybridoma 10-2.16 (BMaMIa), or 5) the mouse hybridoma CBPC-101 (BMaP). The FlRaFer and BMaP served as control stains for the FlRaMμ or FlRaMδ and BMaMIa, respectively, and were used at concentrations equivalent to those used to stain cells with these later reagents. Following this first incubation with one of the directly conjugated Fl or biotinylated antibodies, the cells were washed two times with 3cc of media and incubated for 20 min at 4°C with optimum amounts of "Texas Red" (Molecular Probes, Inc., Plano, Texas) conjugated avidin (Tr).[8] After two additional washes, the cells were resuspended into 0.7 cc of media in preparation for their FACS analysis. The biotinylated antibodies used in the indirect Tr-avidin staining procedure will be referred to as TrRaMμ, TrMaMIa, TrRaFer and TrMaP.

Purification of Antibodies

The affinity purified F(ab')$_2$ fragment of RaMδ was prepared from the sera of rabbits immunized with the IgDκ myeloma protein TEPC-1017.[9] A 50% saturated (NH$_4$)$_2$SO$_4$ cut of 100 ml of this antiserum was dialyzed against 0.1 M acetate buffer, pH 4.5, and digested for 18 hr at 37°C with pepsin (Calbiochem-Behring Corp, La Jolla, Ca.) (enzyme: protein ratio = 1:50), then dialyzed against 0.1 M Tris, pH 8.3 and centrifuged for 1 hr at 100,000 G. The supernatant was sequentially absorbed twice with TEPC-183 (IgMκ) bound to CNBr activated

Sepharose 4B (Pharmacia Fine Chemicals, Piscataway, N.J.) and normal mouse serum—Sepharose, then incubated overnight with 10 ml of normal mouse serum and again centrifuged for 1 hr at 100,000 G. The supernatant was adsorbed to a column containing TEPC-1033 (IgDκ)-Sepharose,[9] that was then washed with 0.1M Tris, pH 8.3 and eluted with 3.5M MgCl$_2$. The eluate was dialyzed against 0.15M NaCl, and passed over a Protein A-Sepharose (Pharmacia Fine Chemicals) to remove undigested rabbit IgG. The column effluent contained greater than 95% F(ab')$_2$ fragment of rabbit IgG, which was specific for mouse δ chain by radioimmunoassay and Ouchterlony analysis. The F(ab')$_2$ fragment of RaMμ antibody was prepared from the sera of rabbits immunized with MOPC-104E (IgMλ) that was (NH$_4$)$_2$SO$_4$ fractionated and pepsin digested, as above, then absorbed with TEPC-1017-Sepharose, Ig-depleted normal mouse serum-Sepharose, and normal mouse IgG-Sepharose. The absorbed pepsin-digested antiserum was adsorbed to and eluted from TEPC-183-Sepharose, dialyzed against 0.15M NaCl, and adsorbed with Protein A-Sepharose. The absorbed affinity purified F(ab')$_2$ fragment was specific for mouse μ chain by RIA and Ouchterlony analysis. The F(ab')$_2$ fragment of affinity purified RaFer was prepared from the sera of rabbits immunized with bovine ferritin (Calbiochem-Behring) that was pepsin digested, adsorbed to and eluted from ferritin-Sepharose, and absorbed with Protein A-Sepharose. This antibody had no detectable reactivity with mouse spleen cell surface molecules. The murine hybridoma 10-2.16[10] obtained from the Salk Institute Cell Distribution Center, (La Jolla, Ca.) was grown in fetal calf serum supplemented RPMI-1640 as previously described.[11] The IgG$_{2a}$ secreted by this cell line, which has specificity for Ia^k, was purified by adsorption to and elution from Protein A-Sepharose.

Fluorescein and Biotin Conjugation of Antibodies

Affinity purified 10-2.16 and affinity purified F(ab')$_2$ fragments of RaMδ and RaFer were labeled with fluorescein isothiocyanate (FITC) by incubating saline solutions of these antibodies in the presence of 0.07 M Na$_2$CO$_3$, pH 9.5 with 2 mg of 10% FITC on celite (Celbiochem-Behring) per 10 mg of protein for two hours at room temperature. Celite was removed from the FITC-labeled antibody by centrifugation, and Sephadex G25 gel filtration was used to separate FITC-antibody from free hydrolyzed FITC. FITC-antibodies prepared in this manner had molar F:P ratio of 2.0-3.5. Affinity purified 10-2.16 and affinity purified F(ab')$_2$ fragments of RaMμ were biotinylated by mixing 1 mg/ml solutions of these antibodies in 0.15 M NaCl/0.1 M NaHlCO$_3$, pH 8.0 with a 10 mg/ml solution of (+)-biotin N-hydroxy-succinimide ester (Calbiochem-Behring) in DMSO (Fisher Scientific Company, Pittsburgh, Pa.). Twenty μl of this solution was added per mg of protein, and the resulting solution was incubated for two hours at room temperature, and then dialyzed against 0.15 M NaCl. A 10 mg/ml solution of Avidin (Sigma Chemical Co., St. Louis, Mo.) was prepared and dialyzed against 0.15 M NaCl. A 10 mg/ml solution of Avidin (Sigma Chemical Co., St. Louis, Mo.) was prepared and dialyzed against 0.15 M NaCl. One ml of this solution was mixed with 4 ml of 0.15 M NaCl and 0.5 ml of 1 M NaHCO$_3$, pH 9.0 plus a solution of 1 mg of Texas Red (8) (Molecular Probes Inc., Plano, Texas) dissolved in 200 μl of acetonitrile (Sigma) that had been made anhydrous by absorption with Davison Molecular Sieves, type 4A, grade 514 (Fisher Scientific). All solutions were cooled to 0°C before mixing, and were incubated at the same temperature for four hours after they were added to each other. Texas Red-avidin was separated from free hydrolyzed Texas Red by sephadex G25 gel filtration. Texas Red-avidin conjugates prepared in this manner had A_{596}/A_{280} ratios of 0.75 to 1.0.

Dual Parameter Fluorescence Analysis

The studies reported in this paper were performed using a FACS (Becton Dickenson, Mt. View, Ca.), modified for dual parameter analysis by the addition of a krypton ion laser and more sophisticated electronic components. In addition, an electronic interface designed by the Division of Computer Research and Technology, Computer Systems Laboratory of the NIH was installed to allow for

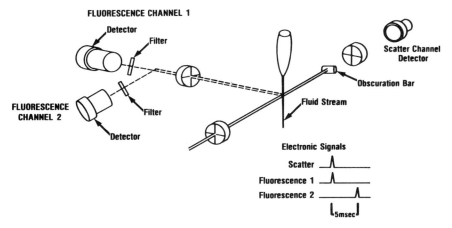

FIGURE 1. A schematic of the dual laser Fluorescence Activated Cell Sorter is shown. Light from argon and krypton ion lasers excites cells at 488 nm and 568.2 nm, respectively, in a sequential manner as the cells tranverse a distance of approximately 350 μm in the fluid sheath. Fluorescence signals 1 and 2 are detected by two different photomultiplier tubes that have filters interposed before them to preclude crossover between signals. The electronic signals generated from the scatter of the laser light by a cell crossing the fluid sheath-laser intersect point, as well as those generated by the excitation of a cell bearing both fluorescein and Texas red probes.

three parameter data processing. This interface permits the operator to gate on one parameter while acquiring the second and third parameters. In all instances, we gated on the scatter signal and acquired the two additional parameters as two single, or one dual fluorescence profile. This enabled us to exclude most nonviable cells, cellular debris and clumps of two or more cells from the fluorescence analysis.[5,6] A detailed explanation of the principles of dual parameter FACS analysis has been published.[11,12] It should be noted however, that the cells passing through the FACS during dual parameter analysis are interrogated by the argon and krypton ion lasers at different points in the fluid stream (FIGURE 1). Thus, the green (argon laser) and yellow (krypton laser) signals (fluorescence 1 and 2) generated from one cell appear as distinct electronic impulses separated in time by 50 msec. These signals are detected by two different photomultiplier tubes which have filters placed before them to exclude signals from the other channel, precluding crossover between the two fluorescence signals. The electronic signals generated by this system are stored and retrieved via a PDP-11 computer (Digital Equipment Corp., Maynard, Mass.) using software developed by the Division of Computer Research and Technology, Computer Systems Laboratory of the NIH.

RESULTS

Characteristics of Dual Parameter FACS Analysis

When adult spleen cells are stained with FlRaMδ or TrRaMμ antibodies and analyzed with the FACS, characteristic fluorescence profiles are generated[5] (FIGURE 2). The single parameter fluorescence profile observed after labeling with anti-δ antibodies is bimodal, and sIgD[−] and sIgD[+] cells are easily distinguished. The fluorescence profile of anti-μ stained cells is different from that of anti-δ labeled cells, since very dull sIgM[+] cells, whose fluorescence intensity is only slightly greater than sIgM[−] cells, represent a large majority of the sIgM[+] cells in

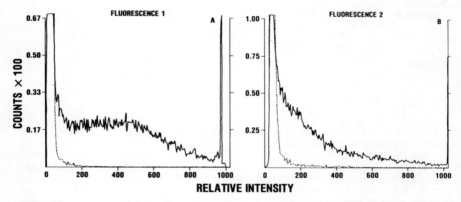

FIGURE 2. The Fluorescence 1 (FlRaMδ) and Fluorescence 2 (TrRaMμ) single parameter profiles (a and b respectively), of spleen cells from a 12-week-old (CBA/N × DBA/2)F₁ female mouse. These profiles were generated from cells stained with both probes, but the data was handled as single parameter. The dashed line in each profile represents the staining of FlRaFer or TrRaFer antibodies.

the spleens of adult mice. In the single parameter analysis shown in FIGURE 2, the X-axis is divided into 1000 linearly increasing channels, so that cells accumulating in channel 15 have tenfold less fluorescence than cells accumulating in channel 150. This provides a great deal of selectivity in determining the channel that distinguishes positively from negatively stained cells. With dual parameter analysis, there being two separate parameters for the instrument to register, the signals generated for each parameter are divided into 64 channels, representing linear increases in fluorescence intensity. Therefore, although a cell can be placed in $64^2 = 4096$ different stations according to its two parameters, the

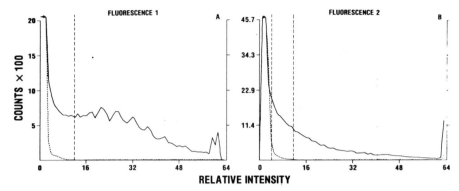

FIGURE 3. The Fluorescence 1 (FlRaMδ) and Fluorescence 2 (TrRaMμ) single parameter profiles (a and b respectively) of spleen cells from a 12-week-old (CBA/N × DBA/2)F₁ female mouse. These profiles were generated by a computer from data acquired as dual parameter. The vertical dotted lines indicate the channels separating the different groups of cells (see text). The dashed line in each profile represents the staining of FlRaFer and TrRaFer antibodies.

selectivity within one parameter is greatly diminished (64 vs. 1000 channels) when compared to single parameter analysis. The fluorescence profiles shown in FIGURE 3 illustrate this point. These profiles were computer generated using a program which draws either of the single parameter fluorescence profiles of a dual parameter analyses.

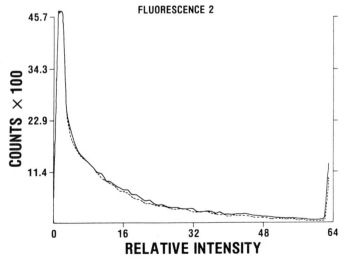

FIGURE 4. The single parameter Fluorescence 2 profiles (TrRaMμ) of two different dual parameter experiments where FlRaMδ or FlMaMIa were used as the Fluorescence 1 stain.

Although the filters and design of the dual parameter FACS make it theoretically impossible for the green (fluorescein) or red (Texas Red) signals to cross outside of their respective channels and detectors, we performed two types of experiments to insure that this was not a problem. Cells stained with one probe were analyzed using the single parameter system and the fluorescence profile generated was compared to the single parameter fluoresence profile of the same population of cells stained with both the Fl and Tr conjugated probes. In no instance did the addition of the second probe influence the fluorescence profile of the individually stained sample (data not shown). Further, the single parameter profiles of cells stained with a reagent such as TrRaMμ were identical whether FlRaMδ or FlMaMIa or no Fl-antibodies was used as a second reagent (FIGURE 4).

FlRaMδ and TrRaMμ Dual Parameter FACS Analysis of Adult Spleen and Bone Marrow Cells

Studies of the sIgM and sIgD on B-cells of developing mice have indicated that the B-cells of immature animals have a high density of sIgM but little or no sIgD.[5,6] With maturation the average density of sIgM decreases while the frequency of sIgD$^+$ cells increases, as does the density of sIgD on these sIgD$^+$ cells. These data, as well as experiments where the functional properties of cells with different densities of sIgM or sIgD were studied,[13-15] suggested that sIgM bright-sIgD dull cells could be considered a distinct subpopulation from a sIgM dull-sIgD intermediate-bright cells. However, there was no direct evidence that such populations actually had these sIg characteristics. This was particularly true in the case of sIg$^+$ spleen cells of immature mice or those found in the bone marrow of adult mice, where the frequency of sIgD$^+$ cells is less than sIgM$^+$ cells. Thus, the sIgD$^+$ cells from these sources could have had any sIgM characteristic, from sIgM$^-$ to sIgM bright. Similarly, although it was presumed that the dull sIgM$^+$ cells of adult mice bore intermediate-high densities of sIgD, this was inferred from studies wherein certain functions of dull sIgM$^+$ and intermediate-high sIgD$^+$ splenic B-cells were shown to be similar, but distinct from bright sIgM$^+$ or dull sIgD$^+$ cells.

FIGURE 3 demonstrates the single parameter fluorescence profiles generated from a dual parameter FACS study of FlRaMδ and TrRαMμ stained 12-week-old mouse spleen cells. Isometric diplays of this data are shown in FIGURE 5. These data can also be displayed in the form of a contour map, with different levels depicting a particular cell number. For example, in FIGURE 6a, which is a dual parameter contour map of the same data presented in FIGURE 3 and 5, four levels of cells are shown, 5, 10, 20 and 30. Level 5 is depicted by a line drawn between points where there are five cells. Points lying outside that line have < 5 cells, whereas points lying inside that line have > 5 cells. Similarly, the lines drawn for levels 10, 20 and 30 have those numbers of cells at the line and less than or greater than those numbers outside or inside those lines.

The cells depicted in the contour map shown in FIGURE 6a appear to be segregated into "islands," representing populations which have different staining characteristics. In the region where sIg$^-$ cells are found (Fluorescence 1, channels 0-4; Fluorescence 2, channels 0-3), large numbers of cells representing T, null and accessory cells are seen. Extending out from this area are two "islands" of sIg$^+$ cells, one with the largest number of cells, encompassing a large area in the lower right portion of the map and with four levels represented, and a second encompassing a smaller area in the upper left portion of the map and with only

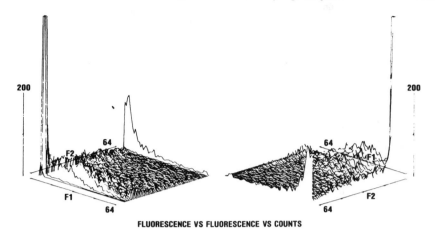

FLUORESCENCE VS FLUORESCENCE VS COUNTS

FIGURE 5. The Fluorescence 1 (FlRaMδ) and Fluorescence 2 (TrRaMμ) dual parameter isometric profiles of spleen cells from a 12-week-old (CBA/N × DBA/2)F$_1$ female mouse. Two views of the same data, rotated by 180°, are shown.

the two lower levels represented. This second grouping of cells can be characterized as being sIgD$^-$, or very low sIgD$^+$ with a heterogeneous distribution of sIgM. (Fluorescence 1, channels 1–12; Fluorescence 2, channels 4–64, see FIGURE 4). The group which is represented in larger numbers has a relatively low-intermediate density of sIgM and a intermediate to high density of sIgD (Fluorescence 1, channels 13–64; Fluorescence 2 channels 4–32, see FIGURES 4 and 7).

The number of cells in these populations was calculated using a computer

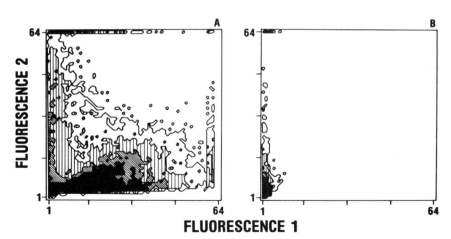

FIGURE 6. The Fluorescence 1 (FlRaMδ) and Fluorescence 2 (TrRaMμ) dual parameter contour map of spleen cells from a 12-week-old (CBA/N × DBA/2)F$_1$ female mouse. Four levels are shown, corresponding to 5, 10, 20 and 30 cells (6a). The control dual parameter contour map using FlRaFer and TrRaFer is also shown (6a). The four levels shown correspond to 5, 10, 20 and 30 cells.

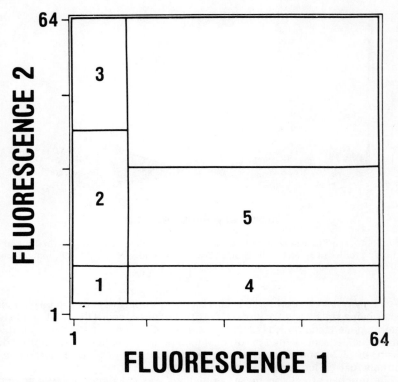

FIGURE 7. The coordinates of the five groups used to determine the frequency of sIgM⁺ cells for FlRaMδ (Fluorescence 1) and TrRaMμ (Fluorescence 2) staining.

program which determines the number of cells within coordinates set on Fluorescence channels 1 and 2. FIGURE 6b is the dual parameter fluorescence profile of the same adult spleen cells depicted in FIGURE 6a, but stained with FlRaFer and TrRaFer antibodies. Very few cells are stained with the FlRaFer beyond Fluorescence 1 channel 6, whereas in the Fluorescence 2 channel, cells

TABLE 1

DISTRIBUTION OF sIgM⁺ CELLS IN THE TWO PARAMETER F1RaMδ AND TrRaMμ
FLUORESCENCE PROFILES OF 12 WEEK OLD SPLEEN AND BONE MARROW CELLS OF A
(CBA/N × DBA/2)F₁ FEMALE MOUSE

Group	Fluorescence 1	Fluorescence 2	Percent of sIgM⁺ Cells Spleen (Figure 6)	Bone Marrow (Figure 7)
1	1–12	4–11	0.0	0
2	1–12	12–40	14.9	45.5
3	1–12	41–64	9.8	13.1
4	13–64	4–11	36.8	19.2
5	13–64	12–32	34.5	21.0
all	1–64	4–11	51.5	12.8

are stained with the TrRaFer reagent out to, and beyond channel 16. This indicates that the Tr avidin-B antibodies tend to interact nonspecifically with spleen cells to a larger extent than the Fl-antibodies. TABLE 1 lists the frequency of cells within a coordinate set, calculated using the number of sIgM$^+$ cells as 100%, and after background subtraction of the number of cells in the equivalent coordinate set of the control (FIGURE 6b). Five coordinate sets were chosen based on our interpretation of the significant group of cells delineated by dual parameter analysis of sIgM and sIgD. Their coordinates are shown in TABLE 1 and Figures 3 and 7 and represent cells with: 1) very low sIgM and negative or low sIgD; 2) low-intermediate sIgM and negative or low sIgD; 3) high sIgM and negative or low sIgD; 4) very low sIgM and intermediate-high IgD; and 5) intermediate sIgM and intermediate-high sIgD. The frequency of sIgM$^+$ cells in each coordinate set, expressed as the percentage of the total sIgM$^+$ cells was determined using the

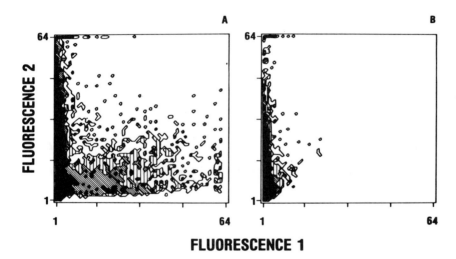

FIGURE 8. The Fluorescence 1 (FlRaMδ) and Fluorescence 2 (TrRaMμ) dual parameter contour map of bone marrow cells from a 12-week-old (CBA/N $\times$ DBA/2)F$_1$ female mouse (8a). Four levels are shown, corresponding to 2, 3, 5 and 8 cells. The control dual parameter contour map using FlRaFer and TrRaFer is also shown (8b). The four levels shown correspond to 2, 3, 5 and 8 cells.

coordinate set defining all sIgM$^+$ cells (Fluorescence 1 channels = 1–64, Fluorescence 2 channels = 4–64). In this experiment 24.7% (0 + 14.9 + 9.8) of the sIgM$^+$ cells have negative or low sIgD (groups 1, 2 and 3) while 71.3% (36.8 + 34.5) have very low-intermediate sIgM and intermediate-high sIgD (groups 4 and 5) (TABLE 1).

In order to determine if the groups of B-cells defined by anti-μ and anti-δ dual parameter analysis were unique to splenic cell populations, we studied the distribution of sIgM and sIgD on bone marrow cells of adult mice (FIGURE 8b). In order to make a direct comparison with the populations found in spleen, the levels used to draw the bone marrow contour map (levels 2, 3, 5, 8) were decreased in proportion to the frequency of sIgM$^+$ cells in the spleen cell population shown in FIGURE 6a. In contrast to the findings with adult spleen cells, the largest number of sIgM⁺ bone marrow cells had negative or low sIgD (groups 1, 2 and 3), representing 58.6% of the sIgM⁺ cells (0 + 45.5 + 13.1), while the very low-intermediate sIgM and intermediate-high sIgD cells (groups 4 and 5) represented 40.2% of the sIgM⁺ cells (19.2 + 21.0) (Table 1).

FlαMδ and TRαMμ Dual Parameter FACS Analysis of Spleen Cells of Developing Mice

The finding that the intermediate-high sIgM, negative or low sIgD cells (groups 2 and 3) are the predominate sIg⁺ bone marrow cells, whereas these cells

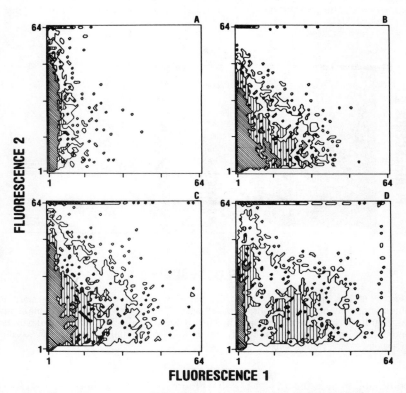

FIGURE 9. The Fluorescence 1 (FlRaMδ) and Fluorescence 2 (TrRaMμ) dual parameter contour maps of spleen cells from 5 day (9a), 2.5 week (9b), 5 week (9c) or 12 week (9d) old C3H/HeN mice. Three levels are shown, corresponding to 7, 14 and 22 (9a), 4, 8 and 12 (9b), 3, 7 and 11 (9c) and 2, 3 and 8 (9d) cells.

represent a minority of the sIg⁺ cells in the spleens of adult mice, suggests that these groups represent earlier appearing B-cells, while groups 4 and 5 are later appearing sIg⁺ populations. This was further studied by analysis of FlRaMδ and TrRaMμ stained spleen cells from 5 day, 2.5, 5 and 12-week-old C3H/HeN mice (FIGURE 9).

TABLE 2

DISTRIBUTION OF sIgM⁺ CELLS IN THE TWO PARAMETER F1RaMδ AND TrRaMμ
FLUORESCENCE PROFILES OF SPLEEN CELLS FROM 5 DAY, 2.5, 5 AND 8 WEEK OLD
C3H/HeN MICE

	Fluorescence		Percent of sIgM⁺ Cells (Figure 8)			
Group	1	2	5 days	2.5 weeks	5 weeks	8 weeks
1	1–12	4–11	20.2	0.0	0.0	0
2	1–12	12–40	58.5	46.7	39.6	20.9
3	1–12	41–64	13.7	5.8	13.5	13.4
4	13–64	4–11	1.5	16.7	15.1	18.9
5	13–64	12–32	3.6	26.2	31.8	46.2
all	1–64	4–64	11.5	20.8	21.2	39.4

The distribution of sIgM⁺ cells in the spleen of 12-week-old C3H/HeN mice is similar to that of 12-week-old (CBA/N × DBA/2)F₁ female mice (compare Figures 6a with 9d), with the majority of cells having a very low-intermediate sIgM and a intermediate-high sIgD density with 66.1% in groups 4 and 5 (TABLE 2). As spleen cells from younger mice are studied, the frequency of sIgM⁺ cells in groups 4 and 5 decreased from 66.1% to 46.9% (15.1 + 31.8), to 42.9% (16.7 + 26.2) to 5.1% (1.5 + 3.6) at 12, 5 and 2.5 weeks and 5 days, respectively. This was associated with an increase in the low-intermediate-high sIgM, negative or low sIgD cells (groups 2 and 3) from 34.3% (20.9 + 13.4), to 53.1% (39.6 + 13.5), to 52.5% (46.7 + 5.8), to 72.2% (58.5 + 13.7) (TABLE 2). Furthermore, whereas there were no very-low sIgM, negative or low sIgD cells (group 1) in the spleens of 2.5, 5 or 12-week-old mice, 20.2% of the sIgM⁺ spleen cells of five-day-old mice were found in this group.

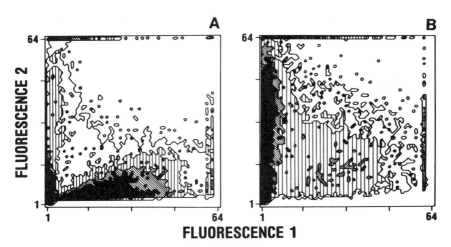

FIGURE 10. The Fluorescence 1 (FlRaMδ) and Fluorescence 2 (TrRaMμ) dual parameter contour maps of spleen cells from a 12-week-old (CBA/N × DBA/2)F₁ female (10a) and a 12-week-old F₁ male mouse (10b). Four levels are shown, corresponding to 5, 10, 20 and 30 (10a) and 3, 5, 10 and 15 (10b) cells.

FlRaMδ and TrRaMμ Dual Parameter FACS Analysis of Adult Spleen and Bone Marrow Cells of (CBA/N × DBA/2)F₁ Male and Female Mice

CBA/N mice have an X-linked immune-defect resulting in a decrease in the frequency and number of sIg^+ cells in their lymphoid organs.[16] The splenic B-cells of these mice, and F_1 males derived from crosses of CBA/N females and immunologically normal male mice, have a higher mean density of sIgM and a lower mean density of sIgD than the B-cells of normal mice, when analyzed by single parameter FACS analysis.[6,17] Furthermore, the time in development when the frequency of $sIgD^+$ spleen cells equals that of $sIgM^+$ cells is delayed in CBA/N mice, when compared to normal mice. It was of particular interest, therefore, to study the sIgM and sIgD of B-cells of these immune-defective mice. FIGURE 10 is a composite of two dual parameter FACS fluorescence profiles of FlRaMδ and TrRaMμ stained spleen cells of 12-week-old immunologically normal (CBA/N × DBA/2)F₁ female and their immune-defective F_1 male littermates. The predominate $sIgM^+$ population of spleen in the immunologically normal F_1 female mouse was cells found in the very low-intermediate sIgM, intermediate-high sIgD population, representing 71.3% (groups 4 and 5), while 24.7% had little or no sIgD (groups 1, 2 and 3) (FIGURE 10a) (TABLE 3). By contrast, these groups represented 41.5% and 50.7% of the $sIgM^+$ spleen cells of F_1 male mice respectively. It should also be pointed out that the largest differences were in the frequencies of the very-low sIgM cells (group 4) which represented 36.8% vs. 10.7% of the $sIgM^+$ cells of F_1 female and male mice respectively.

FlRaMδ and TrMaMIa Dual Parameter FACS Analysis of Spleen Cells of Adult (CBA/N × DBA/2)F₁ Male and Female Mice

The dual parameter fluorescence profiles of FlRaMδ and TrMaMIa stained spleen cells of a 12-week-old (CBA × DBA/2)F₁ female is shown in FIGURE 11a. It is instructive to compare this profile with that shown in Figure 10a, since the cells were derived from the same animal and the Fluorescence 1 portion of both profiles represents FlRaMδ staining. The major difference in these two profiles is the absence of the two distinct "islands" of cells that one sees in the FlαMδ and TRαMμ stained study (FIGURE 10a). The gains at which these studies were performed, i.e., the voltage applied to the Fluorescence 2 photomultiplier tube, were equivalent in these two studies; furthermore, optimum amounts of the

TABLE 3

DISTRIBUTION OF $sIgM^+$ CELLS IN THE TWO PARAMETER F1RaMδ AND TrRaMμ FLUORESCENCE PROFILES OF SPLEEN CELLS FROM 12 WEEK OLD (CBA/N × DBA/2)F₁ MALE AND FEMALE MICE

Group	Fluorescence		Percent of $sIgM^+$ Cells (Figure 9)	
	1	2	F_1 Male	F_1 Female
1	1–12	4–11	0.0	0.0
2	1–12	12–40	30.6	14.9
3	1–12	41–64	20.1	9.8
4	13–64	4–11	10.7	36.8
5	13–64	12–32	30.8	34.5
all			30.2	51.5

TrRaMμ and TrMaMIa antibodies were used. Therefore, the fluorescence intensity of the TRMaMIa stained cells or their sIa density, is relatively homogeneous when compared to the fluorescence intenstiy, or sIgM density of TrRaMμ stained cells.

The FlRaMδ and TrMaMIa dual parameter fluorescence profiles of (CBA/N × DBA/2)F₁ male adult spleen cells is shown in FIGURE 11b. Two comparisons are of interest, the first with the profile shown in Figure 11b, which is a FlRaMδ and TrRaMμ study of the same cells, and the second with Figure 11a, which is that of FlRaMδ and TrMaMIa stained spleen cells. The relative homogeneity of the Fluorescence 2 TrMaMIa staining is much greater than that of the TrRaMμ staining in the cáse of the F₁ male mice, as was seen with the immunologically-normal F₁ female mice. Comparisons of the fluorescence profiles of FlRaMδ and TrMaMIa stained F₁ male and female spleen cells reveals a relative increase in the sIa staining and a decrease in the relative intensity of sIgD staining of the F₁ male spleen cells.

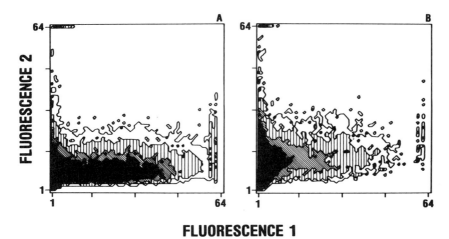

FLUORESCENCE 1

FIGURE 11. The Fluorescence 1 (FlRaMδ) and Fluorescence 2 (TrMaMIa) dual parameter contour maps of spleen cells from a 12-week-old (CBA/N × DBA/2)F₁ female (11a) and a 12-week-old F₁ male mouse (11b). Four levels are shown, corresponding to 5, 10, 20 and 30 (11a) and 3, 5, 10 and 15 (11b) cells.

DISCUSSION

A considerable body of evidence supports the hypothesis that the B-cells of adult mice do not represent a homogeneous population of cells that differ only in the antigen-combining properties of their sIg. Rather, these cells appear to have distinctive surface membrane markers,[3,15] densities of sIgM and sIgD,[5,6,17] and triggering requirements. Two major groups of B-cells have been defined by these characteristics. The first subpopulation appears early in development, and is the predominant B-cell in the spleens of normal mice during their first two–three weeks of life. These B-cells have a relatively high mean density of sIgM when compared to the B-cells in the spleens of adult mice, while their sIgD density is low, when studied with single parameter FACS analysis. Indeed, the frequency of sIgM$^+$ cells is greater than sIgD$^+$ cells during this time of development, indicating that many of the sIgM$^+$ cells lack sIgD. In addition, these cells either fail, or have a very poor capacity to stimulate a Mls determined mixed lymphocyte reaction[13] and do not bear the Lyb 3, 5 or 7 alloantigens.[18-20] These Lyb 5$^-$ cells, which also represent a minority of the B-cells in the spleens of adult mice, can be separated from the late appearing population by mass cytolysis of the later appearing Lyb 5$^+$ cells, using anti-Lyb 5 antiserum.[21] Enriched populations of putative Lyb 5$^+$ cells have been obtained using the FACS to isolate low density sIgM$^+$ cells from FlRaMμ stained adult spleen populations.[13-15] These procedures have demonstrated that the low density sIgM$^+$ cells of adult mice stimulate an Mls determined mixed lymphocyte reaction while the high density sIgM$^+$ or Lyb 5$^-$ cells obtained by cytolysis do not. These two subpopulations are also known to differ in their triggering requirements, since Lyb 5$^-$ cells fail to respond to thymus independent type 2 (TI-2) antigens but do respond to TI-1 antigens, and are unable to accept accessory cell presentation of antigen.[15] Immune-defective CBA/N mice fail to develop Lyb 5$^+$ B-cells, and represent a useful experimental system in which to study the differences between Lyb 5$^-$ and Lyb 5$^+$ B-cells. In fact, much of the stimulus to study the heterogeniety of B-cells came from the finding that CBA/N mice failed to respond to certain TI antigens.[3]

Studies of immature normal mice have indicated that the first class of sIg acquired during development was IgM and that the density of this sIgM increased on B-cells as they matured.[4-6, 17] With continued development, these cells matured, or a distinct subpopulation appeared, so that the sIgM density of adult splenic B-cells was low, and their sIgD density was relatively high. It was presumed that the sIg phenotype of Lyb 5$^-$ and Lyb 5$^+$ B-cells were homogeneous, with Lyb 5$^-$ B-cells having the relatively high sIgM, and negative or low sIgD phenotype, while the Lyb 5$^+$ B-cells were low sIgM, high sIgD bearing cells.[2,15]

This hypothesis was based on indirect studies, which; 1) correlated the functional properties of low vs. high sIgM$^+$ B-cells and high vs. low sIgD$^+$ B-cells, and 2) which demonstrated that the ratio of sIgM to sIgD on Lyb 5$^-$ B-cells of adult mice was high when compared to this ratio on the whole B-cell population of these mice.[3,7,13-15] It was possible however, that B-cells existed which had quite different sIgM and sIgD densities than those hypothesized on the basis of this indirect data. Therefore, we undertook a study to measure the sIgM and sIgD densities of individual B-cells of immature, and mature normal and CBA/N mice as soon as the equipment (Dual Parameter FACS)[11,12] and reagents (Texas Red dye) were available.[8]

Analysis of adult spleen cells of normal mice demonstrated that there were two major populations, as anticipated. The one present in the largest numbers had a heterogeneous distribution of sIgD and a very low-intermediate density of sIgM, while the second had either negative or low sIgD and a heterogeneous distribution of sIgM. These two subpopulations were subdivided into five groups, by dividing the population with negative or low sIgD into three groups, having very-low sIgM, (group 1), low-intermediate sIgM (group 2), and high sIgM (group 3), and by dividing the population with an intermediate-high density of sIgD into two groups, having very-low sIgM (group 4) and low-intermediate sIgM (group 5). When the frequency of cells (number sIgM$^+$ in the group/total number of sIgM$^+$ $\times$ 100) within these groups of adult spleen cells was calculated, and compared to the frequency of cells in these groups of bone marrow on neonatal spleen populations, interesting differences were noted. In general, there was a shift in the frequency of cells in groups 4 and 5 to groups 2 and 3 when cells from adult spleen were compared to adult bone marrow or immature spleen. Thus, the distribution of sIgM$^+$ cells in the bone marrow of 12-week-old (CBA/N $\times$ DBA/2)F$_1$ females was similar to that of 2.5 week old C3H/HeN mice.

However, the frequency of sIgM$^+$ cells in group 3, representing the high sIgM, negative or low sIgD population remained relatively stable in the spleens of mice of different ages during development, during a time when the frequency of cells in group 2 was falling and that of groups 4 and 5 was increasing. These data suggest that the high sIgM, negative or low sIgD cells found in group 3 represents a transitional cell between groups 2 and 4–5. Alternatively, these cells could represent a fully differentiated population that was unable to generate the later appearing intermediate-high sIgD, low-intermediate sIgM bearing cells. The large frequency of group 2 cells in the spleens of five day and 2.5 week old C3H/HeN mice supports the view that many Lyb 5$^-$ cells bear intermediate-high densities of sIgM and negative or low densitites of sIgD, since Lyb 5$^-$ cells represent the predominant B-cells in the spleens of the immature mice.

Group 1 cells were absent from the spleens of C3H/HeN mice at 2.5 weeks of age, but accounted for 20% of the total sIgM$^+$ spleen cells at five days. By contrast, significant numbers of these cells were found in the bone marrow of these animals from birth through two months of age (data not shown). It is presumed therefore, that the population of very-low sIgM, negative or low sIgD bearing cells represents a very immature B-cell population which serves as a progenitor of later appearing and more mature B-cells.

The distribution of cells in the spleens of adult (CBA/N × CBA/2)F$_1$ male immune-defective mice was distinct from that of normals, since the immune-defective mice had an approximate twofold increase in the frequency of cells in groups 2 and 3, and an approximate fourfold decrease in the frequency of cells in group 4. This deficiency in group 4 cells suggests that the majority of Lyb 5$^+$ B-cells in the spleens of adult mice have very-low sIgM and an intermediate-high sIgD density. It must be emphasized, however, that there does not appear to be an absolute deficiency in any of the B-cell groups defined by their sIg phenotype in immune-defective F$_1$ male mice. Thus, although the sIgM and sIgD density of a particular B-cell certainly does give evidence for the stage of its maturation, at least in the CBA/N mouse, it appears that a limited number of Lyb 5$^-$ B-cells can have the sIgM and sIgD phenotype characteristic of the Lyb 5$^+$ B-cells of normal mice.

The dual fluorescence profile of FlRaMδ and TrMaMIa-labeled spleen cells of 12-week-old normal F$_1$ female mice demonstrated a relative homogeneous distribution of sIa$^+$ B-cells, which have a heterogeneous distribution of sIgD. The two major subpopulations defined by FlRaMδ and TrRaMμ staining were not seen in this sIgD, sIa analysis, although it was clear that the B-cells of immune-defective F$_1$ male mice had higher sIa densities than those of the B-cells of immunologically normal stains.[7]

SUMMARY

The dual laser Fluorescence Activated Cell Sorter was used to study the distribution of sIgM, sIa and sIgD on B-cells from the spleens and bone marrow of adult and developing immunologically normal mice and the spleens of adult immune-defective CBA/N mice. Surface IgM and sIgD staining of murine splenic B-cells distinguished two major groups of these cells, comprising negative or low sIgD and intermediate-high sIgD bearing cells. These two groups were subdivided into a total of five different groups depending on their sIg characteristics. Cells with intermediate-high sIgD represented the largest population of sIgM$^+$ B-cells in the spleens of adult mice, whereas those with negative or low sIgD were the largest group in the spleens of immature mice. This later group represented a large fraction of sIgM$^+$ cells in the bone marrow of adult mice when compared to spleen, and they were also seen with higher frequency in the spleens of immune-defective CBA/N mice when compared to the spleens of normals. It was therefore concluded that the population with negative or low sIgD and low-high sIgM predominantly represented the Lyb 5$^-$ B-cells of immature and adult mice, whereas the intermediate-high sIgD and very low-intermediate sIgM cells were predominantly Lyb 5$^+$. Cells with negative or low sIgD and very low sIgM were only found in the spleens of five-day-old mice, suggesting that this group was the most immature B-cell population detected. Surface Ia and sIgD staining did not distinguish the two major populations observed after sIgM and sIgD staining.

ACKNOWLEDGMENTS

We wish to acknowledge the excellent technical support of Alice K. Berning and Pat Acala, and secretarial assistance of Cathy Cameron.

REFERENCES

1. MÖLLER, G. 1961. J. Exp. Med. **114:** 415–434.
2. WARNER, N. L. 1974. Adv. Immunol. **19:** 67–216.
3. SCHER, I. 1982. Adv. Immunol. In press.
4. VITETTA, E. S., J. CAMBIER, J. FORMAN, J. R. KETTMAN, D. YUAN & J. W. UHR. 1977. Cold Spring Harbor Sump. Quant. Biol. **41:** 185–191.
5. SCHER, I., S. O. SHARROW, R. WISTAR JR., R. ASOFSKY & W. E. PAUL. 1976. J. Exp. Med. **144:** 494–506.
6. SCHER, I., A. K. BERNING, S. KESSLER & F. D. FINKELMAN. 1980. J. Immunol. **125:** 1686–1693.
7. MOND, J. J., S. KESSLER, F. D. FINKELMAN, W. E. PAUL & I. SCHER. 1980. J. Immunol. **124:** 1675–1682.
8. TITUS, J. A., R. HAUGLAND, S. O. SHARROW & D. M. SEGAL. 1982. J. Immunol. Methods. In press.
9. FINKELMAN, F. D., S. W. KESSLER, J. F. MUSHINSKI & M. POTTER. 1981. J. Immunol. **126:** 680–687.
10. OI, V. T., P. P. JONES, S. W. GOLDING, L. A. HERZENBERG & L. A. HERZENBERG. 1978. Curr. Top. Microbiol. Immunol. **81:** 115–124.
11. MILLER, M. H., I. S. POWELL, S. O. SHARROW & A. R. SCHULTZ. 1978. Rev. Sci. Instrum. **49:** 1137–1142.
12. SEGAL, D. M., S. O. SHARROW, J. F. JONES & R. P. SIRAGANIAN. 1981. J. Immunol. **126:** 138–145.
13. SCHER, I., A. AHMED & S. O. SHARROW. 1977. J. Immunol. **119:** 1938–1942.
14. SIECKMANN, D. G., I. SCHER, R. ASOFSKY, D. E. MOSIER & W. E. PAUL. 1978. J. Exp. Med. **148:** 1628–1643.
15. SCHER, I. 1982. Immunol. Rev. In press.
16. SCHER, I., A. AHMED, D. M. STRONG, A. D. STEINBERG & W. E. PAUL. 1975. J. Exp. Med. **141:** 788–803.
17. SCHER, I., S. O. SHARROW & W. E. PAUL. 1976. J. Exp. Med. **144:** 507–518.
18. HUBER, B., R. K. GERSHON & H. CANTOR. 1977. J. Exp. Med. **145:** 10–20.
19. AHMED, A., I. SCHER, S. O. SHARROW, A. H. SMITH, W. E. PAUL, D. H. SACHS & K. W. SELL. 1977. J. Exp. Med. **145:** 101–110.
20. SUBBARAO, B., A. AHMED, W. E. PAUL, I. SCHER, R. LIEBERMAN & D. E. MOSIER. 1979. J. Immunol. **122:** 2279–2285.
21. AHMED, A. & I. SCHER. 1979. In B Lymphocytes in the Immune Response. M. Cooper, D. Mosier, I. Scher & E. Vitetta, Eds.: 115–124. Elsevier North-Holland. New York, N.Y.

DISCUSSION OF THIS PAPER BEGINS ON PAGE 224.

ANTI-IgD INDUCED INCREASE IN sIa IS ASSOCIATED WITH AN INCREASE IN B-CELL RECEPTIVITY TO HELP AND/OR INCREASE IN ITS ANTIGEN PRESENTING ACTIVITY

James J. Mond and Fred D. Finkelman

Department of Medicine
Uniformed Services University of the Health Sciences
Bethesda, Maryland 20817

We have recently investigated the change in expression of B-cell aIa (sIa) that occurs after crosslinking of surface immunoglobulin (sIg) with anti-Ig antibodies.[1] Within three hours after injection of anti-δ antibody into adult mice there is a significant increase in expression of sIa and by nine hours after antibody injection the quantity of sIa plateaus at three times that found on control cells. B-cell populations from which T-cells and macrophages have been removed and which are 99% sIg$^+$ cells by (fluorescence activated cell sorter) FACS analysis also show this increase in sIa expression after exposure to anti-δ antibody. Inasmuch as anti-Ig antibodies mimic the action of antigen in crosslinking B-cell sIg, it seems likely that an increase in B-cell sIa occurs early in antigen drive B-cell activation. There is no increase in expression of a number of other B-cell surface determinants examined. The anti-Ig induced increase in sIa is evident both when the expression of sIa is studied by immunofluorescence staining with monoclonal anti-Ia antibodies and when Ia synthesis is quantitated by studying the incorporation of ^{35}S labeled methionine into cell associated Ia. In this latter situation there is an approximately threefold increase in the amount of Ia molecules synthesized by B-cells activated *in vivo* by anti-δ antibody. Unlike heterologous or monoclonal anti-δ antibodies, three monoclonal antibodies with specificity for non-Ig B-cell surface markers do not induce an increase change in expression of sIa.

Since sIa is a critical surface determinant which influences cellular interactions between macrophages, T- and B-cells,[2-6] the observed increase in expression of B-cell sIa might likely influence the function of the B-cell in its subsequent stages of activation. For example, it might enhance its ability to interact with T-cells in MHC restricted antigen responses and/or increase the B-cells' receptivity to various T-cell factors which utilize B-cell sIa as a receptor, as for example, has been postulated for allogeneic effect factor.[7] In addition, the increase in expression of sIa might enhance the ability of the B-cells to function as antigen presenting cells for T-cells. Such an antigen presenting cell function of B-cells has been reported for both normal anti-Ig treated B-cells[8] as well as for B-cell tumor lines.[9]

Experiments by Ryan *et al.*[10] have shown that spleen cells that have their sIa expression increased by treatment with anti-δ antibody are more effective stimulators in an H-2 defined mixed leucocyte reaction (MLR), and to an even greater extent in an Mls defined MLR. Furthermore, this enhanced stimulatory effect of the anti-δ treated spleen cells can be inhibited with anti-Ia, which suggest that Ia plays a role in stimulating T-cell responses even in the Mls defined MLR in which it itself is not the stimulatory molecule.

0077-8923/82/0399-0221/0 $01.75 © 1982, NYAS

We have recently examined whether the anti-Ig induced increase in expression of sIa is associated with an increase in B-cell receptivity to T-cell derived helper factors *in vivo*. The model used makes use of the different *in vivo* effects of the monoclonal anti-δ antibody, 10-4.22 on the immune system of BALB/c and (BALB/c × C57/BL/6)F1, (BCF$_1$) mice. This antibody is a IgG$_{2a}$ immunoglobulin of the b allotype that binds to IgD of the a allotype.[11] Since BALB/C mice have IgD and IgG of the a allotype, their sIgD$^+$ B-cells are bound by 10-4.22 and their T-cells recognize this Ig as a foreign antigen. On the other hand, although 50% of the sIgD$^+$ B-cells from BCF$_1$ mice bear sIgD of the a allotype and thus, are bound by 10-4.22, these mice have serum IgG$_{2a}$ of both the a and the b allotypes and thus fail to recognize 10-4.22 as foreign. Presumably for this reason, while B-cells from both BALB/c and BCF$_1$, mice are induced by 10-4.22 to undergo the direct T-independent anti-δ associated activating effects, including an increase in sIa, the T-dependent B-cell activating effects of anti-δ antibody including the polyclonal activation of antibody secretion are seen in BALB/c but not in BCF$_1$ mice.[12] By providing a source of B-cells that have been activated to increase their sIa but not to differentiate into antibody secreting cells, the 10-4.22 anti-δ injected BCF$_1$ mice can be used to study whether such partially activated cells are more receptive to helper factors than are resting B-cells.

In order to examine this, we induced a parent into F$_1$ graft vs host (GVH) reaction to provide a source of "help" in such mice. BCF$_1$ mice were injected with 200 micrograms of 10-4.22 anti-δ antibody or with the same quantity of antibody together with 5×10^7 C57BL/6 spleen cells. In control groups, the IgG$_{2a}$ immunoglobulin, CBPC101, was injected by itself or together with C57BL/6 spleen cells. Six to eight days later their spleen cells were removed and studied for numbers of cells with large amounts of intracytoplasmic Ig (cIg) as measured by immunofluorescence staining as well as for numbers of Ig secreting cells, as measured by a reverse plaque assay. There was between a three to tenfold increase in the numbers of cIgG$_1^+$ cells in spleens of mice receiving 10-4.22 anti-δ in the face of an ongoing GVH as compared to cells obtained from mice undergoing a GVH reaction only. There was no consistent difference in the numbers of cIgG$_2^+$ or cIgM$^+$ cells between these two groups (FIGURE 1). A similar increase in the number of IgG$_1$ secreting cells was seen using a modified reverse plaque forming cell assay. Thus, there was an approximately fivefold increase in the number of IgG$_1$ secreting plaque forming cells from BCF$_1$ mice injected with the combination of 10-4.22 anti-δ together with C57BL/6 cells as compared to F$_1$ mice injected with C57BL/6 cells only. Thus although injection of 10-4.22 by itself has no effect on antibody secretion by cells from BCF$_1$, mice and induction of a parent into F$_1$ GVH induces an increase in the numbers of IgM, IgG$_1$ and IgG$_2$ immunoglobulin secreting cells (data not shown), the concomitant injection of 10-4.22 anti-δ antibody induces an additional significant increase in the number of IgG$_1$ secreting cells only.

We are aware of three major possibilities that could explain these findings: 1) injection of anti-δ antibody induces an increase in expression of sIa as well as an increase in B-cell receptors for T-cell helper factors[13] which allow for an increase in response to the helper factors generated by the GVH reaction, thus driving the cells into Ig secretion. 2) The increase in sIa on recipient BALB/c cells induced by anti-δ promotes a more vigorous GVH reaction thus generating more helper factors and 3). The GVH reaction leads to the breaking of tolerance of the recipient F$_1$ T cells to the injected 10-4.22 and these 10-4.22 reactive T-cells provoke the T-dependent phase of the differentiation of B-cells into Ig secreting cells; these possibilities are not mutually exclusive. However the fact that 10-4.22 induces a selective increase in IgG_1 secreting cells argues against the exclusive occurrence of the second possibility since, if a more vigorous GVH were stimulated by anti-δ treated cells one would expect 10-4.22 to stimulate propor-

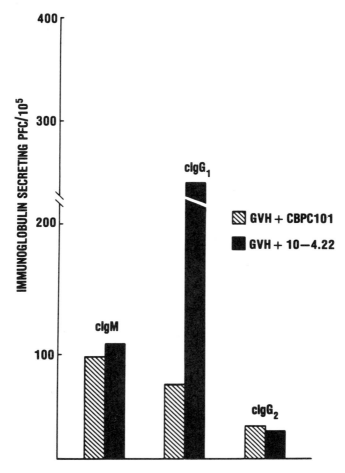

FIGURE 1. Numbers of immunoglobulin secreting PFC in animals injected with anti-δ antibody and C57BL/6 cells.

tionate increases in the number of IgM, IgG_1 and IgG_{2a} secreting cells above those stimulated by the GVH reaction alone.

Since the injection of BALB/c mice with either 10-4.22 anti-δ or a heterologous affinity purified anti-δ antibody stimulates polyclonal antibody production that is predominantly of the IgG_1 isotype, the selective enhancement of antibody production of this isotype by 10-4.22 anti-δ in mice undergoing a parent into F_1 GVH is consistent with possibilities, 1 and 3. That is, the direct B-cell activating effect of anti-δ may predispose to IgG_1 immunoglobulin secretion, either by making B-cells more capable of responding to helper lymphocytes that specifically stimulate IgG_1 antibody production or by making B-cells more likely to secrete IgG_1 immunoglobulin when stimulated by helper factors that have no inherent ability to preferentially stimulate the production of any one Ig isotype. Alternatively, helper lymphocytes produced in response to 10-4.22 anti-δ immunoglobulin either in BALB/c mice or in BCF_1 mice undergoing a GVH reaction, may preferentially stimulate IgG_1 production by B-cells.

REFERENCES

1. MOND, J. J., E. SEHGAL, J. KUNG & F. D. FINKELMAN. 1981. J. Immunol **127:** 881.
2. KAPPLER J. W., & P. C. MARRACK. 1976. Nature **262:** 797.
3. KATZ, D. H., T. HAMAOKA, M. E. DORF & B. BENACERRAF. 1973. Proc. Natl. Acad. Sci. **70:** 2624.
4. ROSENTHAL, A. S. & E. M. SHEVACH. 1973. J. Exp. Med. **148:** 1194.
5. SPRENT, J. 1978. J. Exp. Med. **147:** 1159.
6. ERB, P. & M. FELDMAN. 1975. J. Exp. Med. **142:** 460.
7. DELOVITCH, T. L. & H. O. MCDEVITT. 1977. J. Exp. Med. **146:** 1019.
8. CHESTNUT, R. W. & H. M. GREY. 1981. J. Immunol. **126:** 1075.
9. MCKEAN, D. J., A. J. INFANTE, A. NILSON, M. KIMOTO, C. G. FATHMAN, E. WALKER & N. WARNER. 1981. J. Exp. Med. **154:** 1419.
10. RYAN, J. J., J. J. MOND, F. D. FINKELMAN & I. SCHER. 1981. In B Lymphocytes in the Immune Response. N. Klinman, D. Mosier, I. Scher & E. Vitetta, Eds. **2:** 201. Elsevier/North Holland.
11. OI, V. T., P. P. JONES, J. W. GODING, L. A. HERZENBERG & L. A. HERZENBERG. 1978. In Current Topics in Microbiology and Immunology. F. Melchers, M. Potter & N. L. Warner, Eds. **81:** 115. Springer-Verlag. New York, N.Y.
12. FINKELMAN, F. D., J. SCHER, J. J. MOND, S. KESSLER, J. T. KUNG & E. METCALF. 1982. J. Immunol. In press.
13. YAFFE, L. J., & F. D. FINKELMAN. 1982. Fed Proc. In press.

DISCUSSION OF THE PRECEDING TWO PAPERS

LEN HERZENBERG: These experiments are very provocative and they raise three kinds of questions. Firstly, what is the specificity of the antibodies or immunoglobulins you're producing by GVH plus anti-δ? Are they against the antigen or are they just irrelevant antibodies?

J. J. MOND: I don't know what the specificity is.

L. HERZENBERG: My second point is that controls in that kind of experiment would be more relevant if they had been injected with other antibodies directed against other cell surface determinants to see if they induce an increase in γ-secreting cells? These findings remind me of Ben Pernis' first experiment with monkey, was it? Injecting anti-δ caused a marvelous increase in all sorts of things.

PERNIS: Mostly in IgG, and only about one-third of the increase was absorbed with the injected foreign anti-serum.

F. D. FINKELMAN: Len, let me answer that question, not in the GVH plus anti-δ system where all the controls have not yet been done, but in the system where mice are injected with 200 to 800 micrograms of anti-δ alone. In those mice while you do get an augmented response to the anti-δ antibody, the great majority of the response is polyclonal, probably 95% of the response. I'll go over this in considerable detail in my talk tomorrow. Secondly, while we can't say that anti-δ is unique in its ability to induce this kind of response, it doesn't depend simply on the binding of a foreign immunoglobulins to B-cell, because a rat hybridoma directed against THB absolutely does not activate the humoral immune system.

Further, your question about G2 is very perceptive. By far the greatest polyclonal response gotten is a G1 response, but as the G1 response is going down one gets a G2 response that is probably about tenfold less than the G1 response. This response is also mostly polyclonal, although it is to some extent directed against the immunizing anti-δ antibody.

G. J. THORBECKE: The question I have is about the Lyb5 determinants. In chronically anti-IgD suppressed animals we found a very nice if not enhanced response to TNP-Ficoll, and we therefore looked together with Doctors Skelly and Ahmed whether this went along with the presence of Lyb5 on the B-cells since in normal animals Lyb5 is limited to high IgD$^+$ cells. Indeed among the B-cells that are still there, which are IgD negative and IgM positive, a large proportion is Lyb5 positive. I was wondering if you had a similar experience?

MOND: One can certainly change populations of B-cells in such a way that one can derive what appears to be the typical but stable populations that are IgD$^-$ and and will respond to TNP-Ficoll. By injections of anti-Ia from birth we can chronically suppress mice and thereby generate cells that are IgM$^+$ and IgD$^-$ and Ia$^-$ negative, but that still can respond to TNP-Ficoll.

I. SCHER: These findings support the idea that Lyb5 positive B-cells are not rigidly restricted to a subgroup that can be identified by the surface immunoglobulin.

M. COOPER: Are you saying that anti-δ can stimulate a cell that has a lot of δ on its surface–to then express presumably receptors that allow it to respond much more effectively to a T-cell produced differentiation factor.

SCHER: Yes.

COOPER: Is Kuratani's work similiar? You are in a good position to test that by combining with Bill Paul and Maureen Howard. Can you absorb more of her proliferation factor?

MOND: Lynn Yaffe has a poster that demonstrates that 24 hours after goat anti-δ treatment in vivo the spleen cells are able to absorb a TRFlike component from Con-A induced supernatants. So it's possible that after anti-δ treatment in vivo you induce some sort of T-cell helper receptor on the B-cell that has been able to absorb out the factor from supernatant. In this way the anti-δ treatment improves the ability of B-cells to interact with helper factors. And the absorption data is probably evidence towards that point.

COOPER: Is the reason that the CBA/N doesn't get enhanced IgG production with anti-δ treatment in GVH because there are so few of these high δ positive cells?

MOND: I don't think it relates to the numbers of high δ-positive B-cells. I think the CBA/N's don't seem to increase their expression of Ia very dramatically on exposure of anti-Ig and in some work that Lynn Yaffe has done she also shows that they are not very effective in absorbing out TRFlike factors. I don't think it relates to δ or μ; it relates to the population of cells that may not express an increase in receptors. Does the profile you're looking at change in age since the cells seem to repair some of their deficit if one waits long enough?

SCHER: Well, the answer to that really has two parts. Some of the deficits clearly get better with age, but it's also clear in the CBA/N mouse that they don't really reach their maximum maturity until much later than normal animals. So if you want to study the best that a CBA/N mouse can do, you really have to wait three or four months after birth. In fact you do get a very nice progression of profiles with age in CBA/N mice and each does look more like a normal mouse with age. But some of the functions do not seem to improve with age: there is a conflict between the findings in our laboratory and in Scripps. We don't find that they are able to respond, for example, to TNP-Ficoll with age. In terms of the generation of new receptors or an increase in the density of new receptors after anti-δ stimulation, I should say that if you stimulate CBA/N mice with anti-δ they do not express the MLS determinants whereas normal animals show an enormous increase.

J. CAMBIER: It looks from your data as though anti-μ is perhaps less efficient in inducing this effect as compared to anti-δ.

MOND: That's not really right, John, it may have appeared that way in the slides. The effect *in vivo* is much more dramatic than the effect *in vitro*. *In vivo* one generally sees a three to fourfold increase, *in vitro* it's generally on the order of twofold and there doesn't appear to be a difference between anti-μ and anti-δ.

CAMBIER: Have you looked with hybridoma anti-μ?

MOND: We have with one of the anti-μs of Dr. Sieckmann and it works fine.

E. PURÉ (*Department of Microbiology, Dallas, Texas*): Actually to get to John's questions first, we have done studies in a system similar to David Parker's with both anti-μ and anti-δ. Both adult cells as well as neonatal cells become much more susceptible to T-cell help in the form of a Con-A supernatant or supernatant from T-cell lines and clones. Anti-μ and anti-δ are equally effective.

Secondly, regarding your γ-1 studies, we similarly have stimulated B-cells *in vitro* although in this case with LPS rather than anti-μ or anti-δ and we find with T-cell line supernatants that we selectively increase the γ-1 and we actually inhibit γ-2 since this is *in vitro* which is exactly analagous to what you find, i.e., selective increase in γ-1.

CAMBIER: But again it still would be very hard to answer Len's question because *in vitro* you may be restricted as to the number of days you can keep a cell in culture.

PURIE: This has been done as long as ten days and we actually see a decrease rather than an increase. It really looks like a selective increase in γ-1.

HUMAN T-CELL ACTIVATION IS AUGMENTED BY MONOCLONAL ANTIBODY TO IgD

Denis R. Burger, David Regan, Karen Williams, and Gerrie Leslie

Department of Microbiology and Immunology
Oregon Health Sciences University
and
Immunology Laboratory
Veterans Administration Medical Center
Portland, Oregon 97201

The observations that IgD is usually associated with IgM on the lymphocyte membrane[1-5] and that IgM-bearing lymphocytes appear before IgD-bearing cells ontogenetically[6-8] have been interpreted as indicating a role for the IgD receptor in lymphocyte differentiation.[8] It has also been suggested that cell surface IgD may be an important triggering receptor in monkeys[9] and possibly in mice and rats.[10-14] In support of this concept, Finkelman et al.[15] have shown that the x-linked defect in B-lymphocyte function in CBA/N mice is associated with a decrease in the ratio of IgD to IgM cell surface immunoglobulins. Cell surface IgD also appears to play a role in peripheral lymphocyte activation. We have previously shown that human peripheral lymphocytes become activated when exposed to anti-IgD[16] and that the magnitude of this activation is inversely correlated with the magnitude of PHA-induced proliferation. We predicted that if the functions of IgD-bearing lymphocytes and PHA-responding cells were related, activation of one cell type would exert an influence on the function of the other. We have subsequently presented evidence providing a compelling argument in favor of a synergism between anti-IgD activation and PHA responsiveness.[17] Moreover we showed that F(ab')₂ anti-IgD or supernatant fluids from anti-IgD activated cells were as effective as anti-IgD in augmenting PHA responsiveness.[18,19] The purpose of this work was to investigate the mechanism of augmentation of T-cell activation using a monoclonal antibody to human IgD.

MATERIALS AND METHODS

Mononuclear Cell Isolation and Culture

Mononuclear cells were isolated from peripheral blood cells by Ficoll-Hypaque density gradient centrifugation (Isolymph, Gallard-Schlesinger Chemical Mfg. Corp). The mononuclear cells obtained were cultured in Falcon 96-well plates at 2×10^5 cells/well for five days in RPMI 1640 containing either 10% immunodeficient serum (from patients with combined immunodeficient disease) or 10% IgD serum (from a patient with an IgD myeloma). The cells were cultured in triplicate with PHA (Difco) and Pokeweed mitogen (Gibco) under optimal conditions (PHA, 1 µg/well, PWM 25 µl/well of a 1/5 dilution). In some experiments, cultures contained mouse monoclonal anti human IgD (FC purified, Bethesda Research Labs) at a dose of 0.01 µg., 0.1 µg, 1 µg or 5 µg per well. Cultures were labelled with 1 µCi per well ³H-thymidine (New England Nuclear) 24 hr prior to harvesting on glass filter papers.

0077-8923/82/0399-0227/0 © 1982, NYAS

E-Rosetted Cells

Mononuclear cells from normal donors at 5×10^6 cells/ml were E-rosetted with 10% Neuraminidase-treated sheep red blood cells (SRBC). The final concentration was 2% SRBC/ml of mononuclear cells. This mixture was incubated at 37°C for 10 min. and then centrifuged at 4°C for 8 min. at 800 rpm, and refrigerated for one hour. The supernatant was removed and the mixture gently resuspended. The cells were reconstituted to 5×10^6 cells/ml with fresh RPMI with 10% fetal calf serum then layered over Ficoll-Hypaque and centrifuged at 4°C for 25 min. at 1500 rpm. The interface of B-cells and macrophages was removed, washed, and cultured under the above conditions. To the cellular pellet, 0.83% NH_4Cl was added to lyse the SRBC and the cells washed twice.

Mononuclear Cell Culture for Subsequent Monoclonal Antibody Analysis

Unseparated mononuclear cells, E-rosetted cells and non-E-rosetted cells were cultured for five days in Falcon 3033 tubes at 2.5×10^6 cells/tube prior to staining for monoclonal antibodies. The cells were cultured in the presence of mitogens (PHA 1/100 dilution, 100 μl/tube or PWM 1/3 dilution, 100 μl/tube) or antihuman IgD (2 μg/tube). Some cells were cultured with anti-IgD plus PHA. After five days, the cells were washed twice and reconstituted to 2×10^6 cells/ml in RPMI 1640.

Monoclonal Antibody Staining

Cells (0.2 ml) were combined with various monoclonal antibodies (T_{28}-pan T reagent, OKT 4, OKT8, IgD-BRL, Ia, K and L - BRL). Concentrations of antibodies were used according to previous staining patterns of normal cells. Cells were incubated 30 min. at 4°C and washed twice with RPMI 1640 with 0.2% Na Azide. A goat anti-mouse IgG fluoroscein conjugated F(ab')$_2$ fragment (Cappel Labs.) was added (50 μl) to the cells and incubated for 30 min. at 4°C. The cells were then washed twice as above and fixed in PBS with 1% Formaldehyde (Omega Reagent). The staining was evaluated by flow cytometry using an Ortho Cytofluograf System 50H with 2150 Computer.

RESULTS

Initial experiments were designed to evaluate the effects of monoclonal anti-IgD activation of mononuclear cells on T-cell responsiveness. Lymphocyte transformation of peripheral blood mononuclear cells (MNC) to anti-IgD, PHA, and anti-IgD plus PHA is shown in TABLE 1 for two experiments representative of several that were done. Monoclonal anti-IgD activated the MNC population at 0.1 and 1.0 μg/ml resulting in 2-5 fold stimulation. In agreement with previous findings[16-17] addition of anti-IgD to PHA stimulated cultures resulted in marked augmentation (Exp 1, 47,700 cpm increase at 1.0 μg anti-IgD) when PHA responsiveness was modest, compared to the slight augmentation observed (Exp 2, 23,000 cpm increase) when PHA activation alone was marked (158,000 cpm). These observations were not influenced by the IgD content of the serum used to

TABLE 1

AUGMENTATION OF PHA-INDUCED LYMPHOCYTE PROLIFERATION WITH MONOCLONAL
ANTI-IgD

Culture Stimulant	MC Anti-IgD (μg)	Lymphocyte Activation as CPM of ^{3}H-thymidine Uptake*	
		Exp 1	Exp 2
Control		1,400	600
	0.01	3,400	750
	0.1	3,300	1,150
	1.0	3,200	2,550
	5.0	—	990
PHA		71,200	158,000
PHA+	0.01	84,500	154,000
	0.1	91,600	169,000
	1.0	118,900	181,000
	5.0	—	173,000
PWM		—	38,200

*Culture media was supplemented with serum containing greater than 1 μg/ml IgD. —, not done

supplement the culture media. Cultures supplemented with immunodeficient serum containing less than 1 ng/ml IgD (TABLE 2) exhibited anti-IgD augmentation of PHA responsiveness as did the experiments in TABLE 1 where the serum supplement contained greater than 1 μg/ml IgD.

To investigate which cell types were responding to the anti-IgD augmentation signal, MNC were separated by E-rosetting into T-cells (ER+) and non T-cells (ER−). These cell populations were analyzed for surface markers using a monoclonal antibody screening panel and flow cytometry. TABLE 3 shows the

TABLE 2

AUGMENTATION OF PHA-INDUCED LYMPHOCYTE PROLIFERATION WITH MONOCLONAL
ANTI-IgD

Culture Stimulant	MC Anti-IgD (μg)	Lymphocyte Activation as CPM of ^{3}H-thymidine Uptake*	
		Exp 1	Exp 2
Control		1,600	800
	0.01		1,200
—			
	0.1	—	1,950
	1.0	1,600	1,700
	5.0	—	2,800
PHA		81,300	49,000
PHA+	0.01	69,600	—
	0.1	86,900	35,600
	1.0	120,400	53,500
	5.0	—	77,300
PWM			94,000

*Culture media was supplemented with serum containing less than 1 ng/ml IgD. —, not done

TABLE 3

REACTIVITY OF PERIPHERAL BLOOD MONONUCLEAR CELLS FROM NORMAL HUMAN
DONORS TO A MONOCLONAL ANTIBODY SCREENING PANEL

Monoclonal Antibody	Cell Type(s) Recognized	% Mononuclear Cells (X ± SD)
T28, OKT3	T-cells	63.2 ± 9.1
Leu3, OKT4	T-helper	42.5 ± 7.3
Leu2, OKT8	T-suppressor	22.3 ± 6.9
S33, OKT1, T101	T-cells, malignant B-cells	55.7 ± 9.5
BRL K + L	Ig+ cells	8.1 ± 5.1
BRL IgD	B-cells (IgD+)	2.8 ± 2.8
Ia (2.17)	HLA-DR (Ia) + cells	2.9 ± 1.5
OKM1, BRL D3	Monocytes	10.7 ± 6.7
Mac 120	Macrophage subset/APC	5.2 ± 3.7

markers detected and their distribution on MNC from 20 normal donors. The ER
(+) cells predominantly expressed the T_{28} marker (61%) and IgD (+) or K+L light
chain (+) cells were not detected (0%). The ER (−) cells contained 11% T_{28} (+)
T-cells, 11.8% IgD(+) cells, 18.3% Ia (+) cells and 46.0% K+L light chain positive
cells. It can be seen from the data in TABLE 4 that the ER(+) T-cells proliferated
little if at all to anti-IgD although marked enhancement of PHA responsiveness
was evident. The ER(−) cells (non T-cells) did not respond to anti-IgD and the low
level of activation (1.5-2 fold) of the contaminating T-cells (11%) to PHA was not
augmented with the addition of anti-IgD (TABLE 5).

These data suggested that neither T (ER+) or non- T (ER−) cells responded
significantly to the monoclonal anti-IgD stimulant. Moreover, supernatants from
ER(−) cells stimulated with anti-IgD did not augment PHA-induced T-cell

TABLE 4

ANTI-IgD AUGMENTATION OF PHA-INDUCED PROLIFERATION OF T-CELLS POSITIVELY
SELECTED BY E-ROSETTING

Culture Stimulant	MC Anti-IgD (µg)	Lymphocyte Activation as CPM ^{3}H-thymidine Uptake*	
		Exp 1	Exp 2
Control		12,500	7,600
	0.01	—	9,000
	0.1	5,300	10,200
	1.0	2,800	6,700
	5.0	8,000	4,000
PHA		38,800	14,600
PHA+	0.01	45,400	17,900
	0.1	104,100	21,700
	1.0	47,300	27,300
	5.0	36,500	50,100
PWM		88,700	118,400

*Culture media in experiment one was supplemented with serum containing greater than
1 µg IgD/ml whereas serum in experiment two contained less than 1 ng IgD/ml. —, not
done.

TABLE 5

ANTI-IgD EFFECTS ON PHA-INDUCED PROLIFERATION OF NON T-CELLS NEGATIVELY
SELECTED BY E-ROSETTING

Culture Stimulant	MC Anti-IgD (μg)	Lymphocyte Activation as CPM ^{3}H-thymidine Uptake*	
		Exp 1	Exp 2
Control		8,600	7,200
	0.01	1,700	2,800
	0.1	1,900	2,300
	1.0	6,900	2,200
	5.0	8,600	6,500
PHA		12,900	11,900
PHA+	0.01	8,500	14,200
	0.1	7,500	11,900
	1.0	12,500	13,400
	5.0	11,500	13,200
PWM		7,300	10,400

*Culture media in experiment one was supplemented with serum containing greater than 1 μg/ml IgD whereas serum in experiment two contained less than 1 ng IgD/ml.

activation (data not shown). Since mitogen activation of ER(+) T-cells was augmented by anti-IgD, we entertained the possibility that in the beginning stages of activation T-cells express an Fc receptor (FCR) for IgD and that augmentation is observed when anti-IgD provides a secondary trigger to IgD (+) T-cells. To investigate this possibility, MNC were cultured for five days with various stimulants and analyzed with the monoclonal antibody screening panel for changes in surface markers (TABLE 6). Mitogen stimulation led to increases in T-suppressor (T_S) cells (24.6 to 35.8%) and IgD (+) cells (0 to 0.8%). When anti-IgD was added to the PHA cultures, T_S cells increased to 41.8% and the IgD (+) cells to 3.9%. Although the media in these cultures was supplemented with serum containing IgD, this was not a requirement as similar data was obtained when the serum supplement contained less than 1 ng IgD/ml (data not shown). In order to determine whether the IgD (+) cells were derived from T or non-T populations,

TABLE 6

SURFACE MARKERS ON CULTURED MONONUCLEAR CELLS

MNC Subsets Identified by MC Antibody	Mononuclear Cells (Day 0)	Cells Cultured for Five Days with the Following Stimulants*			
		None	Anti-IgD	PHA	PHA + Anti-IgD
T_{28}	47.0	52.1	50.0	58.7	49.8
T_H	23.4	30.3	30.7	26.3	26.2
T_S	18.3	24.6	25.1	35.8	41.8
IgD	2.4	0	0	0.8	3.9
Ia	6.0	6.7	3.8	2.6	2.3
K + L	16.4	7.5	4.3	5.6	4.7

*Cells were cultured in media supplemented with serum containing greater than 1 μg/ml IgD.

TABLE 7

SURFACE MARKERS ON CULTURED MONONUCLEAR CELLS SELECTED BY E-ROSETTING

MNC Subsets Identified by Monoclonal Antibody	Cells Cultured for Five Days with the Following Stimulants*			
	None	Anti-IgD	PHA	PHA + Anti-IgD
	ER (+) Cells			
T_{28}	63.5	49.5	69.1	69.2
T_H	40.7	46	35.9	38.6
T_S	32.2	31.5	44.2	44.5
IgD	0.4	0.7	2.4	4.0
Ia	3.1	1.3	5.2	2.7
K + L	3.6	5.1	4.0	4.1
	ER (−) Cells			
T_{28}	4.2	4.8	8.2	6.2
T_H	3.2	5.0	9.5	5.8
T_S	28.5	27.3	30.4	29.9
IgD	0.4	0	0	0
Ia	24.2	40.9	41.0	30.8
K + L	53.7	52.9	48.5	45.4

*Cells were cultured in media supplemented with serum containing greater than 1 μg/ml IgD.

this experimental approach was repeated with ER (+) and ER (−) cells in media supplemented with IgD-rich (TABLE 7) and IgD-poor (TABLE 8) serum. In IgD-rich serum 2.4% ER (+) cells expressed IgD (reacted with the monoclonal anti-IgD) after five days' culture with PHA. The IgD (+) cells increased to 4.0% with PHA and anti-IgD in co-culture. Increases in the T_S population (12%) were also observed in the cultures containing PHA. The ER (−) population did not express IgD after five days in culture regardless of the culture conditions. This represented a drop from 11.8% IgD(+) cells at culture initiation. Unexpectedly, although only 4-8% of cells in any culture expressed the pan T-marker (T_{28}), nearly 30% expressed the T_S marker. These cells must have been derived from T_S (−) population since there was only 6.5% T_S (+) in the ER (−) population at the initiation of the five day culture period (data not shown).

In media supplemented with IgD-poor serum, the same trends were observed (TABLE 8). The ER(+) cells expressed IgD (2.2%) after mitogen stimulation whereas the ER(−) cells did not. Again, increases in the T_S (+) and Ia(+) populations were noted with ER(−) cells cultured with mitogen.

DISCUSSION

We have previously shown that anti-IgD activation of human MNC has an enhancing effect on mitogen[16,17] and antigen responsiveness.[19] In previous experiments done with specifically purified goat and rabbit anti-IgD, augmentation was optimal when the cultures responded to anti-IgD alone and if the anti-IgD pulse preceeded mitogen addition. The mechanism of augmentation appeared to involve B-cell products since supernatants from IgD-activated B-cells augmented

T-cell proliferation.[19] The present study was undertaken to investigate further the role of IgD(+) cells in T-cell proliferation. Using monoclonal anti-IgD we have confirmed the anti-IgD augmentation of T-cell activation (TABLES 1, 2). Investigation of the cell types involved suggested that in contrast to the experiments using conventional antibodies, anti-IgD activation was not a requirement for T-cell enhancement (TABLES 4, 5). Moreover supernatants from anti-IgD stimulated ER(−) cells (non T-cells) did not enhance T-cell responsiveness (data not shown). It appears that conventional anti-IgD induces enhancing factors from non-T-cells whereas monoclonal antibody does not. Moreover, in these experiments since T-cell augmentation occurs in the absence of ER(−) non-T-cells or their products, non-T-cells are not required.

During activation with mitogen or mitogen plus anti-IgD, IgD(+) cells were induced from the ER(+) T-cell population only. The magnitude of the induction of the IgD(+) cells appeared to be independent of the concentration of IgD in the serum used to supplement the culture media (TABLES 7, 8).

The basic mechanism of augmentation appears to be that IgD(+) cells react with anti-IgD and directly or indirectly mediate T-cell responsiveness. The IgD(+) cells could be derived from B-cell, macrophage, or T-cell populations since some B-cells express IgD and macrophages and T-cells have Fc receptors for IgD (20). These experiments favor a mechanism involving T-cells although other alternatives have not been ruled out. One possibility is that T-cells express Fc receptors for IgD early during activation and thereby bind IgD from the environment. Subsequent interaction of these IgD(+) T-cells with anti-IgD would then enhance mitogen or antigen activation. If the Fc receptor for IgD was expressed on IL-2 producing cells then triggering of these cells with anti-IgD could result in increased IL-2 release. The increased IL-2 would augment the

TABLE 8

SURFACE MARKERS ON CULTURED MONONUCLEAR CELLS SELECTED BY E-ROSETTING

MNC Subsets Identified by Monoclonal Antibody	Cells Cultured for Five Days with the Following Stimulants*			
	None	Anti-IgD	PHA	PHA + Anti-IgD
	ER (+) Cells			
T_{28}	71.9	71.7	61.0	53.6
T_H	40.3	43.6	33.9	35.5
T_S	28.6	28.6	33.6	33.9
IgD	0	0	2.2	2.0
Ia	0	0.8	1.0	2.5
K + L	0.8	1.4	3.1	2.8
	ER (−) Cells			
T_{28}	3.4	2.6	5.9	7.6
T_H	0	0.5	3.5	3.6
T_S	6.3	5.2	24.9	20.1
IgD	0	0	0	0.7
Ia	9.6	5.7	23.6	21.8
K + L	16	23.8	41.9	35.8

*Cells were cultured in media supplemented with serum containing less than 1 ng/ml IgD.

response of IL-2 dependent blastogenesis to the maximum possible under the culture conditions employed. This type of mechanism would account for our observation that augmentation of T-cell proliferation to antigen occurred predominantly under suboptimal conditions[19] and to mitogen when the mitogen response alone was modest.[16,17]

Because the E-rosette method of dividing cells into T and non-T populations was crude in these experiments, it is not possible to rule out several alternative possibilities involving B-cells. Activated IgD-bearing B-cells or B-cell lymphokines could influence the responsiveness of T-cells. In this regard, Delespesse et al.[21] have shown the enhancing effect of B-cells on the T-cell response to PHA and Con A. Interaction of anti-IgD with the IgD on the B-cell surface may cause conformational changes allowing binding and stimulation by PHA to occur. Clot et al.[22] and Greaves and Janossy[23] have shown that soluble PHA is capable of binding but not stimulating B-cells, whereas insoluble PHA has been shown to increase ^{3}H-thymidine incorporation by B-cells. Thus, the possible epitopic rearrangement of the PHA receptor on B-cells by anti-IgD activation may influence the triggering of B-cells by soluble PHA. Another possibility is that the anti-IgD activated cells and/or their products may in turn activate other components which exert a helper effect on PHA-responding cells. Studies by Gery et al[24] suggest that PHA, or lipopolysaccharide-activated leukocytes release a "potentiating" factor which, possibly through macrophages, enhances the overall T-cell response (IL-1 effect).

The unexpected finding that cells with the T_S marker appeared during culture of ER($-$) cells deserves further investigation as does the concomitant increase in Ia($+$) cells. That these cells could be the same population (phenotypically Tpan$-$, T_S+, Ia$+$) is intriguing.

REFERENCES

1. ROWE, D. S., K. HUG, L. FORNI & B. PERNIS. 1973. Immunoglobulin D as a lymphocyte receptor. J. Exp. Med. **138:** 965.
2. KNAPP, W., R. L. H. BOLUIS, J. RADL & W. J. HIJMANS. 1973. Independent movement of IgD and IgM molecules on the surface of individual lymphocytes. J. Immunol. **111:** 1295.
3. FU, S. M., R. J. WINCHESTER & H. G. KUNKEL. 1974. Occurrence of surface IgM, IgD and free L chains on human lymphocytes. J. Exp. Med. **139:** 451.
4. KUBO, R. T., H. M. GREY & B. PIROFSKY. 1974. IgD: A major immunoglobulin on the surfaces of lymphocytes from patients with chronic lymphatic leukemia. J. Immunol. **112:** 1952.
5. PERNIS, B., J. C. BROUET & M. SELIGMANN. 1974. IgD and IgM on the membrane of lymphoid cells in macroglobulinemia. Evidence for identity of membrane IgD and IgM antibody activity in a case with anti-IgG receptors. Eur. J. Immunol. **4:** 776.
6. VOSSEN, J. M. & W. HIJMANS. 1975. Membrane-associated immunoglobulin determinants on bone marrow and blood lymphocytes in the pediatric age group and on fetal tissues. In Fifth International Conference on Immunofluorescence and Related Staining Techniques. W. Hijmans and M. Schaeffer, Eds. **254:** 262. New York Academy of Sciences. New York, N.Y.
7. UHR, J. W. 1975. The membranes of lymphocytes. In Cell Membranes. G. Weissman and R. Claiborne, Eds.: 223. H.P. Publishing. New York, N.Y.
8. VITETTA, E. S. & J. W. UHR. 1975. Immunoglobulin-receptors revisited. A model for the differentiation of bone marrow-derived lymphocytes is described. Science **189:** 964.
9. MARTIN, L. N., G. A. LESLIE & R. HINDES. 1976. Lymphocyte surface IgD and IgM in non-human primates. Int. Arch. Allergy Appl. Immunol. **51:** 320.

10. ABNEY, E. & R. M. E. PARKHOUSE. 1974. Candidate for immunoglobulin D present on murine B lymphocytes. Nature **252:** 600.
11. MELCHER, U., E. S. VITETTA, M. MCWILLIAMS, M. LAMM, J. M. PHILLIPS-QUAGLIATA & J. W. UHR. 1974. Cell surface immunoglobulin. X. Identification of an IgD-like molecule on the surface of murine splenocytes. J. Exp. Med. **140:** 1427.
12. GOODMAN, S. A., E. S. VITETTA, U. MELCHER & J. W. UHR. 1975. Cell surface immunoglobulin. XIII. Distribution of IgM and IgD-like molecules on small and large cells of mouse spleen. J. Immunol. **113:** 1646.
13. VITETTA, E. S., M. MCWILLIAMS, J. M. PHILLIPS-QUAGLIATA, M. E. LAMM & J. W. UHR. 1975. Cell surface immunoglobulin. XIV. Synthesis, surface expression and secretion of immunoglobulin by Peyer's patch cells in the mouse. J. Immunol. **115:** 603.
14. VITETTA, E. S., U. MELCHER, M. MCWILLIAMS, M. E. LAMM, J. M. PHILLIPS-QUAGLIATA & J. W. UHR. 1975. Cell surface immunoglobulin. XI. The appearance of an IgD-like molecule on murine lymphoid cells during ontogeny. J. Exp. Med. **141:** 206.
15. FINKELMAN, F. D., A. M. SMITH, I. R. SCHER & W. E. PAUL. 1975. Abnormal ratio of membrane immunoglobulin classes in mice with an x-linked B-lymphocyte defect. J. Exp. Med. **142:** 1316.
16. KERMANI-ARAB, V., G. A. LESLIE & D. R. BURGER. 1976. Structure and biological function of human IgD. IX. Anti-IgD activation of human lymphocytes. Int. Arch. Allergy, **54**(1): 1–8.
17. KERMANI-ARAB, V., D. R. BURGER & G. A. LESLIE. 1976. Structure and function of human IgD X. Enhancement of PHA responsiveness by anti-IgD activated lymphocytes. J. Immunol. **117:** 467–470.
18. KERMANI-ARAB, V., G. A. LESLIE & D. R. BURGER. 1977. Anti-IgD and F (ab')₂ Anti-IgD activated B cells enhance PHA responsiveness. *In* Regulatory mechanisms in lymphocyte activation. D. Lucas, Ed. 701–703. Academic Press, New York, NY.
19. CUCHENS, M. A., D. R. BURGER & G. A. LESLIE. 1979. Anti-IgD activated B-cells enhance antigen responses of T-cells. *In* Molecular Basis of Immune Cell Function. J. G. Kaplan, Ed.: 668–670. Elsevier Press, New York, NY.
20. SJOBERG, O. 1980. Presence of Receptors for IgD on human T and non-T lymphocytes. Scand. J. Immunol. **11:** 377–382.
21. DELESPESSE, G., J. DUCHATEAU, P. H. GAUSSET & A. GOVAERTS. 1976. *In vitro* response of subpopulations of human tonsil lymphocytes. I. Cellular collaboration in the proliferative response to PHA and Con A. J. Immunol. **116:** 437.
22. CLOT, J., H. MASSIP & O. MATHIEU. 1975. *In vitro* studies on human B- and T-cell purified populations. Stimulation by mitogens and allogeneic cells, and quantitative binding of phytomitogens. Immunology **29:** 445.
23. GREAVES, M. & G. JANOSSY. 1972. Elicitation of selective T and B lymphocyte responses by surface binding ligands. Transplant. Rev. **11:** 87.
24. GERY, I., R. K. GERSHON & B. H. WAKSMAN. 1971. Potentiation of cultured mouse thymocyte responses by factors released by peripheral leukocytes. J. Immunol. **107:** 1778.

———————◆———————

DISCUSSION OF THE PAPER

B. G. PERNIS: In both hypotheses you have delineated that you require the purified T-cell population to have some B-cells either to produce a factor after anti-δ or to provide δ for the T-cell. You are not postulating the T-cell to provide the δ themselves. They cannot do that because they don't express immunoglobulins.

D. R. BURGER: Correct.

PERNIS: Then what is the nature of the substance produced by the B-cells after anti-δ? One possibility is that it is δ and then the T-cell deals with it, and the other possibility is that the B-cells are producing something which is acting as a stimulus to the T-cells, preparing them to produce more IL-2 after PHA and the nature of these substances is unknown.

BURGER: Correct.

L. HERZENBERG: You say there's an increase in T-cell receptor, i.e., of Fc receptor for δ. Is that specific for δ or does it pick up other immunoglobulins?

BURGER: I think there is a receptor generated that is specific for δ. There may also be other Fc receptors generated in the process, but I don't know about that.

HERZENBERG: When you stain for immunoglobulin on those T-cells don't you pick it up except for the same percentages you get with δ?

BURGER: Yes, you can account for the δ by κ-λ staining.

HERZENBERG: Okay, then just a comment about the Leu 2 staining of the cells that don't bear other T-cell markers. I think those probably are accounted for by cells which also stain with markers for NK cells. Now at least a proportion of NK cells have Leu-2 and they don't have T-cell markers. So it might be worth having a second look with specific antibodies for NK cells which are available.

BURGER: After the five days of culture, with or without mitogen, that population was readily evident.

HERZENBERG: I think it would be quite interesting to look just at that point because they must be activated by all the lymphokines you've got in the cultures.

F. R. BLATTNER: This really is an interesting comment you made because it fits in with the proposal that was made in the talk by Phil Tucker that the secreted form of δ is really predominantly a B-cell product and shuts off when you switch to secretion of μ. The gene arrangement is ideally situated for δ to be a lymphokine. We're starting to call this "the unified field theory" of regulation. Are you saying that there's much more of this so called Fc receptor on T-suppressors?

BURGER: No, I'm not saying that.

BLATTNER: It wasn't stated clearly what those numbers were.

BURGER: They were the percentages of cells that express those markers after culture. The Ts marker appeared on the E rosette negative cells that were cultured, and that's a situation where there isn't anti-δ augmentation of the mitogen response.

BLATTNER: It might be that you just basically have it backwards and that what is happening isn't augmentation at all of the responsiveness of the B-cell but just simply a trapping of the messenger; namely, the IgD secreted form considered as a lymphokine which then would change the amount of T-cell factor produced, by simply avoiding the stimulation of the T-cell by the B-cell lymphokine.

BURGER: The magnitude of the proliferative response can be augmented to a certain level and if the response is low or the culture is done in sub-optimal conditions then the addition of anti-δ augments that response. So it's augmented in terms of the magnitude of proliferation.

BLATTNER: But you can't say whether you think it's a T- helper or a T-suppressor cell that is responding?

BURGER: The T-cell that is responding carries the T-helper cell marker. That's the cell that's proliferating to antigens in this system.

BLATTNER: That's the thing that would be logical according to the unified field theory, but why do you have such high numbers for the suppressors? I still don't understand.

BURGER: That's an observation that we didn't expect and that really has nothing to do with anti-δ augmentation or the anti-δ effect at all. That is simply an observation that fell out of the analysis of the markers of E rosette negative cells when they were cultured for five days.

D. W. SCOTT: Dr. Burger, you mentioned in the beginning of the talk that both anti-δ and anti-μ can cause this effect. Have you tried any other reagents that react with B-cells; for example, monoclonal anti-DR?

BURGER: Yes, anti-μ will augment under certain conditions some of the mitogen responses. It won't augment the antigen responses and it doesn't augment the Con-A response. So I think the anti-μ is quite different. Anti-Ia does not produce the augmentation. The monoclonal antibody, anti-B1, which is a B-cell monoclonal antibody doesn't produce the augmentation. So specific triggering of the δ-receptor is important.

CELL CYCLE DEPENDENCE FOR EXPRESSION OF MEMBRANE ASSOCIATED IgD, IgM AND Ia ANTIGEN ON MITOGEN-STIMULATED MURINE B-LYMPHOCYTES*

John G. Monroe and John C. Cambier

Department of Microbiology and Immunology
Duke University Medical Center
Durham, North Carolina 27710

INTRODUCTION

The majority of B-lymphocytes that populate the spleen and peripheral blood of mature animals express cell surface IgM (mIgM), IgD (mIgD) and Ia antigens (mIa).[1,2] These surface molecules are believed to play critical roles in B-cell activation. MIgM and mIgD bind antigen and may transmit signals for activation or tolerance induction, or they may simply serve as a bridge to focus specific T-cell mediated help which activates the B-cell. MIa antigens function in the collaboration between T- and B-cells during thymus-dependent, antigen-driven B-cell activation.[3-5] This collaboration is genetically restricted[3-5] and has been mapped to the I-region of the murine major histocompatibility complex (H-2)[3], more specifically, the I-A subregion.[6] This restriction is believed to occur at the level of T-cell recognition of Ia antigen on the B-cell surface.[7,8] It has been suggested that an antigen-specific T-cell, or its derived factor, must bind both antigen and mIa in order to transmit its help signal to the B-cell.[9]

Evidence from a variety of sources indicate that during activation, proliferation and differentiation of B-cells, expression mIgM, mIgD and mIa may change. For example, soon after exposure to anti-IgM or anti-IgD antibodies, murine B-cells undergo a period of increased mIa expression.[10,11] MIgD and mIgM expression is effected quite differently by activation. Immunoprecipitation,[12] immunocytoxicity[13] and immunofluorescence[14,15] studies demonstrate that three to five days after mitogen stimulation and before they become secretory cells, B-lymphocytes lose mIgD but not mIgM. Taken together, these data suggest that at some point during activation, proliferation and differentiation of B-cells into antibody secreting cells, Ia expression increases and mIgD expression decreases, while mIgM expression remains constant.

Expression of these markers appear to correlate with functional requirements for them. For example, early after stimulation, presumably as they enter G_1, B-cells appear to lose the requirement for interaction with antigen to drive subsequent proliferation[16] and therefore may have a lessened requirement for mIg correlating with decreased IgD expression. The requirement for antigen-specific, T-cell mediated help and therefore, mIa, is manifest only during or immediately following exposure to antigen, when expression of mIa may peak. I-region restricted help is not required once stimulated B-cells have undergone blastogenesis.[6,16]

*Supported in part by NIH Grants CA 09058-07, AI 16128 and AI 00371. Dr. Cambier is a recipient of a NIH Research Career Development Award.

It is essential to our understanding of the roles of mIgD, mIgM and mIa in B-lymphocyte activation that we rigorously define their expression as a function of position in cell cycle. Here, we report analyses of mIgM, mIgD and mIa expression by B-cells in defined cell cycle phases. To accomplish this we first established a correlation between B-cell diameter and specific cell cycle phase. Utilizing this correlation, we have performed flow cytometric analyses of mIgM, mIgD and mIa-specific immunofluorescence of mitogen-stimulated B-cells as a function of cell cycle phase. Results indicate that when normal B-cells transit from G_0 through G_1, cellular expression of mIgD but not mIgM decreases. In addition, mIa expression increases during transition from G_0 to early G_1. However, by early S phase, mIa expression decreases sharply.

MATERIALS AND METHODS

Culture Conditions

Spleens were removed aseptically from six- to eight-week-old BALB.k ($H-2^k$) mice killed by cervical dislocation. Spleens were teased apart and forced through a fine mesh steel screen. Resulting cells were washed three times with media. T-cells were depleted by treatment with hybridoma T24 anti-Thy1 antibody and guinea pig complement.[17] Resulting B-cells were treated with Gey's solution to lyse erythrocytes and were centrifuged through fetal calf serum to remove dead cells. Cells were washed three times in medium and cultured at 10^6/ml in RPMI 1640 containing 10% fetal calf serum (FCS) (Sterile Systems, Logan, Ut., Lot 100233), 200 mM glutamine, 100 μM/ml streptomycin, 100 μM penicillin and 5 $\times$ 10^{-5} M 2-mercaptoethanol. Mitogen-stimulated cultures also contained 50 μg/ml lipopolysaccaride (LPS) (Difco, Detroit, Mich.) plus 20 μg/ml dextran sulfate (GIBCO, Grand Island, N.Y.). Cells were cultured at 37°C in 7% CO_2.

Antisera

Heterologous anti-IgM was produced in rabbits by injection of the IgM product of the PAF 14 hybridoma, an anti-DNP secretor (Dr. Robert Giles, personal communication). This hybridoma was generously supplied by Dr. Robert Giles (University of Mississippi Medical Center, Jackson, Miss.). The IgG fractions from these antisera were isolated by Staphlococcus Protein A-Sepharose chromatography and absorbed using normal mouse IgG-Sepharose to remove anti-light chain activity.

Heterologous anti-IgD was produced in rabbits by injection of the IgD product of myeloma MOPC 1017 generously provided by Dr. Fred Finkleman (Uniformed Services University of Health Sciences, Bethesda, Md.). The resultant antisera were chromatographed and adsorbed as described for anti-IgM antisera.

Specificity of rabbit anti-IgM and anti-IgD antisera were assessed by immuno-precipitation and polyacrylamide gel analysis of detergent lysates of radiolabeled splenocyte membranes and appear monospecific to the limit of sensitivity by this method (Monroe et al., manuscript submitted).

Monoclonal anti-Ia was obtained from hybridoma 10-2.16[18] obtained from the Salk Institute, San Diego, Ca. The antibody product of this hybridoma recognizes products of the I-A subregion of the H-2 complex in mice with the $H-2^k$ haplotype.[18] The antibody was purified from culture supernatants by adsorption to and elution from Staphlococcal Protein A-Sepharose. The resulting antibody was biotinylated by incubation with biotin succinimide ester.[19,20]

Goat anti-rabbit Ig was prepared by immunization of a goat with normal rabbit Ig purified by Staphlococcal Protein A-Sepharose chromatography. Anti-IgG antibodies were affinity purified using rabbit IgG-Sepharose and fluoresceinated using fluorescein on celite (Sigma, St. Louis, Mo.) as previously described.[21] Fluoresceinated avidin was obtained from Vector Laboratories, Burlingame, Ca.

Immunofluorescence Staining

Cells were washed three times in phosphate buffered saline (PBS), pH 7.4. Approximately 1×10^6 cells were suspended in 100 μl of anti-IgM, anti-IgD or biotinylated anti-Ia appropriately diluted in PBS containing 2% FCS and 0.2% sodium azide. Control cells were cultured in the diluent minus the primary antibody in the case of anti-Ia or in appropriately diluted normal rabbit serum in the case of anti-IgD and anti-IgM. Samples were incubated for 15 minutes at 0–4°C. Following incubation, the cells were washed four times in PBS containing FCS and sodium azide. After washing, the cells were suspended in 100 μl of appropriately diluted fluoresceinated avidin for anti-Ia samples, or fluoresceinated goat anti-rabbit Ig for the anti-IgD and anti-IgM labeled cells. The cells were incubated for 15 minutes at 0–4°C. Following incubation, cells were washed four times as before and suspended in one ml of fresh buffer containing FCS and sodium azide. Cells stained by this procedure were maintained at 0–4°C until analyzed. In some cases, stained cells were fixed by adding 100 μl of formalin per 1 ml of cell suspension. This treatment does not cause detectable alteration in the fluorescence nor the diameter of the cells. If kept at 0–4°C in the dark, cells fixed in this way may be saved for extended periods before analysis.

Cytofluorometric Analysis and Cell Sorting

The size and fluorescence of cells were measured using the Cytofluorograf System 50-H (Ortho Diagnostic Instruments, Westwood, Mass.) equipped with helium-neon and 5 watt argon lasers. For immunofluorescence analysis, log of fluorescence was measured as a function of the pulse width (see below) measurement of size. The log scale of the Cytofluorograf covers three decades. Acridine orange stained cells were analyzed simultaneously for linear red and green fluorescence as described by Darzynkiewicz et al.[22] For acridine orange analysis, a 640 nm bandpass filter (Ditric Optics, Hudson, Mass.) was positioned in front of the red fluorescence detector. For detection and delineation of doublets and higher cell aggregates, integrated red (RNA) fluorescence intensity was measured as a function of the pulse-width of the green fluorescence signal as described by Sharpless et al.[23]

Cell diameter was determined by measuring the "time of flight" or pulse-width of the axial light extinction signal.[24,25] This is a measurement of the length of time that a passing particle blocks any portion of the laser beam. It is a function of particle diameter. Since this is a measurement of time and not a function of the amount of light blocked, latex particles of homogenous size may be used as standards and finite cell diameters determined. In these studies we have used 5, 10 and 15 μm latex spheres (Coulter Electronics, Hialeah, Fla). as markers.

Correlation of B-Lymphocyte Diameter and Position in Cell Cycle

Quantitation of cells in particular phases of the cell cycle has been accomplished with such fluorochromatic DNA binding agents as ethidium bromide,[26] acridine orange[27] and propidium iodide.[28] However, the most exquisite cell cycle analyses to date have been accomplished using the acridine orange (AO) staining procedure developed by Darzynkiewicz *et al.*[29,30]

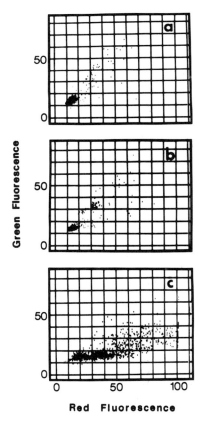

FIGURE 1. Cytograms depicting fluorescence distribution of murine lymphocytes stained with acridine orange. Each dot represents an individual cell; its distance from the origin along the ordinate and abscissa reflects its relative green and red integrated fluorescence, respectively. Each cytogram was constructed using 1000 fresh splenocytes prepared on the day of the analysis (a), B-cells cultured for 48 hr in the absence of LPS or dextran sulfate (b), or, B-cells cultured for 48 hr in the presence of 50 μg/ml LPS and 20 μg/ml dextran sulfate (c).

This procedure relies on differential staining of cellular DNA and RNA. Cellular DNA, which is double-stranded, fluoresces green when stained with AO while single-stranded RNA fluoresces red. Once stained, the cell cycle distribution is determined by simultaneous flow cytofluorometric analysis of green and red integrated fluorescence. FIGURE 1 depicts such an analysis for murine B-lymphocytes. As can be seen, fresh splenocytes (FIGURE 1a) and unstimulated

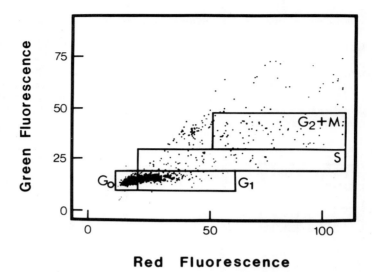

Red   Fluorescence

FIGURE 2. Cytogram depicting two-parameter fluorescence cell cycle analysis of acridine orange stained B-cells stimulated 48 hr with LPS and dextran sulfate. Each dot on the cytogram represents an individual cell, whose distance from the origin along the ordinate and abscissa represent its relative green (DNA) and red (RNA) fluorescence (content), respectively. The demarcations for cell cycle phases were determined as described in the text. The cells exhibiting increased red and green fluorescence intensities but which are excluded from the cycle phases were determined by green pulse-width analysis to be cell aggregates. Dead cells exhibit low levels of red and green fluorescence and were similarly excluded. Analysis depicts 1000 murine B-cells.

B-cells cultured for 48 hours (FIGURE 1b) exhibit very homogeneous staining patterns exhibiting relatively low red (RNA) and green (DNA) fluorescence intensities. Such a staining pattern has been demonstrated to be characteristic of lymphocytes in the G_0 or resting phase of the cell cycle.[30] In both populations there is a cluster of cells exhibiting elevated red and green fluorescence intensities. These cells, when analyzed by green fluorescence pulse-width,[23] have been determined to be cell aggregates. In contrast to the homogeneous staining pattern exhibited by the unstimulated cells, B-cells stimulated for 48 hours with mitogens (FIGURE 1c) exhibit a very heterogeneous staining pattern. A significant but much smaller proportion of cells reside in G_0. Among the mitogen-stimulated B-cells there occurs a large population of cells with increased RNA content relative to G_0 cells, but with no increased DNA content. By definition, these cells are in G_1. Stemming from this G_1 population, are cells exhibiting increased RNA and DNA specific fluorescence. These cells represent S phase cells. Lastly, there appears a population of cells with still higher intracellular RNA and DNA levels. These cells are in G_2 and M. These assignments have been supported using cell cycle inhibitors by us (Monroe and Cambier; unpublished results) and others[31] and are illustrated in FIGURE 2. The group of cells exhibiting G_2 + M and higher levels of DNA which are not included in the designated cell cycle phases represent cell doublets (aggregates), as described previously.

While the AO staining method described above is useful in assigning individual cells to specific positions in the cell cycle it is not amenable to use with

simultaneous immunofluorescence analysis of surface marker expression. Therefore, we have established a correlation between the diameter of stimulated
lymphocytes, determined by pulse-width of axial light extinction, and cell cycle
phase. This parameter is a measurement of cell diameter and is compatible with
simultaneous immunofluorescence analysis. When mitogen-stimulated B-cells
are analyzed by pulse-width of axial light extinction in the Cytofluorograf, they
routinely exhibit a distribution similar to that in FIGURE 3. Unstimulated B-cells
exhibit a restricted, 4.5–5.5 µm diameter distribution. After stimulation by mitogen, the frequency of cells 5.5–12 µm in diameter increases with a simultaneous
decrease in the small cell (4.5–5.5 µm) population. We sorted cells of 4 size
categories from the mitogen-stimulated population and subjected them to AO
cycle analysis. The results are presented in FIGURE 4. Comparing these staining
patterns to that in FIGURE 2, we observed that increased cell diameter correlates
with advancement through cell cycle. Using the cell cycle phase gatings
illustrated in FIGURE 2, we conducted quantitative analysis of the cell cycle phase
distribution of sorted cells. The results are summarized in TABLE 1. The 4.5–5.5 µm
(FIGURE 4a) cells reside in G_0 (99%). Most B-lymphocytes with diameters ranging
from 5.5–7.0 µm (FIGURE 4b) are in early G_1 (68%). This early stage of G_1 has been
designated G_{1A} based upon relative RNA content.[29,32] Only 29% of 5.5–7 µm cells
are in G_0 and 3% in S, G_2 and M. The 7.0–10 µm population (FIGURE 4c) contains
predominantly late G_1 (G_{1B}, 75%) and S phase cells (15%). Only 4% are in G_0 and
we believe these to be G_0 cells which were doublets at the time of sorting. A small
proportion of this population are G_2 and M cells (6%). The 10–12 µm population
(FIGURE 4d) is enriched in S, G_2 and M phase cells (42% and 32%, respectively).
The remaining G_1 cells (23%) are in an extremely late stage of G_1 as evidenced by
their very great red fluorescence intensity. The small percentage (5%) of the
10–12 µm population which appear as G_0 cells are believed to be G_0 doublets
present during sorting.

   These results indicate that a strong correlation exists between cell diameter
and cell cycle position. They further demonstrate the validity of using simulta-

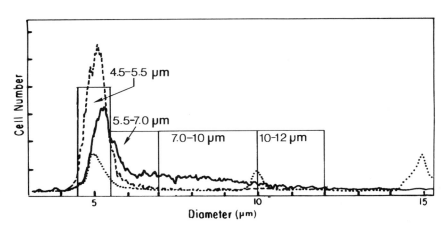

FIGURE 3. Histogram of axial pulse-width analysis of cell diameter of fresh spenocytes
(---) and 48 hr mitogen-stimulated B-cells (—). Finite diameters were determined based
upon 5, 10, and 15 µm diameter latex spheres (· · ·). The areas designated denote regions
sorted for subsequent cell cycle analysis. Each analysis depicts 10,000 lymphocytes.

neous analysis of cell diameter and immunofluorescence to determine marker expression as a function of cell cycle state.

Expression of mIgM, mIgD and mIa as a Function of Position in Cell Cycle

Cells stained for mIgM, mIgD and mIa specific immunofluorescence were analyzed by two-parameter flow cytometry using the parameters axial pulse-width (cell diameter) and log of integrated green fluorescence (marker expression). Results of these analyses are presented in the form of cytograms in FIGURE 5. MIgM-positive fresh (FIGURE 5A) and unstimulated, cultured B-cells (FIGURE 5B) exhibit a homogeneous distribution of cells roughly 4.5–5.5 μm in diameter. The mitogen-stimulated cells (FIGURE 5C) exhibit an increased proportion of large cells (5.5 μm) which bear mIgM. Significant numbers of these large, mIgM bearing cells did not occur in the unstimulated control populations. Therefore, mitogen stimulation of murine B-cells results in an increased frequency of G_1 through M phase cells which bear mIgM. The relative expression of mIgM per unit area of membrane (density) for cells in each cycle phase was calculated and presented in TABLE 2. As can be seen, the density of mIgM remains fairly constant throughout the cell cycle. There is a slight increase during the transition from G_0

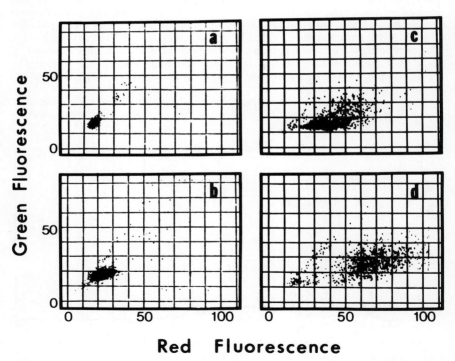

FIGURE 4. Cytograms of acridine orange stained murine B-lymphocytes stimulated 48 hours with LPS and dextran sulfate and sorted on the basis of cell diameter. (A) 4.5–5.5 μm; (B) 5.5–7.0 μm; (C) 7.0–10 μm; and, (D) 10–12 μm. The ordinate and abscissa are identical with those in FIGURES 1 and 2. In all cases, 1000 cells were analyzed. Each dot represents an individual cell.

TABLE 1

CELL CYCLE ANALYSIS OF MITOGEN-STIMULATED B-LYMPHOCYTES SORTED ON THE BASIS
OF CELL DIAMETER

Sorted Population*	$\%G_0$	$\%G_1$	$\%S$	$\%G_2 + M$
4.5–5.5 μm	99	<1	<1	<1
5.5–7.0 μm	29	68	2	1
7.0–10 μm	4	75	15	6
10–12 μm	5	23	42	30

*Sorted from murine B-lymphocytes stimulated for 48 hours with LPS and dextran
sulfate. Comparable results were obtained with B-lymphocytes stimulated with mitogens for
12 hours.

to G_{1A} (.102 units and .146 units, respectively) followed by a slight decrease by late
G_1 (G_{1B}) (.079 units).

When mIgD expression was analyzed in the same manner, quite different
results were obtained. As with mIgM, we observed an increase in the proportion
of large mIgD bearing cells in the mitogen-stimulated population (FIGURE 5F)
compared to fresh B-cells (FIGURE 5D) and B-cells cultured without mitogens
(FIGURE 5E). However, in contrast to the expression of similar or slightly elevated
mIgM expression by B-cells in cycle relative to G_0 cells, expression of mIgD
decreases significantly on cells in G_{1A}. This decrease continues during transition
through S, G_2 and M. The cytograms suggest further that the initial decrease
occurs rather abruptly during the transition from G_0 to G_{1A}. This decrease is much
more pronounced when one compares densities of mIgD expression (TABLE 2).
During the transition from G_0 to G_{1A}, mIgD density decreases sharply by fourfold
(.293 units to .073 units). This decrease continues during the remainder of G_1 and
early S phrase (.035) until by late S, G_2 and M the total decrease is about 13-fold
(.021 units) relative to peak G_0 expression. This decrease is much more than would
be predicted by membrane dilution effects alone. As cells transit from G_0 to late S,
G_2 and M, their surface area increases by only fivefold. The magnitude of the loss
in mIgD density during this time suggests that an active process may mediate this
decrease.

In contrast to mIgD, mIa expression increases as B-cells leave G_0 and enter G_{1A}
(FIGURE 5I). However, by G_{1B} and early S phase there is a sharp decrease in mIa
expression which continues into late S, G_2 and M phases. This modulation in mIa
expression is more obvious when levels are expressed per unit area of membrane
(TABLE 2). As can be seen, during the transition from G_0 (unstimulated) to G_{1A},
density of mIa expression increases from .076 units to .407 units. This translates to
a greater than fivefold increase in mIa density. However, as cells enter G_{1B}, S, mIa
density decreases sharply from peak G_{1A} levels and by late S, G_2 and M the
density of mIa expression is slightly lower than unstimulated G_0 levels. As with
mIgD, this decrease is much more than is expected from membrane dilution
effects alone. The increase in membrane area as B-cells transit from G_{1A} to late S,
G_2 and M is three to fourfold. During this transition there is an eightfold decrease
in mIa density.

Interestingly, unstimulated, G_0 cells (4.5–5.5 μm) exhibit a much lower density
of mIa expression than do 4.5–5.5 μm cells in the mitogen-stimulated population.
This suggests that there is an elevation in mIa expression after stimulation but
prior to when increases in size or RNA production become detectable, presumably during the transition from G_0 to G_1.

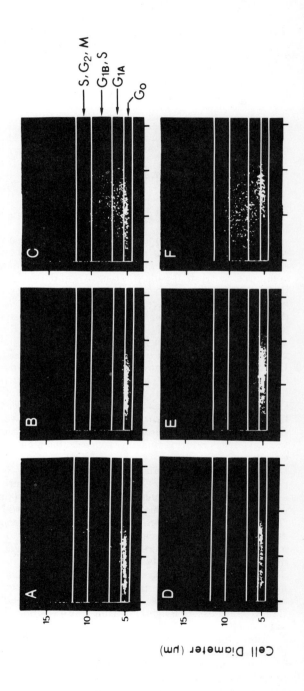

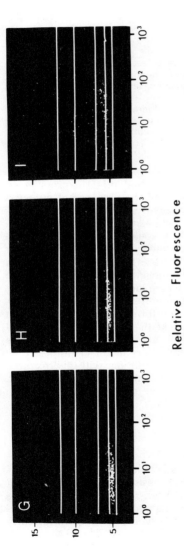

Relative Fluorescence

FIGURE 5. Cytograms demonstrating distribution of murine B-lymphocytes examined simultaneously for surface IgM, IgD or Ia immunofluorescence and cell diameter. The abscissa represents relative log of integrated green fluorescence and the ordinate cell diameter in micrometers, as determined by axial pulse-width measurement. The ordinate was calibrated using 5, 10 and 15 μm latex spheres. Cytograms were constructed using 1000 cells. IgM-specific immunofluorescence of: (A) fresh splenocytes; (B) B-lymphocytes cultured 48 hours in the absence of mitogen; and, (C) B-lymphocytes cultured 48 hours with LPS and dextran sulfate. IgD-specific immunofluorescence of: (D) fresh splenocytes; (E) B-lymphocytes cultured 48 hours in the absence of mitogens; and (F) B-lymphocytes cultured 48 hours with LPS and dextran sulfate. Ia-specific immunofluorescence of: (G) fresh splenocytes; (H) B-lymphocytes cultured 48 hours in the absence of mitogens; and (I) B-lymphocytes cultured 48 hours with LPS and dextran sulfate. Cell cycle gatings were determined from correlation with cell diameter.

TABLE 2

MIgM, MIgD AND MIa EXPRESSION PER UNIT MEMBRANE ON MURINE B-LYMPHOCYTES IN
VARIOUS PHASES OF CELL CYCLE*

Cell Cycle Phase†	Fluorescence Intensity Per Unit Surface Area‡		
	mIgM	mIgD	mIa
G_0 (unstimulated)§	.104	.229	.076
G_0 (4.5–5.5 μm)	.102	.293	.357
G_{1A} (5.5–7.0 μm)	.146	.073	.407
G_{1B}, S (7.0–10 μm)	.079	.035	.088
S, G_2 and M (10–12 μm)	.076	.021	.050

*Performed 48 hours after mitogen stimulation except where noted, 1000 cells per assay.

†Determined by direct measurement of cell diameter correlated with cell cycle as described in text.

‡Determined by dividing relative mean integrated fluorescence intensity by mean surface area for the designated population. Surface area was calculated on the assumption of uniform distribution of cell diameters within the size population.

§Unstimulated cells cultured for 36 hours, 4.5–5.5 μm in diameter.

To further investigate these fluctuations in mIa and mIgD expression on stimulated B-cells, we monitored their expression in the presence of mitogens and the cell cycle inhibitors actinomycin D and hydroxyurea. Actinomycin D, when used at 0.05 μg/ml final concentration, has been demonstrated to block entry of mitogen-stimulated lymphocytes into G_1 by specifically inhibiting rRNA production.[31] Hydroxyurea, on the other hand, allows stimulated cells to enter and transit G_1 but blocks entry into S. FIGURE 6 illustrates the effect of actinomycin D (FIGURE 6A) or hydroxyurea (FIGURE 6B) on mitogen-stimulated changes on mIgD expression. In support of previous results which indicate mIgD is lost in G_1, actinomycin D blocks the observed decrease in mIgD expression while hydroxyurea does not. The same analyses were performed for mIa expression (FIGURE 7A, B). Actinomycin D (FIGURE 7A) blocks the initial increase in mIa expression while hydroxyurea (FIGURE 7B) does not, demonstrating that the elevation in mIa density occurs at some point after the block imposed by actinomycin D but prior to that by hydoxyurea. In addition, with hydroxyurea present, the decrease in mIa expression among cells late in cycle is not evident. These results, in addition to those described previously, suggest that the decrease in mIa expression occurs during early S phase.

DISCUSSION

Polyclonal activation of murine B-cells results in a decrease in mIgD expression as cells transit G_1. The magnitude of this loss suggests that it is mediated by an active process. MIgM expression, on the other hand, remains constant during passage through cell cycle. MIa expression exhibits a sharp increase on stimulated cells transiting from G_0 into early G_1 (G_{1A}). However, beginning during early S phase, mIa expression decreases dramatically until by late S, G_2 and M phase it is lower than that of unstimulated B-cells.

It could be argued that the discussed decreases in mIa and mIgD expression are merely manifestations of selective proliferation by the low mIa and mIgD expressing populations. However, this seems unlikely in view of observations demonstrating that when expression of these markers is monitored at varying time points, an increase in frequency of total low mIa and mIgD expressing B-cells is correlated with a commensurate decrease in cells expressing high levels of the respective markers. This relationship suggests that the cells expressing low levels of these markers are in fact derived from the respective high mIa and mIgD expressing populations. These results are presented in FIGURES 8 and 9, which show the frequency of mIa and mIgD positive cells, respectively, relative to intensity of immunofluorescence marker expression at various time points. For mIa (FIGURE 8), exposure of cells to mitogen results in an increased frequency of high intensity mIa expressing cells relative to unstimulated cells through 36 hours after stimulation (FIGURE 8a–c). However, by 48 hours (FIGURE 8d) there is an increase in the frequency of low mIa expressing cells. This increase is at the expense of frequency of high expressing cells suggesting that low mIa expressors are derived from the high mIa expressors. A similar pattern is exhibited by cells stained for mIgD (FIGURE 9) except one does not observe an initial increase in

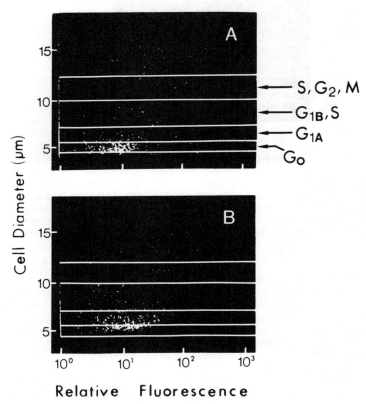

FIGURE 6. Immunofluorescence cytograms demonstrating the effect of cell cycle inhibitors on mIgD expression of LPS and dextran sulfate stimulated murine B-cells. B-cells were cultured with actinomycin D (0.05 μg/ml, A), or hydroxyurea (2 mM, B) plus mitogens for 48 hours before being stained for analysis of IgD expression. In each case 1000 cells were analyzed. Cell cycle gatings were determined from correlation with cell diameter.

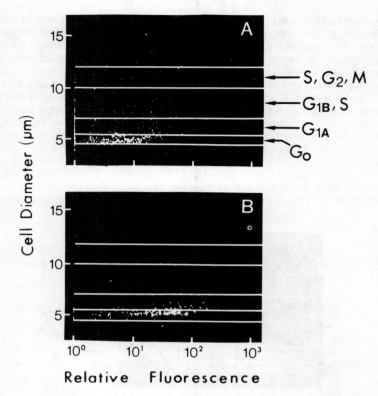

FIGURE 7. Immunofluorescence cytograms demonstrating the effect of cell cycle inhibitors on mIa expression by LPS and dextran sulfate stimulated murine B-cells. B-cells were cultured with actinomycin D (0.05 μg/ml, A) or hydroxyurea (2 mM, B) plus mitogens for 48 hours before being stained for analysis of Ia expression. In each case, 1000 cells were analyzed. Cell cycle gatings were determined from correlation with cell diameter.

frequency of cells expressing, higher level of this marker. The increase in frequency of low mIgD expressors observed occurs earlier than the increase in frequency of low mIa positive cells (36 hours as compared to 48 hours). This is expected since the decrease in mIgD expression occurs earlier in cell cycle than that of mIa. Again, the increased frequency of low mIgD expressors is correlated with a decreased frequency of cells expressing high mIgD levels.

It is interesting that mIgD is removed from the surface of the B-cell while mIgM remains at a relatively constant level. These results suggest differences with respect to mIgM and mIgD regulation and function. Loss of mIgD soon after activation suggests that it may function only during early stages of activation. MIgM is expressed and therefore may function throughout B-lymphocyte activation and clonal expansion. In the case of mIgD, this is consistent with proposals by Melchers et al.[16] that cell surface Ig is only required for stimulation of G_0 B-cell entry into G_1 by antigen and specific T-cell help. After cells become blasts, only nonspecific factors are required for clonal expansion and differentiation into antibody secreting cells.[6,16] MIgM, with its reported propensity for transmitting tolerogenic signals following interaction with haptenated gamma globulins,[33] may function on proliferating cells by binding immune complexes generated during the immune response and transmitting "off" signals to the cells. Thus, the predominance of mIgM on activated cells provides a mechanism by which immune complex feedback regulation may be mediated.[34]

MIa, like mIg, is believed to function during the initial phases of B-cell activation. It has been suggested that mIa influences the interaction of specific T-helper cells or their soluble products with the antigen-specific B cell.[7,8] This

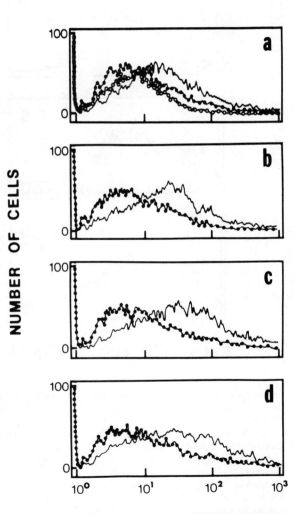

FIGURE 8. Immunofluorescence histograms of murine B-lymphocytes stained for surface Ia. In each case 10,000 cells were analyzed. Fluorescence intensity of fresh splenocytes (O-O-O); unstimulated, cultured B-cells (●-●-●); and mitogen-stimulated B-cells (—). Analysis was conducted 12(a), 24(b), 36(c), and 48(d) hours after initiation of cultures.

NUMBER OF CELLS

RELATIVE FLUORESCENCE

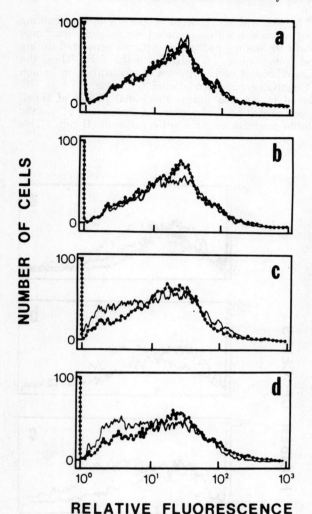

FIGURE 9. Immunofluorescence histograms of murine B-lymphocytes stained for surface IgD. In each case 10,000 cells were analyzed. Fluorescence intensity is expressed as the log of integrated fluorescence intensity. Unstimulated, 48 hour cultured B-cells (●-●-●) and 48 hour cultured and mitogen-stimulated B-cells (—) were analyzed 12(a), 24(b), 36(c), and 48(d) hours after initiation of cultures.

RELATIVE FLUORESCENCE

interaction is believed to occur during the initial stages of B-cell activation (i.e., the G_0 to G_1 transition) since only resting B-cells require Ia-restricted, antigen-specific T-cell help for activation.[6,9] The five to sixfold increase in mIa density which occurs during transition of G_0 cells into G_1, would facilitate more efficient focusing of Ia restricted T-cell help at a time when a requirement for I-region restricted help is manifest. Other studies[6,16] have demonstrated that B-cell blasts, presumably in cycle (i.e., G_1, S, G_2 and M), have no requirements for mIa-restricted, antigen-specific help, instead requiring only nonspecific T-cell help for proliferation and differentiation into antibody secreting cells. Thus, the dramatic decrease in mIa expression we observed at this time is perhaps not surprising.

ACKNOWLEDGMENTS

We wish to thank Drs. Robert Giles and Fred Finkelman for gifts of antigens. We thank Mr. Grant Mills and Ms. Wendy Havran for expert technical assistance. We also thank Ms. Sue Glenn and Ms. Jackie Smith for their secretarial assistance.

REFERENCES

1. GODING, J. 1978. Contemp. Top. Immunobiol. **8**: 203.
2. FRELINGER, J. A., F. J. HIBBLER & S. W. HILL. 1979. J. Immunol. **121**: 2376.
3. KATZ, D. H., M. GRAVES, M. E. DORF, H. DIMUZIO & B. BENACERRAF. 1975. J. Exp. Med. **141**: 263.
4. ANDERSON, J. & F. MELCHERS. 1981. Proc. Natl. Acad. Sci. USA. **78**: 2497.
5. KELLER, D. M., J. E. SWIERKOSZ, P. MARRACK & J. W. KAPPLER. 1980. J. Immunol. **124**: 1350.
6. ANDERSON, J., M. H. SCHREIER & F. MELCHERS. 1980. Proc. Natl. Acad. Sci. USA. **77**: 1612.
7. JONES, B. & C. A. JANEWAY. 1981. Nature **292**: 547.
8. SPRENT, J. 1980. J. Exp. Med. **152**: 996.
9. MELCHERS, F., J. ANDERSON, W. LERNHARDT & M. H. SCHREIER. Biochem. Soc. Symp. **45**: 75.
10. MOND, J. J., E. SEGAL, J. KUNG & F. D. FINKELMAN. 1981. J. Immunol. **127**: 881.
11. FINKELMAN, F. D., J. J. MOND, I. SCHER, S. W. KESSLER & E. S. METCALF. 1981. In Proceedings of the International Conference on B-Lymphocytes in the Immune Response. M. Cooper, D. E. Mosier, I. Scher & E. S. Vitetta, Eds.: **2**. Elsevier/North Holland. New York, N.Y.
12. BOURGOIS, A., K. KITASIMA, I. R. HUNTER & B. A. ASKONAS. 1977. Eur. J. Immunol. **7**: 151.
13. SITIA, R., J. ABBOTT & U. HAMMERLING. 1979. Eur. J. Immunol. **9**: 859.
14. PREUD'HOMME, J. L. 1979. Eur. J. Immunol. **7**: 191.
15. STASHENKO, P., L. M. NADLER, R. HARDY & S. F. SCHLOSSMAN. 1981. Proc. Natl. Acad. Sci. USA. **78**: 3848.
16. MELCHERS, F., J. ANDERSSON, W. LERNHARDT & M. H. SCHREIER. 1980. Immunol. Rev. **52**: 89.
17. DENNERT, G., R. HYMAN, J. LESLEY & I. S. TROWBRIDGE. 1980. Cell Immunol. **53**: 350.
18. OI, V. T., P. P. JONES, J. W. GODING & L. A. HERZENBERG. 1978. Cur. Top. Immunobiol.
19. GREEN, W. M. 1975. Avidin. Adv. Prot. Chem. **29**: 85.
20. POHLIT, H. M., W. HAAS, H. VON BOEHMER. 1979. Haptenation of viable biological carriers. In Immunological Methods. I. Lefkovits & B. Pernis, Eds.: **181**. Academic Press. New York, N.Y.
21. WOFSY, L., C HENRY, J. KIMURA & J. NORTH. 1970. In Selected Methods in Cellular Immunology: 287–304. W. H. Freeman Co. San Francisco, Calif.
22. DARZYNKIEWICZ, Z., D. EVENSON, L. STAIANO-COICO, T. SHARPLESS & M. R. MELAMED. 1979. Proc. Natl. Acad. Sci. USA. **76**: 358.
23. SHARPLESS, T., F. TRAGANOS, Z. DARYZNKIEWICZ & M. R. MELAMED. 1975. Acta Cytologica **19**: 577.
24. CAMBIER, J. C., C. FERNANDEZ DE ALBORNOZ, W. L. HAVRAN & R. B. CORLEY. 1981. J. Immunol. **127**: 1685.
25. MONROE, J. G., W. L. HAVRAN & J. C. CAMBIER. 1982. Cytometry. In press.
26. DITTRICH, W. & W. GOHDE. 1969. Z. Naturforsch **24b**: 360.
27. BRAUNSTEIN, J.D., M. R. MELAMED, Z DARYZNKIEWICZ, F. TRAGANOS, T. SHARPLESS & R. A. GOOD. 1975. Clin. Immunopath. **4**: 209.
28. CRISSMAN, H. A. & J. A. STEINKAMP. 1973. J. Cell Biol. **59**: 766.
29. DARZYNKIEWICZ, Z., T. SHARPLESS, L. STAIANO-COICO & M. R. MELAMED. 1980. Proc. Natl. Acad. Sci. USA. **77**: 6696.

30. DARZYNKIEWICZ, Z., D. EVERSON, L. STAIANO-COICO, T. SHARPLESS & M. R. MELAMED. 1979. Proc. Natl. Acad. Sci. USA. **76**: 358.
31. DARZYNKIEWICZ, Z., F. TRAGANOS, T. SHARPLESS & M. R. MELAMED. 1976. Proc. Natl. Acad. Sci. USA. **73**: 2881.
32. DARZYNKIEWICZ, Z., F. TRAGANOS & M. R. MELAMED. 1980. Cytometry **1**: 98.
33. CAMBIER, J. C., E. S. VITETTA, J. R. KETTMAN, G. M. WETZEL & J. W. UHR. 1977. J. Exp. Med. **146**: 1077.
34. SINCLAIR, N. R. STC. 1980. In Strategies of Immune Regulation. E. Sercarz & A. J. Cunningham, Eds.: 211.

DISCUSSION OF THE PAPER

PARTICIPANT: I thought actinomycin-D inhibited transcription?

J. C. CAMBIER: No, at the level it was used, .05 micrograms per ml, it inhibits production of ribosomal RNA only.

F. D. FINKELMAN: John, do you have any data on what happens to these cells after they've gone through the cycle? Do they stop cycling?

CAMBIER: No. That's a more difficult question to answer because in most instances not all B-cells will go into cycle so it would be necessary to sort the Ss, G2s and Ms, put them back in culture and see what happens when they went back to G1.

FINKELMAN: We have some very preliminary evidence that would suggest that cells that go into cycle as a result of treatment with anti-δ also lose a considerable amount of surface IgM. Have you done any anti-immunogobulin proliferation studies and looked to see if different populations of cells which responded to these different stimuli respond differently with regard to surface Ig isotype?

CAMBIER: No, although this is obviously not physiological we were interested in knowing whether, in the absence of anti-Ig reagents, these kind of effects occurred.

L. HERZENBERG: With all the different commercial instruments you now can get for doing flow cytometry, sorting, and with the different kinds of computer programs for the biologist to play with in which it is easy to press a button and get the apparent amount of fluorescence per surface area after you put all the data in, I was wondering whether this will mislead us because we know that cells are not really plastic spheres. They have very irregular surfaces and that surface area is therefore not dependent necessarily upon the diameter of the cell. We can easily get into trouble by overinterpreting.

CAMBIER: We are limited to the assumption that the cells are smooth spheres and there certainly is evidence that they are villous and not smooth spheres after they undergo blastogenesis. Your point is well taken.

IMMUNOGLOBULIN RECEPTORS REEVALUATED*

Ellen S. Vitetta

Department of Microbiology
University of Texas Health Science Center
Dallas, Texas 75235

INTRODUCTION

Early studies of IgD in the human established that it was a minor serum immunoglobulin (Ig)[1] and a major Ig receptor on B-cells.[2,3] Further studies in the mouse demonstrated that sIgD appeared after sIgM during ontogeny,[4-6] and that the vast majority of B-cells in both humans and mice coexpress both isotypes.[6] This provocative finding of the coexpression of sIgM and sIgD raised questions concerning the necessity for the expression of two receptors with the same antigen-binding specificity[7-9] on a single B-cell from a given clone. Because IgD was not present in significant levels in the serum, it clearly served as a membrane receptor. But, how did it differ from sIgM? Questions concerning the function of sIgD, relative to sIgM, have been studied experimentally for the past several years. While some insight has been gained, a "unique" role for sIgD remains elusive.

IgD: A MODEL

In 1975, Jonathan Uhr and I published a paper in *Science*[10] which postulated a unique role for sIgD. The main features of the model (which encompassed additional aspects of B-cell differentiation as well) were:

1) IgD is a triggering receptor; the interaction of antigen and T-cells with a B-cell bearing both sIgD and sIgM results in either proliferation and/or terminal differentiation into antibody-secreting cells;

2) sIgM is a tolerizing receptor present on immature B-cells which lack sIgD. The interaction of antigen with sIgM$^+$ B-cells results in tolerance.

It was further suggested that sIgM may function univalently with large immunogens, whereas sIgD might function divalently. Thus, triggering *versus* tolerance could depend on the extent of aggregation of receptors by antigens which were either pauci or multivalent.

Reevaluation of the Model

Is IgD a Triggering Receptor?

During the past six yeras, there have been a number of studies which have attempted to test the hypotheses set forth in this model and to determine the ability of sIgM vs. sIgD to deliver a triggering vs. a tolerogenic signal to the B-cell. Data have been accumulated, both in support of the concept that IgD is a triggering receptor, and in disagreement with this suggestion. The pros and cons of this argument are summarized in TABLE 1.

*This study was supported by NIH Grant AI-12789.

255

The major generalizations that I can make from a reevaluation of the different findings are: 1) mature B-cells which are responsive to certain thymus-independent antigens may express IgD but they do not require the presence of IgD for triggering. In contrast, B-cells responding to thymus-dependent antigens appear to require IgD for triggering, at least a certain in vitro systems. This would imply that sIgM on the adult B-cell is capable of generating a positive signal when certain types of antigens are used. The data does not, however, argue against the hypothesis that sIgD is a triggering receptor, but rather limits this hypothesis in the sense that sIgD is required as a triggering receptor when some, but not other, antigens are used. Furthermore, sIgM can also trigger B-cells so sIgD does not appear to be unique in this regard.

The major difficulty with all the experiments described in TABLE 1 is the anti-δ is frequently used to either remove sIgD receptors from cells, sort cells on the FACS, or to alter their function prior to subsequent challenge with antigen. It is therefore possible that the anti-δ reagent itself delivers a signal to the cell. In this regard, it is now established that anti-immunoglobulin antibodies can induce B-cells to proliferate but not to differentiate into antibody-secreting cells.[12,13,23-35] This presents two problems. First, the definition of a "triggering" receptor must be modified to accommodate a more limited type of triggering signal, i.e., proliferation. Secondly, proliferation and differentiation appear to be two different aspects of the activation process,[29-31,33-36] the latter requires T-cell-derived B-cell differentiation factors (BCDF).[30,33-35,37-38] Therefore, it is possible that in cases where anti-δ blocks antibody secretion, there may be an alteration in the ability of the B-cell to receive the second signal, i.e., BCDF. Thus, anti-δ might induce proliferation and at the same time inhibit secretion. If this is the case, it might further imply that sIgD is in some way involved with the receipt of BCDF and that its permanent modulation from the membrane renders the B-cell refractory to the effects of BCDF. Thus, experiments involving anti-δ antibodies must be reevaluated with respect to possible effects of the antibodies themselves.

Is IgM a Tolerizing Receptor?

TABLE 2 summarizes the data bearing on the issue of whether sIgM is a tolerizing receptor.

The original impetus for this hypothesis was the finding that immature B-cells which lack sIgD but express large amounts of sIgM, are easily tolerized in certain in vitro systems. Some experiments designed to investigate the role of sIgM as a tolerizing receptor relied on the use of adult B-cells from which IgD had been

TABLE 1

IgD is a Triggering Receptor

Pro:	1) The major immunocompetent responding B-cell is sIgM+IgD+.[11]
	2) Mitogenic forms of anti-δ induce B-cell proliferation both in vitro[12,13] and in vivo.[14,15]
	3) Anti-δ blocks antibody secretion in vitro (using some TI-2 and TD antigens.)[16-18]
	4) Removal of sIgM from a B-cell renders that cell difficult to tolerize.[19]
Con:	1) Some antibody responses (TI-1) are not blocked with anti-δ.[16]
	2) Cells bearing only sIgM can respond to antigen in adoptive transfer or splenic fragment assays.[20-22]

TABLE 2

IgM IS A TOLERIZING RECEPTOR

Pro:	1) Immature B-cells which bear predominantly sIgM are easily tolerized.[39-44]
	2) Removal of sIgD from an adult B-cell renders that cell more susceptible to tolerance induction.[19,45,46]
	3) If sIgD⁺ cells are removed from a population of adult or neonatal B-cells, the remaining sIgM cells do not respond to antigen *in vitro*.[11]
Con:	1) Sorted sIgD⁻IgM⁺ cells are not readily tolerized.[21]
	2) Sorted sIgD⁻IgM⁺ cells respond in an adoptive transfer assay.[22]
	3) Mitogenic forms of anti-μ induce proliferation of adult B-cells.[12,24,28,32]
	4) Susceptibility to tolerance induction in some systems wanes before sIgD appears.[39]

removed by antibody or proteolytic enzyme. It was assumed that these sIgD⁻ cells were analogous to immature sIgD⁻ B-cells; in retrospect, this was probably an oversimplification. In other experiments, cells were sorted into sIgD⁺ and sIgD⁻ by the use of an anti-δ antibody and these separated populations were tested for susceptibility to tolerance induction. Again, in these experiments, anti-δ itself may have induced a "signal." Taken together, I now reevaluate this issue as follows:

1) IgM on an *adult* B-cell can deliver a proliferative signal when appropriately cross-linked by ligand. Proliferation might imply that the cells subsequently express a receptor for macrophage or T-cell derived B-cell growth factor(s) (BCGF),[47-49] and that binding of BCGF either induces or maintains proliferation. In addition, once the IgM receptors have been cross-linked, the B-cells will express receptors for BCDF. The addition of BCDF will then induce differentiation into antibody-secreting cells. Again, it might be suggested that sIgM and sIgD differ in their ability to be cross-linked by antigen which points to the possibility that sIgM may be univalent and sIgD may be divalent. However, once either or both receptors are cross-linked, proliferation and differentiation would follow.

2) In contrast to the findings with adult B-cells, cross-linking of sIgM on (sIgD⁻) *immature* B-cells does not induce proliferation.[30,31] This might be due to the failure of immature B-cells to express a receptor for BCGF. However, the interaction of sIgM with ligand might lead to expression of receptors for BCDF since the cells may be induced to differentiate (but not proliferate) in the presence of BCDF.[31,35] It might be possible, therefore, to view sIgM-mediated tolerance of the neonatal B-cell as terminal differentiation in the absence of clonal expansion.

The above arguments suggest that the sIgM⁺IgD⁻ neonatal B-cells are different from sIgM⁺ adult B-cells, from which sIgD has been modulated, e.g., the latter can express a receptor for BCGF. This would further suggest that IgM may be a "tolerizing" receptor of the immature B-cell, but only because the neonatal B-cell fails to proliferate in the presence of ligand and instead, terminally differentiates. Thus, some other property of the immature B-cell, rather than the presence of IgM *per se*, may be important in determining the tolerogenic properties of the sIgM.

The Relationship between sIgD and the T-Cell Signal

One interesting finding to emerge from studies with adult B-cells, is that there is an apparent correlation between the T-dependency of an antigen and the requirement for sIgD on the B-cell.[16,18,50] This could be explained by arguments similar to those described above:

1) Most T-dependent antigens are paucivalent. If sIgM is univalent and sIgD is divalent, the presence of both receptors might be necessary for optimal cross-linking. Cross-linking of sIgD or sIgM causes an increase in receptors for BCDF.

2) Thymus-independent antigens which require only sIgM for triggering may interact with a second site on the membrane which either mimics a receptor for BCDF or induces a receptor for BCDF. Such antigens might effectively cross-link the putatively univalent sIgM receptors because they are highly multivalent.

3) Soluble BCDF may bind to sIgD.

Issues to be Resolved

In order to address some of the questions raised in my discussion, I would pose four questions to be explored experimentally:

1) Can immature B-cells bearing *only* sIgM respond to TI-antigens before sIgD appears?

2) What is the functional valency of sIgM vs. sIgD?

3) Does ligand interaction with sIg on an adult vs. neonatal B-cell induce receptors for BCDF and/or BCGF?

4) Do sIgM and sIgD interact differentially with other regulatory molecules in the plasma membrane?

These issues are not mutually exclusive, nor are the answers expected to be universal for all experimental systems employed. Nevertheless, they would serve as a focus for defining a role for sIgM vs. sIgD.

Finally, it should be mentioned that the issues discussed here do not bear on the role of either sIgM of sIgD in generating memory cells. It is possible, for example, that the presence of sIgD on a mature B-cell is in some way involved with the "switch" to IgG and to the generation of IgG memory. Experiments bearing on this issue provide some support for this notion.[51-59] Nevertheless, since both sIgM and sIgD receptors are expressed on mature B-cells, it would be difficult at this time to provide a simple explanation for how they might differ in their ability to mediate either a switch to another isotype or the generation of memory cells. One could perhaps argue that isotype-specific BCDFs secreted by T-cells can bind to one sIg on the adult B-cell and thus generate a signal for a specific switch sequence. To resolve this issue would require purification of such lymphokines and an analysis of their binding to their receptors on the B-cell.

Acknowledgments

While I take sole responsibility for the views expressed in this article, my thinking has been influenced and shaped to a large extent by my collaborative interactions and discussions with Drs. J. Uhr, P. Isakson, E. Puré, J. Layton, J. Cambier, F. Ligler, L. Buck, D. Yuan, J. Kettman, F. Finkelman and J. Mond. I also thank Ms. G. A. Cheek for skillful secretarial assistance.

References

1. Rowe, D. S. & J. L. Fahey. 1965. A new class of human immunoglobulins: II. Normal serum IgD. J. Exp. Med. **121:** 185–188.

Vitetta: Immunoglobulin Receptors 259

2. VAN BOXEL, J., W. E. PAUL, W. D. TERRY & I. GREEN. 1972. IgD-bearing human lymphocytes. J. Immunol. **109:** 648–651.
3. ROWE, D. S., K. HUG, L. FORNI & B. PERNIS. 1973. Immunoglobulin D as a lymphocyte receptor. J. Exp. Med. **138:** 965–972.
4. VITETTA, E. S., U. MELCHER, M. MCWILLIAMS, J. PHILLIPS-QUAGLIATA, M. LAMM & J. W. UHR. 1975. Cell surface Ig. XI. The appearance of an IgD-like molecule on murine lymphoid cells during ontogeny. J. Exp. Med. **141:** 206–215.
5. KEARNEY, J. F., M. D. COOPER, J. KLEIN, E. R. ABNEY, R. M. E. PARKHOUSE & A. R. LAWTON. 1977. Ontogeny of Ia and IgD on IgM-bearing B-lymphocytes in mice. J. Exp. Med. **146:** 297–301.
6. GODING, J. W., D. W. SCOTT & J. E. LAYTON. 1977. Genetics, cellular expression and function of IgD and IgM receptors. Immunol. Rev. **37:** 152–186.
7. PERNIS, B., J. C. BROUET & M. SELIGMANN. 1974. IgD and IgM on the membrane of lymphoid cells in macroglobulinemia. Evidence for identity of membrane IgD and IgM antibody activity in a case with anti-IgG receptors. Eur. J. Immunol. **4:** 776–778.
8. GODING, J. W. & J. E. LAYTON. 1976. Antigen-induced co-capping of IgM and IgD-like receptors on murine B-cells. J. Exp. Med. **144:** 852–857.
9. STERN, C. & I. MCCONNELL. 1976. IgM + IgD as antigen binding receptors on the same cell with shared specificity. Eur. J. Immunol. **6:** 225–227.
10. VITETTA, E. S. & J. W. UHR. 1975. Immunoglobulin receptors revisited. Science. **189:** 964–969.
11. BUCK, L. B., D. YUAN & E. S. VITETTA. 1979. A dichotomy between the expression of IgD on B-cells and its requirement for triggering such cells with two T-independent antigens. J. Exp. Med. **149:** 987–992.
12. PURÉ, E. & E. S. VITETTA. 1980. Induction of murine B-cell proliferation by insolubilized anti-immunoglobulin. J. Immunol. **125:** 1240–1242.
13. ZITRON, I. M. & B. L. CLEVINGER. 1980. Regulation of murine B-cells through surface immunoglobulin. I. Monoclonal anti-delta antibody that induces allotype specific proliferation. J. Exp. Med. **152:** 1135–1146.
14. FINKELMAN, F. D., V. L. WOODS, S. B. WILBURN, J. J. MOND, K. E. STEIN, A. BERNING & I. SCHER. 1980. Augmentation of in vitro humoral immune responses in the mouse by an antibody to IgD. J. Exp. Med. **152:** 493–506.
15. PERNIS, B. 1975. The effect of anti-IgD antiserum on antibody production in rhesus monkeys. In Membrane Receptors of Lymphocytes. M. Seligmann, J. L. Preud'homme & F. M. Kourilsky, Eds.: 25–26. North-Holland Publishing Co. Amsterdam, the Netherlands.
16. CAMBIER, J. C., F. S. LIGLER, J. W. UHR, J. R. KETTMAN & E. S. VITETTA. 1978. Blocking of primary in vitro antibody responses to thymus-independent and thymus-dependent antigens with antiserum specific for IgM or IgD. Proc. Natl. Acad. Sci. (USA) **75:** 432–435.
17. LIGLER, F. S., J. C. CAMBIER, E. S. VITETTA, J. R. KETTMAN & J. W. UHR. 1978. Inactivation of antigen-responsive clones with antisera specific for IgM or IgD. J. Immunol. **120:** 1139–1142.
18. ZITRON, I. M., D. E. MOSIER & W. E. PAUL. 1977. The role of surface IgD in the response to thymic-independent antigens. J. Exp. Med. **146:** 1707–1718.
19. VITETTA, E. S., J. C. CAMBIER, F. S. LIGLER, J. R. KETTMAN & J. W. UHR. 1977. B-Cell tolerance. IV. Differential role of surface IgM and IgD in determining tolerance susceptibility of murine B-cells. J. Exp. Med. **146:** 1804–1808.
20. LAYTON, J. E., B. L. PIKE, F. L. BATTYE & G. J. V. NOSSAL. 1979. Cloning of B-cells positive or negative for surface IgD. I. Triggering and tolerance in T-independent systems. J. Immunol. **123:** 702–708.
21. LAYTON, J. E., J. M. TEALE & G. J. V. NOSSAL. 1979. Cloning of B-cells positive or negative for surface IgD. II. Triggering and tolerance in the T-dependent splenic focus assay. J. Immunol. **123:** 709–713.
22. ZAN-BAR, I., S. STROBER & E. S. VITETTA. 1977. The relationship between surface immunoglobulin isotype and immune function of murine B lymphocytes. I. Surface immunoglobulin isotypes on primed B-cell in the spleen. J. Exp. Med. **145:** 1188–1205.
23. FANGER, M. W., D. A. HART, J. V. WELLS & A. NISONOFF. 1970. Requirement for

cross-linkage in the stimulation of transformation of rabbit lymphocytes by antiglobulin reagents. J. Immunol. **105:** 1484–1492.

24. PARKER, D. C. 1975. Stimulation of mouse lymphocytes by insoluble anti-mouse immunoglobulin. Nature **258:** 361–363.

25. SCRIBNER, D. J., H. L. WEINER & J. W. MOORHEAD. 1978. Anti-immunoglobulin stimulation of murine lymphocytes. V. Age-related decline in Fc receptor- mediated immunoregulation. J. Immunol. **121:** 377–382.

26. SIDMAN, C. L. & E. R. UNANUE. 1978. Control of proliferation and differentiation in B-lymphocytes by anti-Ig antibodies and a serum-derived cofactor. Proc. Natl. Acad. Sci. (USA) **75:** 2401–2405.

27. SIECKMANN, D. G., R. ASOFSKY, D. MOSIER, I. ZITRON & W. E. PAUL. 1978. Activation of mouse lymphocytes by anti-immunoglobulin. I. Parameters of the proliferative response. J. Exp. Med. **147:** 814–829.

28. SIDMAN, C. L. & E. R. UNANUE. 1979. Requirements for mitogenic stimulation of murine B-cells by soluble anti-IgM antibodies. J. Immunol. **122:** 406–413.

29. ISAKSON, P. C., K. A. KROLICK, J. W. UHR & E. S. VITETTA. 1980. The effect of anti-immunoglobulin antibodies on the *in vitro* proliferation and differentiation of normal and neoplastic murine B-cells. J. Immunol. **125:** 886–892.

30. PARKER. D. C. 1980. Induction and suppression of polyclonal antibody responses by anti-Ig reagents and antigen-nonspecific helper factors. Immunol. Rev. **52:** 115–139.

31. VITETTA, E. S., E. PURE, P. C. ISAKSON, L. BUCK & J. W. UHR. 1980. The activation of murine B-cells: The role of surface immunoglobulins. Immunol. Rev. **52:** 211–231.

32. SIECKMANN, D. G., I. SCHER, R. ASOFSKY, D. E. MOSIER & W. E. PAUL. 1978. Activation of mouse lymphocytes by anti-immunoglobulin. II. A thymus-independent response by a mature subset of B-lymphocytes. J. Exp. Med. **148:** 1628–1643.

33. ISAKSON, P. C., E. PURÉ, J. W. UHR & E. S. VITETTA. 1981. Activation of neoplastic B cells by anti-Ig and T-cell factors. Proc. Natl. Acad. Sci. (USA) **78:** 2507–2511.

34. PARKER, D. C., J. J. FOTHERGILL & D. C. WADSWORTH. 1979. B-lymphocyte activation by insoluble anti-immunoglobulin: Induction of immunoglobulin secretion by a T-cell-dependent soluble factor. J. Immunol. **123:** 931–941.

35. PURÉ, E., P. C. ISAKSON, K. TAKATSU, T. HAMAOKA, S. L. SWAIN, R. W. DUTTON, G. DENNERT, J. W. UHR & E. S. VITETTA. 1981. Induction of B-cell differentiation by T-cell factors. I. Stimulation of IgM secretion by products of a T-cell hybridoma and a T-cell line. J. Immunol. **127:** 1953–1958.

36. KISHIMOTO, T., T. MIYAKE, Y. NISLIZAWA, T. WATANABE & Y. YAMAMURA. 1975. Triggering mechanism of B-lymphocytes. I. Effect of anti-immunoglobulin and enhancing soluble factor on differentiation and proliferation of B-cells. J. Immunol. **115:** 1179–1184.

37. SCHIMPL, A. & E. WECKER. 1972. Replacement of T-cell function by a T-cell product. Nature (New Biology) **237:** 15–17.

38. SCHIMPL, A. & E. WECKER. 1975. A third signal in B-cell activation given by TRF. Transplant. Rev. **23:** 176–202.

39. METCALF, E. S. & N. R. KLINMAN. 1976. *In vitro* tolerance induction of neonatal murine B-cells. J. Exp. Med. **143:** 1327–1340.

40. CAMBIER, J. C., J. R. KETTMAN, E. S. VITETTA & J. W. UHR. 1976. Differential susceptibility of neonatal and adult murine spleen cells to *in vitro* induction of B-cell tolerance. J. Exp. Med. **144:** 293–297.

41. BRUYNS, C., G. URBAIN-VANSANTEN, C. PLANARD, C. DE VOS-CLOETENS & J. URBAIN. 1976. Ontogeny of mouse B-lymphocytes and inactivation by antigen of early B-lymphocytes. Proc. Natl. Acad. Sci. (USA) **73:** 2462–2466.

42. ELSON, C. J. 1977. Tolerance in differentiating B-lymphocytes. Eur. J. Immunol. **7:**6–10.

43. SZEWCZUK, M. R. & G. W. SISKIND. 1977. Ontogeny of B-lymphocyte function. III. *In vivo* and *in vitro* studies on the ease of tolerance induction in B-lymphocytes from fetal, neonatal, and adult mice. J. Exp. Med. **145:** 1590–1601.

44. VENKATARAMAN, M. & D. W. SCOTT. 1977. Cellular events in tolerance. VI. Neonatal *vs* adult B-cell tolerance: Difference in antigen-binding cell patterns and lipopolysaccharide stimulation. J. Immunol. **119:** 1879–1881.

45. CAMBIER, J. C., E. S. VITETTA, J. R. KETTMAN, G. M. WETZEL & J. W. UHR. 1977. B-cell tolerance. III. Effect of papain-mediated cleavage of cell surface IgD on tolerance susceptibility of murine B-cells. J. Exp. Med. **146**: 107–117.
46. SCOTT, D. W., J. E. LAYTON & G. J. V. NOSSAL. 1977: Role of IgD in the immune response and tolerance. I. Anti-δ pretreatment facilitates tolerance induction in adult B-cells *in vitro.* J. Exp. Med. **146**: 1473–1483.
47. SREDNI, B., D. SIECKMANN, S. KUMAGAI, S. HOUSE, I. GREEN & W. PAUL. 1981. Long-term culture and cloning of nontransformed human B-lymphocytes. J. Exp. Med. **154**: 1500.
48. FORD, R., S. R. MEHTA, D. FRANZINI, R. MONTAGNA, L. LACHMAN & A. L. MAIZEL. 1981. Soluble factor activation of human B lymphocytes. Nature **294**: 261.
49. HOWARD, M., J. FARRAR, M. HILFILER, B. JOHNSON, K. TAKATSU, T. HAMOAKA & W. PAUL. 1982. Identification of a T-cell derived B-cell growth factor distinct from IL-2. J. Exp. Med. **155**: 914.
50. PURÉ, E. & E. S. VITETTA. 1980. The murine B cell response to TNP-polyacrylamide beads: The relationship between the epitope density of the antigen and the requirements for T-cell help and surface IgD. J. Immunol. **125**: 420–427.
51. YUAN, D., E. S. VITETTA & J. KETTMAN. 1977. Cell surface immunoglobulin. XX. Antibody responsiveness of subpopulations of B-lymphocytes bearing different isotypes. J. Exp. Med. **145**: 1421–1436.
52. ZAN-BAR, I., E. S. VITETTA, F. ASSISSI & S. STROBER. 1978. The relationship between surface immunoglobulin isotype and immune function of murine B-lymphocytes. III. Expression of a single predominant isotype on primed and unprimed B-cells. J. Exp. Med. **147**: 1374–1404.
53. BLACK, S. J., W. VAN DER LOO, M. R. LOKEN & L. A. HERZENBERG. 1978. Expression of IgD by murine lymphocytes. Loss of surface IgD indicates maturation of memory B-cells. J. Exp. Med. **147**: 984–996.
54. LAFRENZ, D., S. STROBER & E. S. VITETTA. 1981. The relationship between surface immunoglobulin isotope and the immune function of murine B-lymphocytes. V. High affinity secondary antibody responses are transferred by both IgD-positive and IgD-negative memory B-cells. J. Immunol. **127**: 867–872.
55. HERZENBERG, L. A., S. J. BLACK, T. TOKUHISA & L. A. HERZENBERG. 1980. Memory B-cells as successive stages of differentiation. Affinity maturation and the role of IgD receptors. J. Exp. Med. **151**: 1071–1087.
56. ZAN-BAR, I., S. STROBER & E. S. VITETTA. 1979. The relationship between surface immunoglobulin isotype and immune function of murine B-lymphocytes. IV. Role of IgD-bearing cells in the propagation of immunologic memory. J. Immunol. **123**: 925–930.
57. BLACK, S. J., T. TOKUHISA, L. A. HERZENBERG & L. A. HERZENBERG. 1980. Memory B-cells at successive stages of differentiation: Expression of surface IgD and capacity for self renewal. Eur. J. Immunol. **10**: 846–851.
58. COFFMAN, R. L. & M. COHN. 1977. The class of surface immunoglobulin on virgin and memory B-lymphocytes. J. Immunol. **118**: 1806–1815.
59. OKUMURA, K., M. H. JULIUS, T. TSU, L. A. HERZENBERG & L. A. HERZENBERG. 1976. Demonstration that IgG memory is carried by IgG-bearing cells. Eur. J. Immunol. **6**: 467–472.

DISCUSSION OF THE PAPER

LEE HERZENBERG: When we take B-cells from a given source and then discuss what happens to them, we can come up with different results because we may be dealing with different cell populations. So it seems to me what's in front of us now is to find out what the individual cell populations do.

E. S. VITETTA: I've been just as involved in sub-set analysis and function as you have and I really feel at this point that your point is valid. However, unless we can shorten the assay system, so we know the phenotype of the cell the day it's triggered, we're in trouble. When you take a cell that expresses a particular array of markers, inject it into an animal and wait three weeks, that cell can change. I think we have to shorten the assays to know what's on the cell when it's triggered.

LEE HERZENBERG: I think you are absolutely right but then we are all limited by the existing culture assays.

VITETTA: That's why I think that it's difficult to make unique interpretations using the sub-set approach. And, of course, you've got to add back the correct T-cells and adherent cells in the right ratios.

FINKELMAN: One can trigger the cell very nicely with either anti-μ or anti-δ, and one can trigger in a T-dependent way if you add T-factors to either anti-μ or anti-δ treated cells.

Second, anti-μ and anti-δ can both block in vitro antibody responses but anti-μ tends to block a great deal better than anti-δ. If anti-μ or anti-δ can block, and yet the other immunoglobulin isotype is sufficient by itself to trigger, that would indicate to me that the combining of ligands to either surface immunoglobulin can give a negative signal as well as a positive signal: the negative signal being the one responsible for blocking. I would conclude that the main difference between antigen binding to IgM and to IgD is a quantitative difference in this negative signal. I think that since '74 the main shift has been away from the idea that one isotype is black and the other is white. They are both tones of gray but IgM is a darker immunoglobulin than IgD.

VITETTA: I think that one thing we have to take into account is that when we talk about triggering with an antibody against an isotype we're talking about proliferation. When we're talking about blocking with an antibody against an isotype we're talking about differentiation, and we know now that those two phases of B-cell activation are rather independently controlled and may have different requirements. It may be very possible that if you take a receptor off a cell an anti-δ antibody that cell will proliferate, but if you keep that receptor off the cell you can't receive the second part of the cascade to go on to differentiate. So you can see where it could proliferate and yet be inhibited at the same time. I think we have to put these blocking experiments into that kind of context.

FINKELMAN: I think it's hard to accept that context when you have experiments to show that anti-δ+ factor or anti-μ+ factor will give you differentiation. I agree there may well be quantitative differences. In vivo this is supported also by the idea that anti-δ, when there's a T-cell response to the anti-δ molecule, can give you polyclonal activation. Yet, if you remove IgD positive cells and seem at least to have only IgM positive cells by neonatally suppressing with anti-δ, you can still get a response to just about any antigen you can think of.

VITETTA: With neonatal suppression the IgD molecule is hit with an anti-δ. My problem with this experiment is that I am uncertain as to the outcome.

G. J. THORBECKE: I agree with your "negative" hypothesis that there is no essential difference between the B-cell triggering via IgD, IgM, or antigen on the surface. The in vivo experiments, in which suppression from birth with anti-IgD is obtained, and the animals have a continuous absence of the δ receptor, show the presence of very few B-cells in such mice. The differences between such mice and normal mice are explained primarily on a quantitative basis. Those differences that don't seem to be explained on a purely quantitative basis have something to do with the recirculating ability of the IgD cells, such that B-cells are almost completely absent in the lymph nodes. From such experiments we should come away with the strong message that there is the ability of anti-IgD to inhibit the development of the B-cell, but certainly not to inhibit the ability of B-cells to respond.

VITETTA: I think the *in vivo* studies will be discussed at greater length tomorrow.

D. W. SCOTT: Ellen, I agree with most of what you said; however, I do take issue with one point which has to do with the proposal that in the neonate an interaction with the IgM receptor, in the presence of T-cell factors, leads to terminal differentiation without proliferation. Now that to me seems to be a very testable hypothesis.

VITETTA: Ellen Puré in my lab did such experiments and she did get terminal differentiation in the absence of proliferation.

SCOTT: I think there are some alternative results obtained by others.

D. PARKER: I guess David is talking about my experiments in which we didn't see much of a response from the very young B-cells in a similar protocol.

VITETTA: We looked at your data, and we read it as a positive response so we have a question of interpretation.

PARKHOUSE: In 1974 there was a great feeling of euphoria that IgD must do many things. Today we're discussing IgM versus IgD, but really you haven't solved a unique function for any class of surface immunoglobulin and we haven't discussed whether IgG and IgA do or do not do anything in particular. I suspect that they don't.

VITETTA: Presumably, they are all divalent.

PARKHOUSE: They are receptors for B-lymphocytes, I think it will be a mistake to consider as functional receptors either in a positive or a negative sense only the IgM and IgD. You have to expand it to every known immunoglobulin class.

LEN HERZENBERG: In 1974, there was evidence, and certainly there now is absolutely airtight evidence, that there are IgG membrane molecules as well as IgA and IgE. They are all, therefore, receptors for antigen on the appropriate cells and they all must be taken into account. Here's an experiment which you might like to do. You say the difference between M and D is rigidity versus flexibility. Well, if you look at IgG then you know that γ-1 versus γ-2 have these different properties, γ-1 being inflexible and γ-2 being flexible. How about doing an experiment of the same sort as you've now done with IgM and IgD, where it's very complicated to explain, because they are on the same cell sometimes and there are different sub-sets, but it looks like there's much less of a problem if you'd look at the Gs. So I would suggest an experiment to reevaluate immunoglobulin receptors which would be to compare the response of γ-1 versus γ-2 on memory cells to polyvalent versus univalent antigens.

VITETTA: The problem with that approach is that you have such tight regulation by T-cells once you get B-cells to γ responses that I'm not sure one can really dissect out the epitope effect in a unique way.

LEN HERZENBERG: Maybe by analogy it's exactly as valuable as having looked at IgM and IgD in that way with different antigens. I think what is absolutely clear now, though, is that all these immunoglobulins can serve as receptors which I think is the big difference in reevaluating that 1974 paper now. If all the immunoglobulins have that same terminal amino acid intra-cytoplasmic extension maybe they all give the same signal and if some of them, such as was suggested for G are different, then maybe they all give different signals.

J. UHR: One reason to concentrate in the valency aspect of μ and δ is because of the old findings with regard to serum IgM. Serum IgM was distinguished from

IgG for a decade by sensitivity to 2-mercaptoethanol and what clearly happened when one reduced a molecule of the polyvalent ten or five to one, was that the univalent antibody is very ineffective at causing all the things that we looked at, including, surprisingly enough, phage inactivation. So there was every reason for thinking basically that any type of monomeric IgM was univalent. Further, what about the time element necessary for ligand receptor actions to result in imparting the signal to the cell? That time dimension, if not kept in mind, might make us misinterpret the data. I don't think we should talk about these interactions as not having that time element. It's not just a few seconds of interaction and cross linking and the results are fixed but rather, from studies with mitogens and anti-Ig, there's a significant time element. If this is true then immediately one has to be concerned about the possibilities that the dynamics of metabolism of the cell surface molecules might make a difference. With regard to neonatal cells, we can't forget about the older studies of Raff showing that they are fairly incapable of replenishing surface IgM after it's been removed by two or three rounds of capping.

FINKELMAN: I just couldn't pass up the point Len Herzenberg was making that because an immunoglobulin had the SIg gene structure and the proteins were on a membrane, that they had to serve as a receptor. It could be up there simply to tell the outside world what type of antibody this cell will make if it's triggered. It may not be serving as a receptor to tell the cell anything, so much as to just announce what kind of cell it is. So it's in the same sense that I would like to switch the IgD story and emphasize the role of the secreted form as an efferent signal. I think that some of these membrane forms might not be there primarily as antigen-recognizing units, but simply as more lymphocyte surface markers to tell the world what kind of cell it is.

VITETTA: There are known isotype specific T-cells factors and that might be the other rationale for having an IgE or an IgG-1 on the membrane.

LEN HERZENBERG: If you think the molecules are on there only to say what isotype and what idiotype they have and you want to discard the importance of antigen, then we could go along with you. Otherwise it is, as a minimum, the immunoglobulin molecule in the cell surface particularly because it's immuno-globulin that has got to find antigen. That's the definition of an antigen receptor.

COOPER: Theories aren't right or wrong, they are either useful or not useful. Early on I heard Bob Good say that so often that I began believing it. One could elaborate or debate that for awhile but to someone who has had a lot of disagreements with that particular theory, that you and Jon Uhr put forth, I'd just like to say that it's been in that sense an enormously useful hypothesis and model. Much of what we're discussing here has arisen by many of us trying to either shoot it down or support it but at least we were stimulated by it.

SURFACE IgD AS A FUNCTIONAL RECEPTOR ON MURINE B-LYMPHOCYTES*

Ian M. Zitron

Department of Biochemistry
Jefferson Medical College
Thomas Jefferson University
Philadelphia, Pennsylvania 19107

INTRODUCTION

The high representation of immunoglobulin D (IgD) on lymphocyte membranes compared to the low concentration at which IgD is found in serum has led to the suggestion that the principal function of this isotype is as a cell-bound receptor.[1] Over the past five years experimental evidence in support of this postulate has become available. The evidence has been obtained from two types of experiments, one type providing indirect support and the other providing a more direct and convincing demonstration of an active signalling function for surface IgD (sIgD).

The indirect evidence comes from studies in which anti-δ antibodies have been used to block immune responses in vitro. It has been shown that responses to type 2 thymic-independent (TI-2)[2] and thymic-dependent (TD)[3] antigens are susceptible to suppression by anti-δ antibodies while, in contrast, responses to type 1 thymic-independent (TI-1) antigens are resistant. Such experiments have been interpreted as showing the obligatory involvement of sIgD in the elicitation of responses to TI-2 and TD antigens; responses to TI-1 antigens would then presumably be induced either via sIgM alone, or via sIgM and a receptor for polyclonal B-cell activation (PBA). The mechanism by which anti-δ antibodies suppress responses is open to a variety of interpretations. While the simplest mechanisms to propose are the steric hindrance or capping away of sIgD, neither of these require that the interaction of ligand (whether anti-δ or antigen) with sIgD results in the active delivery of transmembrane signals. Blocking studies, therefore, can provide only inferential evidence for an active, signalling role for sIgD.

More direct and compelling evidence comes from studies in which anti-δ antibodies can be shown to induce B-cells to synthesize DNA, as measured by the incorporation of tritiated thymidine (^{3}H-TdR).[4-7] Several groups have reported this as, indeed, have there been reports of anti-μ antibodies activating cells to DNA synthesis.[8-10] Such studies are difficult to interpret in any way other than demonstrating an active signalling function for the surface immunoglobulin (sIg) isotype to which the antibodies are directed.

The aim of the experiments described in this paper was to investigate the signals delivered through sIgD. To do this, the purified Ig product of a monoclonal hybridoma which secretes an anti-δ antibody[4] was used. The study was designed to investigate the further consequences of stimulation through sIgD. The results provide a clearer view of B-cell activation through this isotype and indicate that even responses to TI-1 antigens can be affected by signals delivered to the B-cell by sIgD.

*Supported by RO1 AI-17989 from the National Institutes of Health

0077–8923/82/0399–0265 $01.75/0 © 1982, NYAS

METHODS

The B.C8 and C57BL/Ka mice used in these experiments were bred in the animal facility of the Biochemistry Department, Jefferson Medical College, from breeding stocks originally obtained from Litton Bionetics (provided under NCI contract NOI-CB-94326).

The monoclonal anti-δ, Hδ^a/1, which was used throughout, has been previously reported.[4] Priming with antigen or anti-δ was performed in Costar 3524 plates with cells at 5×10^6/ml in RPMI 1640 plus 1% fresh normal mouse serum (nms) (C57BL/Ka, heat-inactivated). After the indicated duration of priming culture, cells were harvested, washed and viable cells counted using either fluorescein diacetate or trypan blue. Challenge cultures were performed in Costar 3596 plates, using RPMI 1640 plus 10% foetal calf serum (fcs) for the induction of plaque-forming cells (pfc) or 2.5% fcs for ^{3}H-TdR incorporation. Hapten-specific pfc were assayed after three days of challenge culture, using the appropriately coupled sheep erythrocytes as indicator cells. ^{3}H-TdR incorporation was measured by pulsing challenge cultures after 48 hours with 1μCi ^{3}H-TdR and harvesting 16–18 hours later.

Limiting dilution analysis[11-13] in response to LPS was performed by diluting viable cells recovered from priming cultures into irradiated (1500r) thymocytes from young C57BL/Ka mice. Each microwell in the analysis contained a constant (5×10^5) irradiated thymocytes.

Elimination of cells by the use of 5-bromodeoxyuridine (BUdR) and the bis-benzimidazole dye Hoescht 33258 was performed as described by Maryanski et al.[14]

The data presented are the geometric means of triplicates, with the relative standard error shown in parentheses. ΔCPM is calculated as (stimulated-control) and the standard error of the difference (SEdiff) calculated as described previously.[2] Regression lines are calculated by the least squares method.

RESULTS

Hapten-coupled Ficolls are potent TI antigens but not polyclonal B-cell activators (PBAs). Moreover, Ficoll itself shows no immunogenicity; prior immunization of mice with undervitalized Ficoll has no apparent effect on anti-hapten responses to hapten-Ficoll. In experiments designed to investigate whether TI-2 antigens could generate B-cell memory, it was shown[15] that, while long-term B-cell memory could not be generated, a transient effect could be obtained. The effect, of increased response in vitro to TNP-Ficoll and TNP-Brucella abortus (TNP-BA) was shown using spleen cells from mice which had been immunized in vivo with low doses of DNP-Ficoll. The short-lived nature of the effect–optimal at three days after immunization and gone by 10 days–argued against memory generation in the generally understood sense, but rather in favor of a mechanism whereby the B-cells were activated from a resting state to a partially-activated state, which was reflected by greater responsiveness in vitro. In order to make the effect more amenable to study, I attempted to perform both the priming (for the sake of convenience, prestimulation whether in vivo or in vitro is referred to as priming) and challenge phases in vitro. The data from one such experiment is shown in TABLE 1.

The priming phase is carried out in medium supplemented with nms and the challenge phase in medium containing fcs. Preliminary experiments showed that

TABLE 1

In Vitro Priming with Hapten-Ficoll Compounds Is Hapten-Dependent, Hapten-Specific and Sensitive to Cytosine Arabinoside (Ara-C)

| 1st culture priming antigen | Anti-hapten IgM pfc/culture on challenge | | | |
| | anti-TNP pfc | | anti-FL pfc | |
	Medium	TNP-BA	Medium	FL-BA
AECM.Ficoll	8 (1.14)	168 (1.06)	41 (1.26)	241 (1.41)
TNP-AECM.Ficoll	76 (1.47)	1,693 (1.08)	16 (1.06)	298 (1.34)
FL-AECM.Ficoll	5 (1.59)	92 (1.26)	10 (1.10)	1,959 (1.06)
FL-AECM.Ficoll + Ara-C	6 (2.00)	66 (1.58)	5 (1.59)	378 (1.01)

1% nms was incapable of supporting pfc generation; and the use of fcs in both phases led to unacceptably high backgrounds when ^{3}H-TdR incorporation was used to assay the challenge cultures (data not shown). The data in TABLE 1 show that in vitro priming is both hapten-dependent and -specific and appears to involve the cells undergoing DNA synthesis, since priming is largely prevented by the inclusion of cytosine arabinoside (Ara-C) in the priming phase. This system of in vitro priming is essentially identical to that described by Scott.[16]

The question immediately arises as to the sIg isotype through which the priming effect operates. Scott et al. have also considered this question[16] and concluded that sIgD is not involved. However, given the evidence of inhibition studies that TI-2 antigens appear to require sIgD, and the availability of a monoclonal alloanti-δ which could be shown to activate B-cells, the ability of sIgD to induce priming was investigated directly. The data shown in TABLE 2 indicate quite clearly that stimulation in vitro through sIgD alone is capable of mimicking the antigen-driven priming seen with TI-2 antigens. In common with Scott's antigen-driven system, responses to both TI-1 and TI-2 antigens are increased. One can legitimately conclude, therefore, that sIgD may be involved in the priming process, though this in no way precludes a role for sIgM.

Ideally one would like to pursue these studies using permanently established, antigen-specific B-cells bearing both sIgM and sIgD. Since these are as yet unavailable, the alternative approach of using a polyclonal B-cell stimulus, lipopolysaccharide (LPS) (E. coli 0111:B4), has been adopted. The data which will be presented in the rest of this paper employs ^{3}H-TdR incorporation as the challenge assay. The results obtained using this assay have been unexpectedly interesting and are important as they provide a clearer picture than previously available of the events set in train by stimulating B-cells through sIgD.

The initial observation giving rise to these studies is shown in TABLE 3. The priming system was as described and three separate groups were set up. In this experiment the anti-δ and anti-group A carbohydrate (GAC) were ascitic fluids used at a final 10^{-3} dilution. In addition, LPS (10 μg/ml) was used for priming. The

TABLE 2

Stimulation of Cells via sIgD Alone Mimics Antigen-Driven Priming

| 1st culture stimulus | Anti-FL IgM pfc/culture on challenge | | |
	Medium	FL-BA	FL-ACEM. Ficoll
Anti-group A carbohydrate	19.1 (1.36)	444.6 (1.17)	20.8 (1.35)
Anti-δ	24.4 (1.36)	1,868.1 (1.06)	283.2 (1.16)

TABLE 3

STIMULATION THROUGH sIgD INCREASES SUBSEQUENT RESPONSIVENESS TO LPS

1st culture addition	³H-TdR incorporation in challenge culture			
	Medium	LPS	anti-δ	anti-GAC
anti-GAC	5,198 (1.11)	50,064 (1.03)	18,026 (1.02)	6,335 (1.09)
anti-δ	5,645 (1.11)	139,088 (1.06)	16,723 (1.04)	9,054 (1.01)
LPS	9,269 (1.08)	65,166 (1.03)	27,090 (1.08)	11,112 (1.05)

same three reagents, as well as medium (RPMI 1640 plus 10% fcs in this experiment) were used in the challenge cultures, which contained 5×10^5 viable cells recovered from the priming cultures plus an equal number of syngeneic, irradiated spleen cells as fillers. The only effect of substantial magnitude observed is when one compares the LPS-induced responses of cells from control (anti-GAC) and sIgD-stimulated cultures: the response of the stimulated cells is approximately three-fold greater than the control cells. Interestingly, the inclusion of an LPS-driven group shows no effect upon subsequent response to LPS.

The data in TABLE 3 are from an experiment in which the priming culture was of four days duration and the challenge culture performed at only a single responding cell number, 5×10^5. To ask whether this duration of priming was optimal, a kinetic experiment was performed. A single pool of B.C8 spleen cells was used, half being cultured in the presence of anti-δ and half in its absence. One, two and four days later, cells were harvested and recultured in a limiting

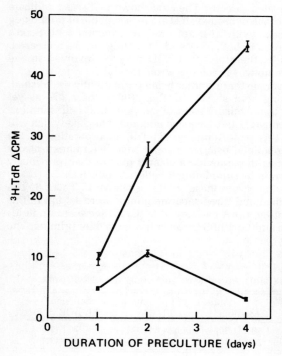

FIGURE 1. The kinetics of sIgD-restricted in vitro priming. Spleen cells from B.C8 mice were cultured for the indicated times in the presence (▲) or absence (●) of monoclonal anti-δ. The ordinate shows the responses (ΔCPM ± SE diff) to LPS (10 µg/ml) of 1.25×10^4 recultured viable cells. Cultures were pulsed at 48 hr and harvested 18 hr later.

dilution analysis, the assay being the incorporation of ^{3}H-TdR induced by LPS. The data from part of this experiment are shown in FIGURE 1. The points shown are the responses of 1.25×10^4 precultured cells in the presence of 5×10^5 irradiated thymocyte fillers. It is clear that one day of priming gives rise only to a small effect. Two days of priming give a significantly greater effect and four days give a greater effect still. Subsequent experiments have been performed with four days of priming culture, more extended times not having been investigated.

One possible, trivial explanation might be increased survival of B-cells cultured in the presence of anti-δ, compared to its absence. This is, in fact, not the case. Viable cell recoveries are comparable, averaging 20–25% of the starting viable cells after four days of preculture under the conditions described. If

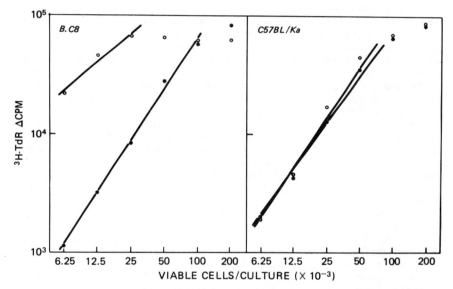

FIGURE 2. Priming through sIgD is allotype-specific. Spleen cells from B.C8 (left panel) and C57BL/Ka (right panel) mice were cultured for four days in the presence (open circles) or absence (solid circles) of monoclonal anti-δ. The data shown are the limiting dilution analyses of the recovered, viable cells in response to LPS (10 μg/ml).

anything, the recovery of viable cells from cultures containing anti-δ is slightly lower than the controls.

The experiment to examine the duration of priming also contained an allotype-specificity control. In parallel, throughout the whole experiment, a pool of spleen cells from C57BL/Ka mice was included. The data in FIGURE 2 confirm the allotype-specificity of the priming effect. In both panels, the open symbols show the responses of cell precultured in the presence of anti-δ; the closed symbols are the responses of cells cultured in its absence. These data result from four days of priming.

Several points can be made from these results. The priming effect is seen only in cells from B.C8 mice and not C57BL/Ka. This is consistent with the previously demonstrated allotype specificity of the anti-δ antibody. Thus priming is likely to be a direct result of the anti-δ, rather than resulting from a hitherto unrecognized contaminant. Cell recoveries after four days of priming were similar in all four pools of cells.

Two major types of quantitative information are obtainable from such limiting dilution analyses. The slope of the dilution curve indicates the number of cell types which are being diluted out; theoretically, then, the slopes should be integers. And if one obtains a priming effect such as that seen here, one can calculate the change in precursor frequency by asking how many cells for each pool are needed to obtain a comparable response. For this to be an accurate estimate, the lines should be parallel.

First, considering the slopes of the regression lines, three of the four lines show very similar slopes: BC8 control, m = 1.45; C57 control, m = 1.38; C57 anti-δ, m = 1.55. The slope of the fourth line, BC8 anti-δ, does not fall with the others, m = 0.81. This final slope is the least accurate of the four, since only three points were used to calculate the regression, so the value for m may be too low, because the assumption is made that the Δcpm value corresponding to 2.5 × 10⁴ cells is either off the plateau, or right at its edge. If one omits this point and just uses the data from the two lowest cell numbers, then m = 1.05. Regardless of the precise values of the slopes, it is clear from this and other experiments that the slopes of the regression lines obtained with LPS stimulation of precultured cells which have not been stimulated by anti-δ, either because of its absence from the culture or because the cells do not bear the allotypic determinant recognized by this antibody, have values around 1.4. I interpret this as indicating the requirement for another cell type. In contrast, the slopes of the regression lines obtained with cells which have been successfully primed with anti-δ are far closer to a value of 1, suggesting either that the need for this additional cell type has been obviated by prior activation, or that the rapidly dividing cells in the challenge culture have a medium-conditioning effect.

Given the differences in slopes, any estimate of the increase in LPS-responsive precursors must be approximate. However, if one performs the calculations using the responses of the two lowest doses of anti-δ-primed B.C8 cells and compares these to the regression line of the control B.C8 population, the increase in precursors is approximately sevenfold.

The T-dependence of anti-δ-driven priming has been investigated using monoclonal anti-Thy1.2 and rabbit complement (C). A pool of B.C8 spleen cells was divided into two aliquots, one being treated with anti-Thy1.2 followed by C and the other with medium followed by C. Each aliquot was then cultured for four days as described, one half of the cells in the presence of anti-δ, the other half in its absence. The challenge assay was as described and the data are shown in FIGURE 3. Treatment with anti-Thy1.2 plus C clearly did not affect the ability of the cell population to be primed. In this experiment, the precursor increase of the T-depleted population was 11-fold; the increase in the undepleted population was 14-fold. Therefore priming through sIgD appears to be operationally T-independent. To demonstrate the complete lack of a requirement for T-cells would require the use of a mixture of antibodies, and this has not been pursued.

The final point investigated was to ask whether DNA synthesis was involved in the priming phenomenon. The monoclonal anti-δ used in these experiments has been shown to stimulate ³H-TdR incorporation. However, since no increase in cell numbers as a result of anti-δ-induced priming was seen, despite an apparent seven to tenfold increase in the frequency of precursors responsive to LPS, it was possible that the cells induced to go through S phase by anti-δ and those which manifested the priming effect were different subpopulations of sIgD-positive cells. The experimental method used was the incorporation of BUdR into newly-synthesized DNA, followed by exposure to light. In order to improve the efficiency of killing, the bisbenzimidazole dye H33258 was also used both alone and in conjunction with BUdR.

Two pools of anti-Thy1.2 plus C-treated B.C8 spleen cells were cultured as described. One of these contained anti-δ, the other did not. After two days, BUdR

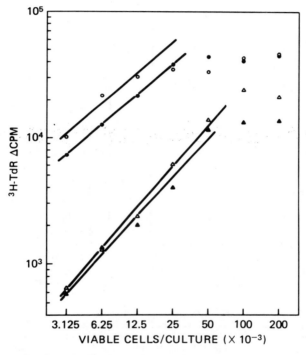

FIGURE 3. Priming through sIgD is resistant to pretreatment of the starting spleen cell population with monoclonal antiThy1.2 and complement. Spleen cells from B.C8 mice were treated with monoclonal anti-Thy1.2 and complement (closed symbols) or complement alone (open symbols) and then cultured for 4 days in the presence (O and ●) or absence (Δ and ▲) of anti-δ. The data shown are the limiting dilution analyses of all four populations in response to LPS.

was added to half of the cultures in each group to a final concentration of $10^{-6}M$. After a further two days, 33258 was added to half of the cultures to a final concentration of 5 μg/ml. There were now a total of eight distinct groups: medium or anti-δ, with for each of these two primary conditions, no additional treatment, BUdR only, 33258 only and BUdR plus 33258. After the addition of 33258, the cultures were incubated for a further two hours to allow incorporation of the dye, then all the groups were harvested, and exposed to light for 30 minutes at 23°C.

After further washing, viable cells were counted by trypan blue exclusion and all groups recultured in a limiting dilution analysis to measure their responses to LPS. The data are shown in FIGURE 4.

The left panel simply shows the full dilution curves obtained with cells which had been exposed to light only. Priming has obviously been successful, since the

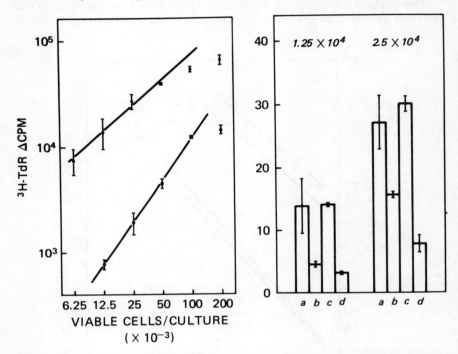

FIGURE 4. *In vitro* priming through sIgD activates cells to go through S phase. Anti-Thy1.2 + C-treated spleens cells from B.C8 mice were cultured for two days in the presence or absence of anti-δ. BUdR was then added to half of the cultures. After a further two days, Hoescht 33258 was added to half of each of the BUdR$^+$ and BUdR$^-$ cultures. Two hours later, all groups of cells were exposed to fluorescent light then washed and recultured for limiting dilution analysis in response to LPS. The left panel shows the full dilution curves for the populations exposed to light alone. The presence of anti-δ during the four day priming culture has resulted in an approximate 10-fold increase in precursor frequency to LPS. The right panel shows the responses of cells which had been primed with anti-δ; the data are ΔCPM ($\times 10^{-3}$) ± SEdiff and are abstracted from the full dilution curves and show only the responses of 1.25×10^4 and 2.5×10^4 viable cells. The letters a, b, c and d indicate the treatment groups: a–light exposure only, b–BUdR + light, c–Hoescht 33258 + light, and d–BUdR + Hoescht 33258 + light.

presence of anti-δ has resulted in an approximately tenfold increase in precursor frequency. The right panel shows data abstracted from the full dilution curves of cells which had been cultured in the presence of anti-δ; incorporation of ^{3}H-TdR is shown for two levels of input viable cells, 1.25×10^4 and 2.5×10^4. For both sets of data, block a shows the effect of light exposure only; block b shows the effect of BUdR plus light; block c, 33258 plus light; and block d BUdR + 33258 + light. The results are consistent for the two cell concentrations shown and also for the other points on the curves. BUdR plus light results in a significant depression of subsequent LPS responses. 33258 plus light in the absence of BUdR has no effect, but the combination of BUdR + 33258 + light clearly has an effect greater than BUdR + light. The priming effect therefore must be in large part a function of those cells which go through S phase during the latter half (days two–four) of the priming culture and not simply a subpopulation of sIgD-bearing cells which can become activated, but which do not go on to synthesize DNA.

Discussion

Models involving one,[17] two[18] or three[19] signals, to drive a resting B-cell all the way to high-rate antibody secretion, have been proposed. The "One Non-Specific Signal" model is unlikely to be correct, since both sIgM and sIgD are capable of delivering signals which result in DNA synthesis. Both of the other models postulate an active role for sIg.

The system of *in vitro* priming used in this work is very similar to the 'cross-priming' system of Scott et al.[16] The data which I have obtained is in general agreement with Scott with one exception, that being the role which sIgD might play in the priming event. The data in TABLE 2 demonstrate quite clearly that a B-cell population activated through sIgD alone during the priming phase gives greatly enhanced responses to both TI-1 and TI-2 antigens in the challenge assay. The claim that sIgD was not involved[16] was based upon experiments in which the addition of an alloanti-δ antiserum to priming cultures failed to inhibit priming. Those data must now be reinterpreted in the light of the evidence presented here. The interpretation which accommodates both sets of data is that both sIgM and sIgD can be responsible for priming. Thus blocking or removing sIgD simply diverts the priming signal to sIgM. In further support of sIgM being capable of priming are data from preliminary experiments in which anti-μ antibodies have been shown to prime for proliferative responses to LPS (I.M.Z. unpublished observations). Scott's demonstration that the same anti-δ which failed to abrogate priming was inhibitory to the primary p.f.c. response to Fl-Ficoll suggests that the mechanism by which anti-δ inhibits responses to TI-2 antigens is simply removal of sIgD or steric hindrance, rather than the ability of this isotype to deliver inhibitory signals.

In the context of models for B-cell triggering, while sIg is clearly not simply a passive focussing device, it might have been possible that in the response to mitogenic TI-1 antigens, such as hapten-coupled LPS and BA, that the signal delivered through sIg was largely unimportant, the principal stimulus being conveyed through the PBA receptor. The pfc data in TABLE 2 and the ^{3}H-TdR incorporation data shown in the rest of this paper indicate that this is, in fact, not the case. Rather, the response to mitogenic stimuli is profoundly affected by changes in the cells induced by signals delivered through sIgD.

The principal focus of this paper has been the effect of sIgD-mediated priming on the proliferative response to LPS. The effect is quite striking, giving rise to an apparent tenfold increase in precursor frequency as measured by limiting dilution analysis, in the face of no difference in the number of viable cells recovered from cultures which contained anti-δ compared to controls. The process appears to be the result of direct interaction of anti-δ with B-cells, since depletion of T-cells has no effect. Also, since B-cells appear to lose sIgD when they enter cycle,[20-22] the target cell is presumably a small, resting B-cell in G_0. The cells are activated from G_0 to G_1 and a significant fraction of these go through S, as indicated by the effect of BudR and light (FIGURE 4). The failure to observe an increase in the number of viable cells recovered from anti-δ-containing cultures can be the result of any three possible mechanisms.

The first is that the cells which have gone through S phase, enter G2 and become blocked prior to M. Subsequent stimulation with LPS in the challenge phase would allow them to undergo immediate mitosis and to continue in cycle without any lag period such as has been reported to occur in cells taken directly from mice and stimulated immediately with LPS.[23] The most direct evidence to support this mechanism would be cell cycle analysis, the prediction being that an anti-δ-primed population would contain a very high percentage of cells with 2C DNA, compared to control cells, which would presumably show a random distribution around the cycle. Finkelman et al.[24] have published data showing an increased frequency of cells with 2C DNA when the donor animals had received anti-δ in vivo. Cell cycle analysis of in vitro primed and control populations is in progress and the results should provide a direct demonstration of a G_2 block if this is the case. There is, however, evidence which can be used to support the model proposed and this comes from experiments in which challenge cultures were pulsed with ^{3}H-TdR at times earlier than the 48 hours time-point used in the experiments shown here. Both anti-δ-primed and control cells require LPS to transit S phase again; in the presence of LPS, the anti-primed cells enter S very rapidly (within the first six–seven hours), while control cells show a lag period of at least 18 hours. This would explain the apparently increased precursor frequency seen in the challenge assay, when the ^{3}H-TdR pulse is added at 48 hours: during that time the anti-δ-primed B-cells would have completed their first mitosis and continued to cycle, there being sufficient time to complete at least two more rounds of division.

The second mechanism which would successfully explain the data does not call for a G_2 block. Instead, cells put into cycle by the anti-δ would complete mitosis, their progeny possibly continuing in cycle and undergoing more divisions. This increase in cell numbers would, however, be balanced by death of some cells in the anti-δ-driven cultures. Parker[6] has reported the death of cells shortly after the addition of anti-δ antibodies. One might go even further and propose that there is a subset of sIgD-positive cells which do not respond to LPS and it is these which are preferentially lost, thereby reducing the number of cell divisions necessary to obtain the observed increase in precursor frequency.

The third alternative explanation is that the reported frequency[25] of B-cells capable of being activated by LPS is too high. While it has been suggested[26] that LPS can activate G_0 cells, while anti-Ig antibodies might stimulate only cells already in G_1, it seems possible that LPS is relatively inefficient at the initial activation step. Cross-linking of sIg might be the most crucial first step in making B-cells receptive to other regulatory signals. Given the clonal nature of the immune response, this is not unreasonable.

The physiological relevance of the priming process seems quite clear in terms of the immune response. B-cells would bind antigen via sIg, be put into cycle and thus rendered susceptible to other regulatory signals, in the case of these experiments the mitogenic signal delivered by LPS. One would predict that susceptibility to other signals, such as macrophage and T-cell-derived factors would also be increased. While experiments have not been performed with in vitro anti-δ-primed cells to demonstrate increased responses to TD antigens, cells primed in vivo[15] and in vitro[16] with haptenated-Ficoll do show increased responses to TD antigens on challenge. It is also noteworthy that Anderson and Melchers[19] have reported that their B-cell replication and maturation factor requires that the sIg on the target B-cell be occupied in order for division to occur.

Howard et al.[27] have recently reported the successful long-term growth of murine B-cells, using a protocol which begins with culture of the cells with LPS for a substantial period of time. If, in fact, stimulation through sIgD enables B-cells which would otherwise not be able to respond to LPS to do so, then a priming protocol involving stimulation via sIg prior to LPS might be a more efficient method of generating long-term lines of murine B-cells.

ACKNOWLEDGMENTS

I wish to thank Dr. Michael Potter for providing the breeding pairs of B.C8 and C57BL/Ka mice from which the animals used in these studies were derived. I thank Drs. Michael Cancro and Carol Cowing for helpful discussion, Ms. Kerri Pratt for excellent technical assistance and Ms. Susan Hanson for the preparation of the manuscript.

REFERENCES

1. VAN BOXEL, J. M., W. E. PAUL, W. D. TERRY & I. GREEN. 1972. J. Immunol. **109:** 648.
2. ZITRON, I. M., D. E. MOSIER & W. E. PAUL. 1977. J. Exp. Med. **146:** 1707.
3. CAMBIER, J. C., F. S. LIGLER, J. W. UHR, J. R. KETTMAN & E. S. Vitetta. 1978. Proc. Nat. Acad. Sci. USA. **75:** 432.
4. ZITRON, I. M. & B. L. CLEVINGER. 1980. J. Exp. Med. **152:** 1135.
5. PURÉ, E. & E. S. VITETTA. 1980. J. Immunol. **125:** 1240.
6. PARKER, D. C. 1980. Immunol. Rev. **52:** 115.
7. SIECKMANN, D. G. 1980. Immunol. Rev. **52:** 182.
8. WEINER, H. L., J. W. MOOREHEAD & H. CLAMAN. 1976. J. Immunol. **116:** 1656.
9. SIECKMANN, D. G., R. ASOFSKY, D. E. MOSIER, I. M. ZITRON & W. E. PAUL. 1978. J. Exp. Med. **147:** 814.
10. PARKER, D. C., D. C. WADSWORTH & G. B. SCHNEIDER. 1980. J. Exp. Med. **152:** 138.
11. COPPLESON, L. W. & D. MICHIE. 1966. Proc. Roy. Soc. (London) Ser. B. **163:** 555.
12. MOSIER, D. E. & L. W. COPPLESON. 1968. Proc. Nat. Acad. Sci. USA. **61:** 542.
13. TSE, H. Y., R. H. SCHWARTZ & W. E. PAUL. 1980. J. Immunol. **125:** 491.
14. MARYANSKI, J. L., J. C. CEROTTINI & K. T. BRUNNER. 1980. J. Immunol. **124:** 839.
15. ZITRON, I. M. & D. E. MOSIER. 1976. Fed. Proc. **35:** 862.
16. SCOTT, D. W., J. TUTTLE & C. ALEXANDER. 1979. In B-Lymphocytes in the Immune Response. M. Cooper, D. E. Mosier, I. Scher & E. S. Vitetta, Eds.: 263. Elsevier/North Holland.
17. COUTINHO, A. & G. MOLLER. 1973. Nature New Biol. **245:** 12.
18. BRETSCHER, P. & M. COHN. 1970. Science **169:** 1042.
19. ANDERSSON, J. & F. MELCHERS. 1981. Proc. Nat. Acad. Sci. USA. **78:** 2497.
20. BOURGOIS, A., K. KITAJIMA, I. R. HUNTER & B. A. ASKONAS. 1977. Eur. J. Immunol. **7:** 151.
21. PREUD'HOMME, J. L. 1977. Eur. J. Immunol. **7:** 191.
22. CAMBIER, J. C. 1982. Ann. N.Y. Acad. Sci. This volume.
23. WETZEL, G. D. & J. R. KETTMAN. 1981. J. Immunol. **126:** 723.
24. FINKELMAN, F. D., J. J. MOND, I. SCHER, S. W. KESSLER & E. S. METCALF. 1981. In B Lymphocytes in the Immune Response: Functional, Developmental and Interactive

Properties. N. Klinman, D. E. Mosier, I. Scher and E. S. Vitetta, Eds.: 201. Elsevier/North-Holland.

25. ANDERSSON, J., A. COUTINHO, F. MELCHERS & T. WATANABE. 1977. Cold Spring Harbor Symp. Quant. Biol. **41:** 227.

26. ANDERSSON, J., A. COUTINHO, W. LERNHARDT & F. MELCHERS. 1979. *In* B Lymphocytes in the Immune Response. Eds. M. Cooper, D. E. Mosier, I. Scher and E. S. Vitetta, Eds.: 257. Elsevier/North Holland.

27. HOWARD, M., S. KESSLER, T. CHUSED & W. E. PAUL. 1981. Proc. Nat. Acad. Sci. USA **78:** 5788.

IgD AS A RECEPTOR IN SIGNALING THE PROLIFERATION OF MOUSE B-LYMPHOCYTES*

Donna G. Sieckmann, Fred D. Finkelman, and Irwin Scher

Naval Medical Research Institute
and
Department of Medicine
Uniformed Services University of the Health Sciences
Bethesda, Maryland 20814

INTRODUCTION

The majority of lymphocytes present in the adult mouse or human express antigen specific immunoglobulin receptors of both IgM and IgD isotypes[1-4] which display identical idiotypes.[5-7] Although the role of IgM as humoral antibody has been firmly established, the function of IgD in the immune system is unknown. Only minor amounts of IgD are found in the circulation of humans and mice[8-10] and IgD is primarily present on the plasma membrane of mature lymphocytes.[11] Since IgD appears as membrane (m) immunoglobulin (Ig) on neonatal lymphocytes much later in ontogeny than IgM, it was postulated that IgD functions as a "triggering" receptor, while tolerance is expressed upon binding of antigen to the IgM receptor.[12]

One approach to the study of the role of membrane Ig in lymphocyte activation has been to investigate the consequences of binding of antigen to mIg or of binding mIg by antibodies directed at antigenic determinants on mIg. Such studies of the latter type have shown that mouse B-lymphocytes can be induced to proliferate when cultured *in vitro* with anti-Ig antibodies.[13-16] More specifically, anti-μ antibodies have been shown to be B-cell mitogens,[14-16] supporting the hypothesis that mIgM serves as a receptor for induction of mitogenesis. It was thus of immediate importance to access the role of mIgD in activation of B-lymphocytes to mitogenesis, particularly since anti-μ activates a B-cell subset, which has been characterized as having high amounts of mIgD, but low amounts of mIgM.[17]

Our laboratory[18,19] and others[20,21] have recently reported that mouse B-lymphocytes can be induced to proliferate when cultured *in vitro* with anti-δ antibodies. This phenomenon has also been demonstrated by *in vivo* injection of anti-δ antibodies.[22] Taken together, these findings would suggest that both mIgM and mIgD can serve as receptors for induction of mitogenesis in B-cells. In this communication, we wish to review the parameters of activation of mouse lymphocytes to proliferation *in vitro* by anti-δ antibodies.

*This work was supported by the Naval Medical Research and Development Command Research Task No. MR041.20.01-0439 and the Uniformed Services University of the Health Sciences Research Nos. R08307 and R08308. The opinions and assertions contained herein are the private ones of the writers and are not to be construed as official or reflecting the views of the Navy Department or the naval service at large. The experiments reported herein were conducted according to the principles set forth in the current edition of the *Guide for the Care and Use of Laboratory Animals,* Institute of Laboratory Animal Resources, National Research Council.

0077-8923/82/0399-0277 $01.75/0 © 1982, NYAS

Experimental Methods

Animals

(C57Bl/6 × DBA/2N)F$_1$ (BDF$_1$) mice were obtained from the Division of Research Services, National Institutes of Health, Bethesda, Md. (C57Bl/6 × DBA/2)F$_1$ (BDF$_1$) and DBA/2 mice were purchased from the Jackson Laboratory, Bar Harbor, Me. Mice were used at two to four months of age unless noted otherwise.

Anti-immunoglobulin Antibodies

Antisera that react with mouse lymphocyte membrane IgD were prepared by immunizing goats or rabbits with a mouse IgD myeloma protein, TEPC 1017.[23] The anti-δ antibodies were isolated by passage of the serum through an affinity column of a second IgD myeloma, TEPC 1033.[23] A complete description of these preparations can be found elsewhere.[23] The mouse hybridoma alloanti-δ (10-4.22)[24] was purified from culture supernatants by passage over a Protein A-Sepharose column and elution with 3.5M MgCl$_2$. Affinity purified goat anti-μ and goat anti-$\gamma\kappa$ were prepared as previously described.[15]

Cell Culture and Assay for Proliferation

Proliferative responses by mouse spleen cells were obtained by culturing 2–5 × 10^5 cells in microtiter plate cultures (Cluster 96, Costar No. 3596, Cambridge, Mass.) in 0.2 ml of a minimal essential medium containing 10% fetal calf serum, 16-mM Hepes buffer, 5 × 10^{-5}M 2-mercaptoethanol and appropriate concentrations of soluble anti-Ig as previously described.[15] After 48 hr, DNA synthesis was measured by a 16–18 hr pulse of methyl-[^{3}H]-thymidine (^{3}H-TdR). Cell cultures were harvested onto glass fiber filters and counted in a β-scintillation counter. Results are expressed as the geometric mean of triplicate cultures ± standard error of the mean.[15]

Other mitogeneic agents used were lipopolysaccharide (LPS, *Escherichia coli* 0111:B4, Westphal preparation, Difco Laboratories, Detroit, Mich.) and concanavalin A (Con A, Pharmacia Fine Chemicals, Uppsala, Sweden) and phytohemagglutinin (PHA, Lot K1954, Welcome Research Laboratories, Beckenham, England).

Preparation of Ig$^+$ Spleen Cells and of Cell Populations Depleted of T-Lymphocytes or Macrophages

Spleen cells were depleted of T-cells by treatment with a rabbit anti-mouse thymocyte serum (ATS, Microbiological Associates, Walkersville, Md.) and guinea pig complement as previously described.[16] Spleen cells were depleted of macrophages by passage through two 30-ml columns of Sephadex G-10[25] (Pharmacia Fine Chemicals, Uppsala, Sweden) at 37°C. Depletion of macrophages was assessed by testing for uptake of latex particles (1.091 μm diameter, Dow Chemical Co., Indianapolis, Ind.)[16] and the ability of the macrophage depleted spleen cells to stimulate across an H-2 and Mls defined histocompatibility difference[26,27] (kindly performed by Dr. John Ryan, Naval Medical Research Institute, Bethesda, Md.). Peritoneal exudate cells (PEC) were isolated from normal syngeneic mice and were given 2000 R in a CS-137 irradiator (Mark I, Model 68A, J. L. Shephard and Assoc., Glendale, Ca.).

Separation of spleen cells into surface Ig⁻ and Ig⁺ populations bearing various amounts of surface Ig was accomplished with the FACS II (Becton, Dickenson and Co., Mountain View, Ca.), as previously described.[17]

RESULTS

Affinity purified rabbit and goat anti-δ antibodies were found to be mitogenic for adult mouse spleen cells when added to cultures in concentrations ranging from 1 to 200 μg/ml. FIGURE 1 shows a comparison of the dose-response curves for anti-δ, anti-μ and anti-γκ in cultures stimulated with these antibodies for 48 hr. A

TABLE 1

ABILITY OF SPLEEN CELLS TO RESPOND TO ANTI-δ AFTER TREATMENT WITH
ANTI-THYMOCYTE SERUM (ATS) AND COMPLEMENT (C)*

Stimulant	Concentration (μg/ml)	Normal Spleen Cells	ATS and C-treated Spleen Cells
None	–	1,210 ± 101	1,670 ± 190
Anti-δ	10	14,924 ± 52	24,131 ± 439
Anti-μ	100	27,887 ± 667	58,112 ± 1,145
Anti-γκ	50	11,791 ± 34	23,259 ± 1,114
LPS	50	68,213 ± 2,780	89,608 ± 2,017
Con A	2	244,518 ± 8,591	1,489 ± 109

*Cultures of 2 × 10⁵ normal BDF₁ spleen cells or cells treated with a rabbit anti-thymocyte serum and complement, were incubated with the designated concentrations of rabbit anti-δ, goat anti-μ, goat anti-γκ, LPS, and Con A for 48 hr, followed by a 16 hr pulse with ³H-TdR.

noteworthy feature of the dose response curve for anti-δ, is the vigorous response obtained at concentrations of 1–10 μg/ml, as compared with anti-μ or anti-γκ, which were only stimulatory at >10 μg/ml. In multiple experiments, goat anti-δ antibodies induced proliferative responses which were less than or equal to those induced by goat anti-μ, however, the level of stimulation attained by rabbit anti-δ was much less than that induced by goat anti-μ. The stimulatory activity of rabbit anti-δ was found to be enhanced by removal of the Fc portion of the molecule. Thus, F(ab)₂ fragments of rabbit anti-δ were more stimulatory than intact molecules of rabbit anti-δ at higher concentrations (Sieckmann, Finkelman, and Scher, unpublished results). These data formed the basis for concluding that mIgD could serve as a mitogenic receptor for activation of B-cells.

FIGURE 2 demonstrates the kinetics of the proliferative response to anti-δ. Similar to the response of anti-μ antibodies, spleen cells respond to anti-δ after remaining in culture with anti-δ for 48 hr. The response occurs maximally on day 3, and is down to background levels by day 5.

Cellular Requirements for an Anti-IgD Induced B-Cell Proliferative Response

The proliferative response to anti-δ was shown to be the property of Ig⁺ B-lymphocytes responding without help of T-lymphocytes or macrophages. TABLE 1 demonstrates the effect of prior removal of T-cells on anti-δ induced proliferation of spleen cells treated with anti-thymocyte serum and complement. The proliferation induced by anti-δ as well as anti-μ was actually enhanced in proportion to the increased number of B-cells in the culture, while the Con A response was completely eliminated by such treatment. These data support the notion that few, if any, T-lymphocytes are required for the proliferative response induced by anti-δ.

The requirement for accessory macrophages was investigated by passing spleen cells over Sephadex G-10 or by incubation of spleen cells with carbonyl

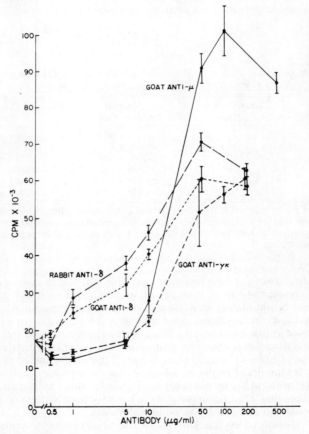

FIGURE 1. Proliferative response of mouse spleen cells to anti-δ, anti-μ, or anti-γκ. Spleen cells from DBA/2 mice were cultured at 5×10^5 cells per microwell in 0.2 ml medium containing the indicated concentrations of affinity purified goat anti-δ, rabbit anti-δ, goat anti-μ, and goat anti-γκ for 48 hr, followed by a 16 hr pulse of ³H-TdR. (From Sieckmann.[19])

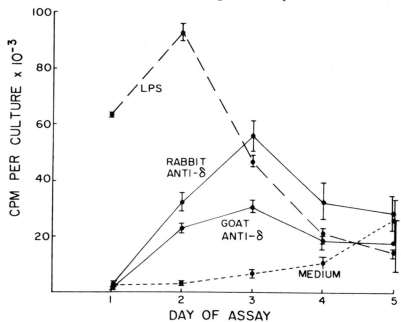

FIGURE 2. Kinetics of the proliferative response to anti-δ. The stimulation of BDF_1 spleen cells by rabbit anti-δ (50 μg/ml), goat anti-δ (100 μg/ml) or LPS (50 μg/ml) was measured each day after a 4 hr pulse of ^{3}H-TdR.

iron. Neither procedure was effective in diminishing or removing the ability of spleen cells to respond to anti-δ. As shown in TABLE 2, the proliferative response to either goat or rabbit anti-δ or goat anti-μ is enhanced after passage of spleen cells over Sephadex G-10, while the response to Con A, which is adherent cell dependent, is depleted by 77%. Addition of peritoneal washout cells (PEC) to G-10 passed cells restored the Con A response, while suppressing both the anti-δ and anti-μ responses. It should be noted that more PEC are required to suppress the anti-δ response than to suppress the anti-μ response. Similar results were obtained when spleen cells were treated with carbonyl iron and cells adherent to iron were removed by a magnet. The efficiency of adherent cell removal was monitored during each procedure by latex bead phagogtosis. Normal spleen cell preparations containing 5-6% latex positive cells were decreased to 1% or less latex positive cells. Cells passaged over Sephadex G-10 were also found to be totally depleted of their ability to stimulate across an H-2 and Mls defined histocompatibility difference. Stimulation across both of these barriers have previously been shown to be dependent upon an adherent cell population.[26,27] The data suggest that accessory adherent cells are not required, at least within the limits of the ability of G-10 passage to remove adherent cells.

To further demonstrate the dependence of the response on an Ig^+ B-lymphocyte, adult spleen cells were sorted on the Fluorescence Activated Cell Sorter (FACS) on the basis of amount of staining with a fluorescenated anti-Ig. Only the Ig^+ lymphocyte fraction responded to anti-δ (data not shown). Ig^- cells

TABLE 2

EFFECT OF SEPHADEX G-10 REMOVAL OF ADHERENT CELLS ON THE ANTI-δ RESPONSE*

Stimulant	Normal Spleen	G-10 Passed Spleen	G-10 Passed Spleen and 5×10^4 PEC	G-10 Passed Spleen and 1×10^5 PEC
	Δ CPM per Culture ± S.E.			
Goat anti-δ	88,805 ± 3,682	120,326 ± 5,418	123,474 ± 13,668	59,814 ± 1,806
Rabbit anti-δ	26,219 ± 573	33,312 ± 1,553	31,354 ± 4,235	10,583 ± 692
Goat anti-μ	120,379 ± 8,486	150,923 ± 12,034	94,351 ± 3,295	38,955 ± 1,968
LPS	73,026 ± 12,534	76,020 ± 768	53,673 ± 2,698	29,553 ± 2,008
Con A	173,734 ± 12,340	40,556 ± 4,386	167,717 ± 3,936	167,036 ± 11,571
PHA	84,717 ± 2,091	53,135 ± 719	118,538 ± 8,339	104,037 ± 4,359

*BDF$_1$ spleen cells were passed over Sephadex G-10 as described in the MATERIALS AND METHODS section. They were cultured at 5×10^5 cells per microwell with either goat anti-δ (50 μg/ml), rabbit anti-δ (10 μg/ml), goat anti-μ (100 μg/ml), LPS (50 μg/ml), Con A (2 μg/ml), or PHA (1 μg/ml) for 48 hr followed by a 16 hr pulse with ^{3}H-TdR.

were unresponsive to anti-δ and anti-μ. When spleen cells were sorted on the basis of amount of mIgD, only δ$^+$ cells responded to anti-δ (data not shown). The bright δ$^+$ cells responded best, while dull δ$^+$ cells were minimally responsive. These findings suggest that cells which respond to anti-δ are of the same subset which respond to anti-μ and are phenotypically IgD bright, IgM dull on the FACS, corresponding to a cell with a high mIgD:mIgM expression.

The type of B-lymphocyte responsible for this phenomenon was also investigated by testing for the appearance of this cell type in various ages of mice. TABLE 3 shows a representative experiment in which spleen cells from mice of various ages were stimulated in vitro with anti-δ, anti-μ or LPS. Similar to previous findings for the anti-μ induced response[16] spleen cells from mice younger than four weeks of age were unresponsive to anti-δ in vitro, while they were significantly stimulated to proliferate by LPS.

In support of the above was the finding that spleen cells from immune

TABLE 3

ONTOGENY OF THE PROLIFERATIVE RESPONSE TO ANTI-δ AND ANTI-μ*

Age	Anti-δ	Anti-μ	LPS
	Δ CPM per culture ± S.E.		
4 days	0 ± 154	1,965 ± 259	15,407 ± 610
3½ weeks	970 ± 640	2,476 ± 611	44,054 ± 929
4½ weeks	6,337 ± 780	23,176 ± 3,204	43,344 ± 929
6½ weeks	18,114 ± 1,199	54,331 ± 3,904	93,260 ± 316
7½ weeks	25,167 ± 819	80,294 ± 5,781	89,195 ± 9,783
11½ weeks	29,207 ± 1,075	63,474 ± 1,746	87,564 ± 1,966
21 weeks	39,924 ± 1,015	68,289 ± 3,110	96,068 ± 3,801
36 weeks	44,904 ± 1,404	94,228 ± 5,108	103,898 ± 306

*BDF$_1$ spleen cells from mice of various ages were cultured in the presence of rabbit anti-δ (10 μg/ml), goat anti-μ (100 μg/ml), or LPS (50 μg/ml), for 48 hr followed by a 16 hr pulse with ^{3}H-TdR.

defective (CBA/N × DBA/2)F$_1$ male mice were unable to respond to anti-δ (data not shown). Taken together, these results suggest that a more mature or later developing B-cell subset, which is absent in the CBA/N defective mouse, is the cell type which is activiated by anti-δ, as has been previously shown for anti-μ induced proliferation.[16]

Complementation in the Response Induced by Anti-μ and Anti-δ

In stimulating mouse spleen cells with either anti-μ or anti-δ, one hopes to mimic the effect of antigen in binding mIgM and mIgD receptors, the advantage being, the possibility of stimulating mIgM receptors separately from mIgD, and vice versa, for purposes of dissecting out the unique functions of each receptor. However, during antigenic stimulation these two receptors function in unison, since antigen will hypothetically crosslink IgM with IgD as well as IgM with IgM

TABLE 4

PROLIFERATIVE RESPONSE INDUCED BY ANTI-μ AND ANTI-δ TOGETHER IN
SPLEEN CELL CULTURES*

Antibody (μg/ml)	ΔCPM/Culture ± S.E.	
	Exp. 1	Exp. 2
Anti-μ (100)	131,445 ± 3,158	55,681 ± 3,761
Anti-δ (100)	109,127 ± 2,571	71,523 ± 2,695
Anti-μ (100) and Anti-δ (100)	129,703 ± 5,183	85,148 ± 3,040
Anti-μ (50)	121,168 ± 9,710	55,021 ± 1,965
Anti-δ (50)	105,871 ± 1,745	53,221 ± 2,930
Anti-μ ba0) and Anti-δ (50)	109,911 ± 1,450	56,711 ± 1,819
Anti-μ (10)	37,460 ± 691	34,078 ± 418
Anti-δ (10)	81,315 ± 2,186	17,251 ± 734
Anti-μ (10) and Anti-δ (10)	64,961 ± 637	32,266 ± 1,591

*BDF$_1$ spleen cells were cultured at 5 × 10^5 per microwell with the indicated additions of either goat anti-μ or goat anti-δ. Cultures were pulsed with ^{3}H-TdR at 48 hr and harvested 16 hr later.

and IgD with IgD. In order to study the effect that the simultaneous interactions of mIgM and mIgD with ligand has on B-cell activation, spleen cells were exposed to equivalent amounts of a goat anti-μ and goat anti-δ, and the proliferative response was compared with that of cultures stimulated with either reagent alone. As shown in TABLE 4, the response from cultures receiving both stimulants was no greater than the response by either stimulant acting alone. This was true for a range of concentrations of anti-Ig from 10 to 100 μg/ml. These data suggest that anti-μ and anti-δ are stimulating the same population of B-cells, since the mixture of the two stimulants does not induce more proliferation than either stimulant alone, as measured within the plateau range of the dose response curve. Thus, the susceptible B-cell can be activated by crosslinking either its IgM or IgD, and there are apparently no B-cells which require crosslinkage of both receptors to be activated. The reason for lack of an additive effect at lower concentration of anti-Ig remains unclear. One possibility is that the binding of mIgM or mIgD regulates the functioning of the other receptor. The other possibility is that triggering can only be effected by a certain threshold of crosslinkage or binding of only one class of receptors. Thus, any cell not sufficiently crosslinked by anti-μ to cause triggering, could not be triggered by additional crosslinkage of mIgD.

In further experiments the relationship of the anti-μ signal to the anti-δ signal was investigated by sequentially incubating spleen cells with different stimulants. These experiments demonstrate that signals received through mIgM or mIgD on one cell can compliment each other. A representative experiment is shown in TABLE 5, in which spleen cells were cultured for 24 hr in normal medium or in medium containing goat anti-μ or goat anti-δ. The cultures were then washed and either normal medium or medium containing anti-μ or anti-δ was added, and the cultures were incubated for another 24 hr. The results demonstrate that, (1) the anti-μ or anti-δ had to be present in the culture for both 24 hr pulse periods to obtain a response at 48 hr, and (2) the two antibodies were interchangeable in stimulating the suseptible cell population. Thus, cells which were initially stimulated with anti-μ for 24 hr could be completely triggered by adding optimal concentrations of either anti-μ or anti-δ. Finally, the magnitude of the response in the double pulse experiment was determined by the order of pulsing. That is, the

TABLE 5

PULSE STIMULATION WITH ANTI-μ OR ANTI-δ*

0–24 Hour Pulse	24–48 Hour Pulse	CPM per Culture ± S.E.
–	–	3,235 ± 341
Anti-δ	–	3,403 ± 323
Anti-μ	–	3,936 ± 215
–	Anti-δ	3,137 ± 7
Anti-δ	Anti-δ	16,256 ± 1,152
Anti-μ	Anti-δ	15,910 ± 859
–	Anti-μ	4,721 ± 141
Anti-δ	Anti-μ	30,719 ± 1,763
Anti-μ	Anti-μ	33,874 ± 931

*BDF$_1$ spleen cells were incubated in microtiter plate cultures with goat anti-μ (100 μg/ml) or rabbit anti-δ (1 μg/ml) or medium for 24 hr at 37°C, followed by two washs and readdition of either normal medium, anti-μ or anti-δ, and cultured for another 24 hr. The cultures were pulsed with ^{3}H-TdR the last 4 hr of incubation.

magnitude of the response to anti-μ alone was more equal to the response derived by anti-δ followed by anti-μ and not by anti-μ followed by anti-δ. This polarity of response potential may suggest that the crosslinkage or binding which occurs in the first 24 hr generates a qualitatively different signal than that which occurs during the second 24 hr.

DISCUSSION

The experiments presented in this study demonstrate that lymphocytes from adult mice can be activated to synthesize DNA by culture with affinity purified heterologous antibodies specific for mouse δ heavy chain determinants. Thus, mIgD as well as mIgM can serve as a receptor for activation to blastogenesis. The characteristics of the response to anti-δ are similar to those for activation by anti-μ.

Both antibodies seem to be stimulating an Ig^+ B-lymphocyte which is relatively late appearing and is absent in the immune defective CBA/N mouse. The responsive B-cell subset is characterized as being a μ^+ δ^+ cell which has a low $\mu{:}\delta$ ratio of surface Ig. It is interesting to note that relatively smaller concentrations of anti-δ will trigger mitogenesis in mouse spleen cells in comparison with the concentrations of anti-μ which are required (FIGURE 1). It is unclear whether the ability of relatively smaller concentrations of anti-δ to stimulate is related to the relative amounts of μ and δ determinants on the cell surface. Thus, smaller amounts of anti-δ may be required to stimulate this B-cell subset because they have relatively large amounts of surface δ, while larger concentrations of anti-μ are required to stimulate these cells which display small amounts of surface μ. An alternate view is that the concentrations of surface Ig are inherent in the differentiation state of the cell and that the relative concentrations of anti-μ and anti-δ that are required are related to the individual affinities of the two antibody preparations.

The heterologous anti-δ antibodies used in this study were mitogenic in soluble form, in contrast to other studies[20] in which anti-Ig insolubilized on beads was required. The Fc portion of the molecule was not required for stimulation, but appeared instead to be inhibitory for the rabbit anti-δ response (Sieckmann, Finkelman, and Scher, unpublished data). Inhibitory effects of Fc on anti-Ig stimulation have been noted previously by other investigators.[28,29]

The contrast to the mitogenic heterologous anti-δ antibodies, the hybridoma 10-4.22 anti-δ antibodies are nonmitogenic.[18,21] Thus, binding of anti-Ig to mIg alone is insufficient to trigger mitogenesis. However, another hybridoma anti-δ antibody, also directed at allotypic determinants, has been shown to be mitogenic.[21] The differential ability of these antibodies to trigger mitogenesis may be related to their relative binding affinities or their individual binding sites on membrane bound IgD.

The response to anti-δ was shown to be independent of need for the presense of T-lymphocytes or adherent cells and in fact, was enhanced by the elimination of T-cells or adherent cells from these cultures. Similar results have previously been shown for the response to anti-μ.[16] The response to a hybridoma allo-anti-δ antibody has also been found to be T-cell independent.[21] In the present study, removal of adherent cells on Sephadex G-10 or using carbonyl iron was not able to decrease or deplete the anti-δ proliferative response. These results suggest that the proliferative response to anti-δ is relatively T-cell and macrophage independent; however, we cannot determine whether the few contaminating T-cells and macrophages remaining in these cultures after treatment might be required for optimal B-cell viability via secretion of growth factors, or that they might be necessary for B-cell activation by anti-Ig antibodies via a direct interactive mechanism.

This study indicates that both mIgM and mIgD can serve as triggering receptors for induction of mitogenesis. There appear to be few if any differences in the triggering of the cell through its IgM receptor vs. triggering through the IgD receptor when viewed by anti-Ig stimulation. Experiments directed at studying the relationship of the IgM receptor to the IgD receptor have led to the conclusion that (1) one cell type is being activated by either anti-μ or anti-δ and (2) the effects of incubation with both anti-Ig are complimentary. The results of pulsing experiments, in which, anti-μ and anti-δ are added sequentially, show that the two stimulants compliment each other. This suggests that these two receptors, although isotypically different, interact via similar biochemical pathways in signal generation, leading to the initiation of DNA synthesis by the cell. The results further show that to initiate cell division, the cells must receive continuous or closely spaced signals for the 48 hr preceeding initiation of cell division.

In summary, this study concludes that both mIgM and mIgD can serve as triggering receptors for induction of DNA synthesis. A select subpopulation of B-lymphocytes which is $\mu^+ \delta^+$ and has a low $\mu{:}\delta$ ratio of mIg can be activated by either anti-μ or anti-δ antibodies. Finally, the signals received through the IgM and IgD receptor which lead to mitogenesis are complimentary.

ACKNOWLEDGMENTS

The authors wish to thank Dr. William E. Paul for many helpful discussions; Dr. John Ryan for performing Mls assays; HMC Edward Benigno, Mr. Alfred Black, and Mr. Steven Allen for expert technical assistance; and Mrs. Cathy Cameron for secretarial and editorial assistance in preparation of this manuscript.

REFERENCES

1. MELCHER, U., E. S. VITETTA, M. MCWILLIAMS, M. E. LAMM, J. M. PHILLIPS-QUAGLIATA & J. W. UHR. 1974. Cell surface immunoglobulin. X. Identification of an IgD-like molecule on the surface of murine splenocytes. J. Exp. Med. **140:** 1427–1431.
2. ABNEY, E. R. & R. M. E. PARKHOUSE. 1974. Candidate for immunoglobulin D present on murine B lymphocytes. Nature **252:** 600–602.
3. VAN BOXEL, J. A., W. E. PAUL, W. D. TERRY & I. GREEN. 1972. IgD bearing human lymphocytes. J. Immunol. **109:** 648–651.
4. FU, S. M., R. J. WINCHESTER & H. G. KUNKEL. 1974. Occurrence of surface IgM, IgD and free L chains on human lymphocytes. J. Exp. Med. **139:** 451–456.
5. FU, S. M., R. J. WINCHESTER & H. G. KUNKEL. 1975. Similar idiotypic specificity for the membrane IgD and IgM of human lymphocytes. J. Immunol. **114:** 250–252.
6. GODING, J. W. & J. E. LAYTON. 1976. Antigen-induced cocapping of IgM and IgD-like receptors on murine B cells. J. Exp. Med. **144:** 852–857.
7. GODING, J. W., D. W. SCOTT & J. F. LAYTON. 1977. Genetics, cellular expression, and function of IgD and IgM receptors. Immunol. Rev. **37:** 152–186.
8. ROWE, D. S. & J. L. FAHEY. 1965. A new class of human immunoglobulins. II. Normal serum IgD. J. Exp. Med. **121:** 185–199.
9. FINKELMAN, F. D., V. WOODS, A. BERNING & I. SCHER. 1979. Demonstration of mouse serum IgD. J. Immunol. **123:** 1253–1259.
10. BARGELLESI, A., G. CORTE, E. COSULICH & M. FERRARINI. 1979. Presence of serum IgD and IgD-containing plasma cells in the mouse. Eur. J. Immunol. **9:** 490–492.
11. VITETTA, E. S., U. MELCHER, M. MCWILLIAMS, J. PHILLIPS-QUAGLIATA, M. LAMM & J. W. UHR. 1975. Cell surface immunoglobulin. XI. The appearance of an IgD-like molecule on murine lymphoid cells during ontogeny. J. Exp. Med. **141:** 206–215.
12. VITETTA, E. S. & J. W. UHR. 1975. Immunoglobulin receptors revisited. Science **189:** 964–969.
13. PARKER, D. C. 1975. Stimulation of mouse lymphocytes by insoluble anti-mouse immunoglobulius. Nature (Lond.) **258:** 361–363.
14. WEINER, H. L., J. W. MOORHEAD & H. CLAMEN. 1976. Anti-immunoglobulin stimulation of murine lymphocytes. I. Age dependency of the proliferative response. J. Immunol. **116:** 1656–1661.
15. SIECKMANN, D. G., R. ASOFSKY, D. E. MOSIER, I. M. ZITRON & W. E. PAUL. 1978. Activation of mouse lymphocytes by anti-immunoglobulin. I. Parameters of the proliferative response. J. Exp. Med. **147:** 814–829.

16. SIECKMANN, D. G., I. SCHER, R. ASOFSKY, D. E. MOSIER & W. E. PAUL. 1978. Activation of mouse lymphocytes by anti-immunoglobulin. II. A thymus-independent response by a mature subset of B lymphocytes. J. Exp. Med. **148:** 1628-1643.

17. SIECKMANN, D. G., R. HABBERSETT, I. SCHER & W. E. PAUL. 1981. Activation of mouse lymphocytes by anti-immunoglobulin. III. Analysis of responding B lymphocytes by flow cytometry and cell sorting. J. Immunol. **127:** 205-211.

18. SIECKMANN, D. G., F. FINKELMAN & I. SCHER. 1980. Induction of DNA synthesis by heterologous anti-δ in mouse spleen cell cultures. Fed. Proc. Fed. Am. Soc. Exp. Bio. **39:** 806 (abstr).

19. SIECKMANN, D. G. 1980. The use of anti-immunoglobulins to induce a signal for cell division in B lymphocytes via their membrane IgM and IgD. Immunol. Rev. **52:** 181-210.

20. PURÉ, E. & E. VITETTA. 1980. Induction of murine B cell proliferation by insolubilized anti-immunoglobulins. J. Immunol. **125:** 1240-1242.

21. ZITRON, I. M. & B. L. CLEVINGER. 1980. Regulation of murine B cells through surface immunoglobulin. I. Monoclonal anti-δ antibody that induces allotype-specific proliferation. J. Exp. Med. **152:** 1135-1146.

22. FINKELMAN, F. D., I. SCHER, J. J. MOND, J. KUNG & E. S. METCALF. 1982. Polyclonal activation of the murine immune system by an antibody to IgD. I. Increase in cell size and DNA sythesis. J. Immunol. Submitted for publication.

23. FINKELMAN, F. D., S. W. KESSLER, J. F. MUSHINSKI & M. POTTER. 1981. IgD-secreting murine plasmacytomas: Identification and partial characterization of two myeloma proteins. J. Immunol. **126:** 680-687.

24. OI, V. T., P. P. JONES, J. W. GODING, L. A. HERZENBERG & L. A. HERZENBERG. 1978. Properties of monoclonal antibodies to mouse Ig allotypes, H-2, and Ia antigens. Curr. Top. Microbiol. Immunol. **81:** 115-129.

25. LY, I. A. & R. I. MISHELL. 1974. Separation of mouse spleen cells by passage through columns of Sephadex G-10. J. Immunol. Methods **5:** 239-247.

26. AHMANN, G. B., P. I. NADLER, A. BIRNKRANT & R. J. HODES. 1979. T cell recognition in the mixed lymphocyte response. I. Non-T, radiation-resistant splenic adherent cells are the predominant stimulators in the murine mixed lymphocyte reaction. J. Immunol. **123:** 903-909.

27. AHMANN, G. B., P. I. NADLER, A. BIRNKRANT & R. J. HODES. 1981. T cell recognition in the mixed lymphocyte response. II. Ia-positive splenic adherent cells are required for non-I region-induced stimulation. J. Immunol. **127:** 2308-2313.

28. SCRIBNER, D. J., H. L. WEINER & J. W. MOORHEAD. 1978. Anti-immunoglobulin stimulation of murine lymphocytes. V. Age-related decline in Fc receptor-mediated immunoregulation. J. Immunol. **121:** 377-382.

29. TONY, H.-P. & A. SCHIMPL. 1980. Stimulation of murine B cells with anti-Ig antibodies: Dominance of a negative signal mediated by the Fc receptor. Eur. J. Immunol. **10:** 726-729.

DISCUSSION OF THE PAPER

PARTICIPANT: Your question about whether macrophages and T-cells are required for proliferation is a fundamental one, so I wonder if you have any additional information, other than the experiment you showed on the depletion of macrophages, to substantiate that they are unnecessary for the triggering?

D. SIECKMANN: We've done repetitive experiments on this and come up with the same results all the time. These cultures are depleted of responsiveness for mixed lymphocyte reactions. They have 1% neutral red or latex phagocytic cells. That's about the best we can do.

PARTICIPANT: Are they particularly dependent on the batch of fetal calf serum needed?

SIECKMANN: We screen all our fetal calf serum for endotoxin content. If you have too high a background you wouldn't see a response.

PARTICIPANT: In the macrophage depletion experiments, do you have data showing that they were depleted for con-A responsiveness?

SIECKMANN: They were lowered for the T-cell mitogens.

F. FINKELMAN: (to Zitron) With regard to the hypothesis that anti-immunoglobulin treated cells may get stuck in S phase, Tony De Franco and Bill Paul have done some experiments in which they treated small B-cells in vitro, predominantly with anti-μ but I think in some experiments also with anti-δ. They compared the number of cells they got at various times which had greater than 2CDNA, when they cultured with anti-immunoglobulin and/or colcimid (which as you know will stop cells in M-phase). If anti-immunoglobulin was pushing cells up to but not beyond G2 then the addition of colcimid would not increase the percent of cells in M phase. However, they find a very substantial increase in the percent of cells in M phase when they add colcimid at the time of anti-immunoglobulin. And thus the anti-immunoglobulin must make cells go all the way through the cell cycle and back to G1.

I. ZITRON: I had heard some time ago about Tony De Franco's data from Bill Paul that short exposure to anti-δ increased cell size. I wasn't aware of the data that you just mentioned. I think it's very interesting.

FINKELMAN: It brings up the alternative hypothesis that, as the two-signal people said a long time ago, the cell that gets signal one but doesn't get signal two is not going to stay happy for very long periods of time.

ZITRON: Absolutely, you know we could be looking at a situation where we are getting a lot of death in the stimulated cells.

VITETTA: We know however that if you leave an anti-δ antibody in the whole time while the antigen is present you block the response and I think that single observation suggests that the receipt of the second signal for terminal differentiation requires the reexpression of the receptor on the surface, maybe in conjunction with something else. I don't think that's a trivial point if you look at these different systems. Maybe it explains why we get proliferation on the one hand and on the other hand we block antibody secretion.

ZITRON: I think you are absolutely right.

VITETTA: Another technical point I'd like to make is, I think Donna Sieckmann has been very successful with intact antibodies in doing some of these things but I think many of us have to make F(ab')$_2$s or put these antibodies on particles or we have trouble. That's why I asked whether anti-Ia had been used as a F(ab')$_2$; I think it's an important point. Not to belabor an old issue, but it is still a problem in many labs using intact antibody to induce proliferation.

M. PARKHOUSE: If you are hitting the same cell population with either anti-μ and anti-δ and if both anti-μ and anti-δ cause this increased representation of Ia, and if you can substitute sequentially, i.e., you have a little spell in anti-δ, pull it out, then a little spell in anti-μ. I don't see why anti-Ia shouldn't do the same thing whichever specificity of isotype the antibody is.

VITETTA: What he's asking is, why does the anti-Ia work with one isotype and not the other if they are interchangeable in terms of stimulation. Isn't that the essence of what your question?

SIECKMANN: It's inhibiting both. It either inhibits the anti-δ or anti-μ response.

PARKHOUSE: But didn't you say the inhibition was 90% when you provoked it with anti-δ and only about 30–40% with anti-μ?

SIECKMANN: Yes. There's greater inhibition of the anti-δ response and we don't know the reason for that yet.

PARKHOUSE: So when you did the sequential experiment, what happens? If you do the mixed sequential experiment in the two ways: which is anti-δ, wash out, followed then with anti-μ and then the other way around. And then you look for inhibition with anti-Ia.

SIECKMANN: Yes, we have incorporated anti-Ia in both pulse periods and it's inhibitory in both pulse periods, to a certain extent. It seems to be additive.

PARKHOUSE: What happens with Ia, does it go up in the B-cell population when you do a modulation either with anti-μ or anti-δ?

FINKELMANN: Yes, that seems to be precisely the B-cell population that responds with proliferation and also responds with an increase in Ia. It goes up equally with anti-μ and anti-δ, but I'm not sure that it's been done at the same time with the same subpopulation.

B. G. PERNIS: Well, the real question was raised by the fact that anti-Ia inhibits effects of anti-μ and anti-δ. Is Ia a functional molecule in a triggering process started by cross linking membrane immunoglobulins? It would appear that this is the case but not in all the cells and this is why you have only a partial inhibition. There are cells which instead of using Ia or instead of having Ia as a limiting element have a different pathway.

With regard to the direct observations concerning the involvement of Ia molecules in cross-linked membrane immunoglobulins I remember many years ago we were looking for cocapping of Ia and membrane immunoglobulins. We never observed complete cocapping. At about the same time (1974), a paper was published saying there was no cocapping, and it was absolutely correct. We have been looking again at this phenomenology recently with the monoclonal anti-Ia. There is no question you can cap out your IgM or your IgD and there's still plenty of Ia left, but we don't know if some Ia interacts with the complex.

In other words saying there is no cocapping on the basis of the fact that we have not cleared the surface of the second component doesn't show that there is no interaction. It only shows there is an excess of this second component. So there must be other ways to look for this interaction in a positive way, not just in the negative, in the sense of a complete cocapping. I'm convinced that there is some interaction and still believe in my old observation that some Ia goes into the cap.

If you cap IgM you cocap the Fc receptor totally. If you cap the Fc receptor, IgM does not move. It's a unidirectional interaction and at that time what we saw with Ia was certainly unidirectional and we have repeated the experiment with a monoclonal anti-Ia. The problem is that the anti-Ia doesn't cap at all.

ROLE OF IgD IN TOLERANCE AND CROSS-PRIMING: IgD-RELATED SIGNALS IN B-CELL GROWTH, DIFFERENTIATION AND TOLERANCE

David W. Scott, Jane Tuttle, P. S. Pillai, and Margaret Piper

Department of Microbiology and Immunology
Duke University Medical Center
Durham, North Carolina, 27710

Despite extensive studies, the exact functions of B-lymphocyte membrane IgM and IgD remain an enigma. Although early pioneering studies by Uhr and Vitetta et al.[1] suggested opposing signalling roles for IgM and IgD, more recent data has suggested that both surface receptors can transmit positive as well as negative signals to the B-cells.[2,3] Our laboratory has been interested in the functional role played by IgM and IgD, especially with regard to B-cell growth and differentiation. We have focused on three systems of in vitro functional analysis: tolerance induction in B-cells from young adult mice, antigen-induced clonal expansion ("cross-priming"), and direct B-cell growth in agar.[4-7] The last system has been especially useful in analyzing separately the events related to B-cell growth and their subsequent differentiation into antibody secreting cells (PFC).

ROLE OF IgD IN TOLERANCE

Initially, we and others[8,9] reported that membrane IgD played an important role in the resistance to tolerance induction of adult B-cells. As reported earlier in the meeting, the removal of IgD by several methods led to an increase in tolerance susceptibility in the treated spleen cell populations.[8,9] These data suggested that acquisition of resistance to tolerance induction should correlate with the appearance of surface IgD during the ontogeny of splenic B-cells. Moreover, analogous rules were also drawn for the effect of anti-IgD on PFC responses induced by different antigens. While some correlations existed, a number of exceptions were noted.[4,10] For example, using a variety of thymus-independent (TI) and thymus-dependent (TD) antigens, all coupled with the same fluorescein (FL) hapten, we found that certain FL-antigens triggered B-cells which were relatively susceptible to tolerance induction, while others triggered subsets which were relatively resistant.[4] However, this tolerance susceptibility did not correlate either with the presence of IgD on these putative B-cell subsets[4,11] or with the ability of anti-IgD reagents (allo-anti-δ or monoclonal anti-δ) to inhibit the PFC responses elicited by these antigens. We have reexamined this question especially with regard to the exact conditions of tolerance induction.

As previously described, we attempted tolerance induction in vitro and then challenged the washed cells with various FL-antigens. The data presented in FIGURE 1 show that the susceptibility to tolerance induction can be related firstly to the epitope density of the haptenated-tolerogen, as recently reported by Nossal and coworkers.[12] Secondly, different tolerance susceptibility curves were obtained with 24 vs. 48 hour preculture (tolerance induction) steps, as shown in FIGURE 2. These experiments emphasize that different results obtained by several

290

0077-8923/82/0399-0290$01.75/0 © 1982, NYAS

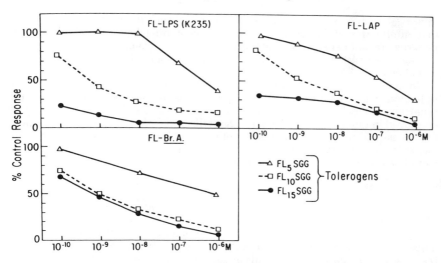

FIGURE 1. Effect of epitope density of FL-tolerogens on the dose response curves generated upon challenge with various FL-antigens. Splenocytes were cultured for 40–80 hours with FL-SGG preparations, harvested, washed and then challenged with the indicated FL-antigens. FL-LPS, FL-conjugated to *E. coli* K-235 lipopolysaccharide; FL-LAP, FL-conjugated to lipid-A associated protein of LPS; FL-BrA, FL-conjugate to *Brucella abortus* organisms.

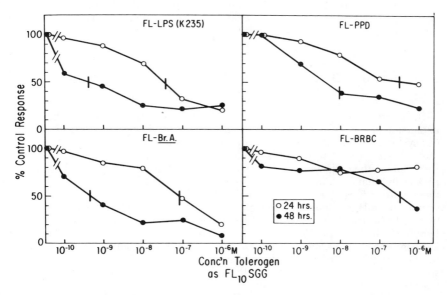

FIGURE 2. Kinetics of tolerance induction with FL-$_{10}$SGG. Protocol as in FIGURE 1 using moderately haptenated FL-$_{10}$SGG and the challenge antigens indicated. Abbreviations as in FIGURE 1: FL-PPD, FL-conjugated to purified protein derivative of *M. tuberculosis*; FL-BRBC, FL-conjugated burro RBC.

investigators may be due in part to different experimental protocols. We suggest that efforts should be made to unify these approaches. Nonetheless, some patterns are still evident. As originally observed, for example, the TD responses are the most resistant to tolerance induction and most readily inhibitable by anti-δ (data not shown).

In contrast to reported results, we have not been able to facilitate tolerance induction by pretreating normal adult spleen cells with monoclonal anti-δ and the same challenge antigens as used in our prior studies. Since allo-anti-δ was employed in those experiments, we suggest that monoclonal anti-δ does not cause the cross-linking and cocapping of other membrane receptors necessary to facilitate tolerance induction. Experiments with mixtures of monoclonal reagents would be useful in resolving this question.

Role of IgD in Cross-Priming

It has been previously reported[5,13] that exposure of B-cells to a single haptenated antigen can prime multiple subsets such that the subsequent PFC responses to that hapten on several carriers are greatly expanded. This effect has been termed "cross-priming." Because this phenomenon was first described with neonatal B-cells,[13] it was felt that cross-priming occurred via an antigen:IgM interaction independent of IgD. We have tested whether IgD plays a role in this cross-priming process by including various concentrations of either allo-anti-δ or monoclonal anti-δ (10-4.22) during the initial priming culture. Our data indicate that cross-priming at optimal doses of haptenated ficoll is relatively insensitive to inhibition by anti-δ at least with certain TI antigens (FIGURE 3) although it can occur (see FIGURE 4 in reference 4). Whether cross-priming for an augmented TD response is anti-δ sensitive is unknown.

Role of IgD in Agar Clonal Growth and in the Subsequent Differentiation of B-Cell Colonies

Most recently, we have investigated the role of IgD and IgM in the clonal expansion of B-cells using the agar cloning system of Metcalf, Kincade et al.[14,15] In our system, hapten-specific B-cells are first purified as described earlier[6] and are then cloned in agar in the presence of growth potentiators such as SRBC and LPS.[15] Since the cells which we cloned are hapten-specific, we can subsequently pick individual colonies after six to seven days in vitro, and attempt to stimulate them with different FL-antigens.[6] Moreover, we can investigate the effect of various ligands, including tolerogens,[7] on the growth and subsequent differentiation of these B-cell colonies (CFU-B). Earlier studies in our laboratory,[6] established that hapten-specific B-cell colonies could be triggered by both TI and TD antigens at a high responsive frequency (1 in 3 to 1 in 10 colonies gave rise to PFC in three-day microculture). This system allowed us to analyze the effect of specific tolerogen on CFU-B growth and this antigen-induced differentiation with respect to different B-cell subsets.[7]

Recently, Margaret Piper has compared the effect of anti-μ and anti-δ on CFU-B growth and differentiation. Hapten-specific B-cells are cloned in agar as described earlier.[6,7] Subsequently, individual clones are picked and stimulated with FL-POL to generate PFC. As previously reported by Kincade and coworkers using whole normal B-cells, the inclusion of affinity-purified anti-μ in the cloning stage reduced colony formation.[16] This inhibition is more complete with B-cells grown in the presence of either SRBC or LPS alone. However, when B-cells are grown with both SRBC and LPS, CFU-B numbers are reduced only 50% in the presence of anti-μ. The same is true with hapten-purified B-cells (TABLE 1). Interestingly, when those colonies, which can be grown in the presence of anti-μ are picked and cultured with FL-POL to stimulate PFC formation, very few, if

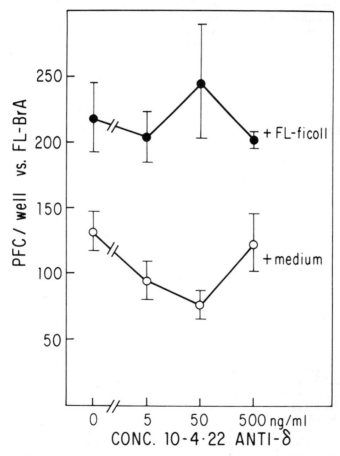

FIGURE 3. Effect of monoclonal anti-δ on cross-priming. Spleen cells were preincubated with the indicated concentrations of anti-δ overnight, washed and then cultured for 40 hours with 1 ng FL-ficoll as a cross-priming stimulus. The cells were then harvested, washed, and challenged with FL-*Brucella* organisms.

any, colonies are able to differentiate. This suggests that anti-μ is delivering a negative signal affecting the growth of the majority of B-cells which we clone in agar. Moreover, those B-cells which grow in the presence of anti-μ are unable to differentiate in response to antigen. These results are analogous to data previously reported using FL-SGG as a B-cell tolerogen in agar cloning system; in contrast, however, B-cells grown with LPS or SRBC alone were resistant to the effect of tolerogen in terms of B-cell growth.[4]

When monoclonal anti-δ (10-4.22) is included in the agar cultures, CFU-B numbers are reduced up to 60%. However, when those colonies which grow in the presence of anti-δ, are challenged *in vitro* with FL-POL, they respond with an equal or greater clonal precursor frequency compared to normal colonies (TABLE 1). These data suggest that anti-δ is able to inhibit a substantial portion of those B-cells which grow in the presence of LPS plus SRBC, but that those cells which are resistant to this effect are highly responsive to the antigen FL-POL. It will be interesting to determine the frequency of responsive colonies grown in the presence of anti-δ and subsequently challenged with other FL-antigens, especially thymus-dependent antigens. These studies are now in progress.

TABLE 1

EFFECT OF ANTI-IgD AND ANTI-IgM ON GROWTH
AND DIFFERENTIATION OF HAPTEN-SPECIFIC B-CELL COLONIES

	μg anti-Ig	% Control Response*	% Stimulable Colonies
Exp. 1	0	100	14.6
	25μg $\alpha\mu$†	34	0
	5μg $\alpha\delta$‡	52	30.2
Exp. 2	0	100	6.5
	1μg $\alpha\mu$	73	ND
	10μg $\alpha\mu$	51	3.2
	25μg $\alpha\mu$	56	ND
	5μg $\alpha\delta$	45	13.4
	10μg $\alpha\mu$ + 5μg $\alpha\delta$	14	ND

*Average control response = 250 CFU-B/10^4 FL-specific cells.
†$\alpha\mu$ = affinity purified goat anti-μ.
‡$\alpha\delta$ = 10-4.22 monoclonal anti-δ. Note: Monoclonal anti-H-2 reagents did not inhibit CFU-B growth.

DISCUSSION

Our studies suggest that B-cell subsets cannot be easily delineated on the basis of sensitivity to tolerance induction nor on their ability to be inhibited by anti-IgD in their terms of triggering to PFC. Nonetheless, using B-cell colony formation in agar, we have been able to grow hapten-specific B-cells that may represent distinct subsets. Our data suggest that both anti-μ and tolerogen deliver negative signals to most B-cells. Thus, in the presence of anti-μ, the subsequent differentiation of CFU-B, which are able to respond to the mitogens in our colony formation system, is subsequently impeded. In contrast, the anti-δ resistant B-cell colonies are highly responsive to one of our TI FL-antigens.

Our studies further indicate that both anti-μ and anti-δ can deliver negative signals with respect to B-cell clonal growth. Since both ligands have been shown to induce B-cell proliferation when appropriately presented to the lymphocyte, we would agree with the hypothesis that both IgM and IgD can provide positive triggering stimuli or negative signalling depending on the conditions of the exposure. Differential signalling would then be dependent on the dose and period of exposure to antigen (ligand), the relative IgM:IgD ratio of individual

B-cells, and the associated markers which may be cocapped with either Ig receptor. While the exact function of IgD and mechanism of signalling by this receptor remain to be elucidated, it is clear that this surface molecule plays an important role in regulating B-cell growth and its subsequent differentiation into antibody forming cells.

REFERENCES

1. CAMBIER, J. C., F. S. LIGLER, J. W. UHR, J. R. KETTMAN & E. S. VITETTA. 1978. Proc. Nat. Acad. Sci. (USA) **75:** 432.
2. SIECKMANN, D. 1980. Immunol. Rev. **52:** 181.
3. PARKER, D. 1980. Immunol. Rev. **52:** 115.
4. SCOTT, D. 1981. Cell. Immunol. **53:** 375.
5. SCOTT, D. & C. ALEXANDER. 1981. Cell. Immunol. **53:** 376.
6. PILLAI, S. & D. SCOTT. 1981. J. Immunol. **127:** 1883.
7. PILLAI, S. & D. SCOTT. 1981. J. Immunol. **127:** 1603.
8. SCOTT, D. W., J. E. LAYTON & G. J. V. NOSSAL. 1977. J. Exp. Med. **146:** 1473.
9. VITETTA, E. S., J. C. CAMBIER, F. S. LIGLER, J. R. KETTMAN & J. W. UHR. 1977. J. Exp. Med. **146:** 1804.
10. ZITRON, I. M., D. E. MOSIER & W. E. PAUL. 1977. J. Exp. Med. **146:** 1707.
11. SCOTT, D. W., J. TUTTLE & C. ALEXANDER. 1979. Proceedings, International Conference on B Lymphocytes in the Immune Response. M. Cooper *et al.*, Eds.: 263. Elsevier, North-Holland. New York N.Y.
12. NOSSAL, G. J. V. & B. PIKE. 1980. Prog. Immunol. (Paris) **4:** 136.
13. MOSIER, D. E. 1978. J. Immunol. **121:** 1453.
14. METCALF. D. *et al.* 1979. J. Exp. Med. **142:** 949.
15. KINCADE, P. *et al.* 1976. J. Exp. Med. **143:** 1265.
16. KINCADE, P. & P. RALPH. 1976. Cold Spring Harbor Symp. **41:** 245.

DISCUSSION OF THE PAPER

PARTICIPANT: Do you have any information on the Fc dependence of the inhibitory effects, particularly with the anti-μ?

D. W. SCOTT: No, I don't have any information on the Fc dependence of these phenomena. If I can extrapolate from Paul Kincade's experiments, F(ab')$_2$ anti-μ will inhibit B-cell colony formation quite efficiently. I think the interesting results will come out of the tolerogen story. I think the differences between intact immunoglobulin tolerogens and their F(ab')$_2$ fragments may be critical, as suggested by Ellen Vitetta and some of our own experience. Clearly, other kinds of tolerogens ought to be tried.

APPARENT DIFFERENCES IN B-LINEAGE DIFFERENTIATION OCCURRING IN FETAL AND ADULT LIFE*

Paul W. Kincade,† Kenneth S. Landreth, and Grace Lee

Sloan-Kettering Institute
145 Boston Post Road
Rye, New York 10580

INTRODUCTION

B-lymphocytes first appear in fetal liver and spleen of mammalian embryos whereas bone marrow is the principal site for their formation in adults. Studies of embryos and neonates provide a unique perspective on early events in B-lymphocyte differentiation, but there is reason to suspect that there may be fundamental differences in the fetal and adult models. Not only do populations of B-cells in fetal/neonatal tissues differ from those which predominate in adult marrow and spleen but recent observations indicate that the immediate precursors of B-cells in these tissues may differ as well. Expression of cell surface IgD (sIgD) coincides with acquisition of "adult" characteristics by the humoral immune system and the general question of whether B-cells are formed through similar processes in fetal and adult life can be considered in that context.

GENERAL CHARACTERISTICS OF B-CELLS

A considerable amount is known about the properties of B-cells in fetal and adult tissues. One of the earliest findings was that fetal and neonatal B-cells were uniquely sensitive to exposure to anti-Ig antibodies, and this provided an explanation for the block in B-lineage development in anti-Ig treated animals.[1,2] Presumably related is the susceptibility of these cells to "clonal abortion" tolerance.[3,4] With either anti-Ig or tolerogen treatment, sIg receptors must be cross-linked and extended exposure is required for complete population inactivation.

Only a subpopulation of the B-cells in adult marrow are tolerogen/anti-Ig sensitive and one can assume that these represent recently formed cells.[4] The length of time that a differentiating B-cell is tolerance susceptible is not known. However, it has been estimated that less than 48 hr is required for the majority of B-cells in marrow to be turned over and the average half-life of splenic B-cells in adult animals was recently suggested to be only one day.[5-7] In contrast, in one study virtually *all* newborn splenic B-cells were tolerizable and did not become adult in this respect before one week of life.[4] Ig-bearing cells can be found in that organ from at least two days prior to birth.

Similar differences have been seen in expression of cell surface markers. Ia is expressed on very few neonatal B-cells and then only in very small amounts.[8,9]

*Supported by N.I.H. Grants AI-12741, CA-09190 and Research Career Development Award AI-00265.

†Present address: Oklahoma Medical Research Foundation, 825 N.E. 13th Street, Oklahoma City, Oklahoma 73104.

296

Virtually all B-cells in spleen acquire Ia by eight days of age but more than three weeks is required for the average density of Ia to equal that of adult splenic B-cells. Studies employing immunofluorescence or cytotoxicity suggest that while sIg⁻ precursors of B-cells in adult marrow lack Ia; this is acquired by young marrow B-cells almost as soon as sIg and functional capability.[10,11]

The Qa-2 alloantigen is especially interesting because it is found on both undifferentiated and fully mature cells of adults, but its display is dependent on the chronological age of the animal.[11,12] That is, it cannot be demonstrated on any cells of fetal and newborn animals and longer than four weeks are required for full expression on all tissues. This may suggest that some type of systemic and age-dependent control regulates display of certain cell surface receptors. If this were true, a lymphocyte taken from an immature animal might quickly acquire such markers after being placed in an adult environment.

Flow cytometric analyses have revealed that the average density of sIgM molecules on newborn splenic B-cells is very high and then falls to adult values by five weeks after birth.[13] On the other hand, newly formed B-cells in adult marrow are thought to have a low density of surface IgM which then gradually increases.[14] This could indicate that a majority of the B-cells in newborn spleen are not recently formed and/ or that the sIgM density on these cells is high because the cell surface is sparsely occupied with other markers (e.g., Ia, Qa-2, IgD).

B-cells of immature animals are uniquely unresponsive in particular functional assays and this is believed to be an intrinsic characteristic. For example, they fail to proliferate in anti-IgM containing cultures under circumstances where adult splenocytes are fully responsive.[15] Furthermore, they do not make antibody to the hapten TNP presented on particular carriers (Ficoll, soluble polyacrylamide, lightly conjugated polyacrylamide beads), whereas these were good immunogens for B-cells from nature animals.[16] Unresponsiveness of young animals can also result from the fact that their repertoire of antibody specificities may not be sufficiently diverse.[17]

All of these findings might be used to argue either that the process of B-cell maturation in neonates is unusually slow or that cells in their tissues are intrinsically different from those in adult marrow. However, this could be specious because the composition of B-cell populations in organs of young animals is probably a complex function of migration of B-cell precursors as well as formation, death, and emigration of B-cells. For example, we do not know how rapidly the newly formed cells in neonatal spleen are exported to other organs and whether their average lifespan is equivalent to that of B-cells produced in adults.

IgD EXPRESSION DURING DEVELOPMENT

Many reports have documented the acquisition of sIgD by B-lymphocyte populations during development.[8] Our own studies in this area were motivated by the desire to characterize murine B-cell sets that are capable of mitogen-dependent clonal proliferation and to use IgD expression as a milestone in our studies of B-lymphocyte differentiation. We found by separating cells on anti-δ coated dishes that clonable B-cells were typical of B-cells in general in adult spleen, i.e., over 90% were sIgD⁺. However, two major subsets could be distinguished on the basis of their sensitivity to anti-δ added directly to the semisolid cultures. One was prevented from clonal proliferation by as little as 50 ng/ml of anti-δ whereas the other was unaffected by 1000 times more antibody. Calculations indicated that antibody-resistant but IgD$^+$ B-cells are most prevalent in lymph nodes and spleen. Bone marrow IgD-bearing cells, which presumably would have recently acquired sIgD, seemed to be exclusively anti-δ sensitive.[18]

An experiment of this kind is shown in TABLE 1. Monoclonal 10-4.2 antibody is specific for the IgH-5a allele[19] and therefore did not bind to control C57BL/6 cells in the immunofluoresence assay. Clonable B-cells were neither removed by incubation in 10-4.2 coated dishes nor inhibited by addition of the antibody to the cultures. In contrast, most of the B-cells in CBA/H spleen were labeled and 98%

TABLE 1

CLONABLE sIgD$^-$ LYMPHOCYTES DO NOT BECOME ANTI-δ SENSITIVE DURING CULTURE

| | | Clonable B-Cells | | | |
| | | Present Initially | | Recovered After 72 hr Preculture | |
	sIgD$^+$ Cells	Total	Anti-δ Resistant	Total	Anti-δ Resistant
19-Day Fetal Liver					
Unseparated	<0.5%*	13†	25	350	412
δ Depleted		31	33	1,464	1,595
2-Day Neonatal Spleen					
Unseparated	2.5%	7,790	7,710	13,608	13,136
δ Depleted	<0.5%	5,730	5,730	8,959	8,780
Adult CBA/H Spleen					
Unseparated	46.4%	36,450	22,950	23,025	14,063
δ Depleted	<0.2%	677	763	418	416
Adult C57BL/6 Spleen					
Unseparated	<0.5%	98,167	102,417	19,368	19,368
δ Depleted	<0.5%	125,113	127,890	23,716	23,475

*The incidence of IgD-bearing cells was determined by immunofluorescence with biotin-labeled 10-4.2 monoclonal antibody specific for the Igh-5a allele and fluorochrone-labeled avidin.

†Data are colonies obtained per 10^6 initial nucleated cells. Sensitivity to anti-δ was tested by including 5 µg/ml of anti-δ in the semisolid agar cultures. Separations were done as previously described[18] before placing cells directly into semisolid cultures or before liquid preculture and subsequent plating.

of the colony-forming cells specifically bound to the antibody-coated dishes. Direct addition of 10-4.2 to the cultures only diminished clonal proliferation by 37% in this experiment. Cells bearing IgD were infrequent in neonatal spleen and not demonstrable in fetal liver. Adherence to antibody-coated plates and colony inhibitions were correspondingly low.

Previous studies have shown that semisolid agar cultures do not provide optimal conditions for maturation of sIg$^-$ precursors of B-cells.[20,21] In this experiment there was no evidence that sIgD$^-$ cells in any of the separated suspensions became sensitive to anti-δ during semisolid agar culture. Most of the δ$^-$ cells in adult spleen might represent memory B-cells which had shed sIgD[22] but some immature cells in neonatal spleen might have the potential for sIgD expression. It seemed reasonable to ask if this maturation step could occur during 72 hr of incubation in conventional liquid medium as these conditions were previously found to permit the pre-B to B-cell transition.[20] Immunofluorescence examination of the cells recovered at this time did not provide evidence that sIgD was acquired in the liquid culture period (not shown); nor did any of the immature B-cells become sensitive to anti-δ in the combined preculture and semisolid culture interval (TABLE 1).

This experiment does not necessarily prove that "immature" B-cells from neonatal spleen are incapable of IgD synthesis and display. It would be necessary to prove that substantial numbers of newly formed B-cells with the phenotype sIgM+, sIgD− from adult marrow can undergo this maturation step during this interval and with these particular culture conditions. Others have suggested that LPS promotes the maturation of sIgD− cells obtained from older spleen and bone marrow and the effect of LPS addition to the liquid precultures should be tested.[23,24] However, if sIgD expression were to be demonstrated under any of these culture circumstances, one could question if "adult" type precursors were acquiring *both* IgM and IgD. A more stringent test of the maturation potential of neonatal B-cells would be to transfer positively selected sIgM+, sIgD− cells to immunodeficient CBA/N mice and subsequently determine their phenotypes. However, the known sensitivity of neonatal B-cells to manipulation via their sIg receptors might pose both practical and theoretical problems to such an approach.

B-CELL PRECURSORS

A number of cell transfer and culture assays have been developed in recent years which permit the detection of precursors of B-cells, and it has also become apparent that such cells may display distinctive markers. Sometime ago we noticed that cells from fetal liver which could quickly restore clonable B-cells to irradiated mice were more rapidly sedimenting than cells with equivalent potential from adult marrow.[25] It also appeared that fetal B-cell precursors more readily colonized the bone marrow of unirradiated, immunodeficient CBA/N mice than did normal adult marrow precursors.[26] Adult type precursors were absolutely dependent on adherent cells for their maturation in culture but it was not possible to demonstrate this for fetal liver precursors and the latter seemed also to be uniquely sensitive to LPS.[20] In addition to the differential expression of Qa-2 mentioned above, we noted that fetal but not adult precursors resisted lysis with anti-Lyb-2 plus complement.[11] All of these studies were performed with complex mixtures of cells where the only separations involved depletion of sIg+ and adherent cells. It is entirely possible that the differences were more apparent than real and reflect differences in total cellular compositions of fetal and adult hemopoietic tissues rather than intrinsic differences in the precursor cells.

Advances in our understanding of cell surface antigens should make it possible to address the question of differences in B-cell precursor populations with more precision. Cells capable of quickly giving rise to functional B-cells after transfer to irradiated or immunodeficient recipients and similar cells which can mature in culture may be recognized by monoclonal antibodies directed to a high molecular weight cell surface antigen.[11] This marker is displayed on virtually all cells of the B-lineage from a very early stage of embryonic life. In addition, subsets of peripheral T-cells can also express small amounts of this antigen. Lymphocyte precursors can be enriched from adult bone marrow by first depleting B-cells, allowing the remaining cells to adhere to monoclonal 14.8 antibody-coated dishes, and then gently removing the specifically bound cells. This yields almost pure lymphocyte suspensions of which approximately half synthesize but do not display μ heavy chains of IgM.[27] Similar separations have been performed with fetal liver suspensions, and this permits a direct comparison of characteristics of putative B-cell precursors from the two sites. In both cases essentially all of the $c\mu^+$ cells are included in the positively selected suspensions. However, only 0.5% of the selected fetal precursors synthesized detectable μ chains and we assume that this marker is displayed prior to Ig gene activation.

There were other notable differences in the enriched fetal and adult B-cell precursors. The fetal cells commonly had an irregular nuclear outline and cytoplasmic basophilia. Direct measurements on cytocentrifuge smears revealed that while there was great size heterogeneity in both preparations, fetal cells were on average larger. Transmission and scanning electron microscopy also revealed morphologic differences. Fetal cells were more likely to bear blebs and microvilli and had more abundant polyribosomes (E. S. Medlock, unpublished observations).

The possibility remains that fetal and neonatal B-cells and their precursors represent relatively rare intermediate stages of adult B-cell differentiation. Direct comparisons of the fate of highly enriched cells from these sites may provide support for that notion. Alternatively, we may learn that the early waves of B-cell formation that occur in fetal tissues take place through processes somewhat different from and perhaps simpler than those that occur in adult life. Until this question is resolved, it would be wise to avoid equating the events which occur in adult marrow with the population changes that can be observed in tissues of developing animals.

REFERENCES

1. RAFF, M. C., J. J. T. OWEN, M. D. COOPER, A. R. LAWTON, M. MEGSON & W. E. GATHINGS. 1975. Differences in susceptibility of mature and immature mouse B lymphocytes to anti-immunoglobulin-induced immunoglobulin suppression *in vitro*: Possible implications for B-cell tolerance to self. J. Exp. Med. **142:** 1052-1064.

2. LAWTON, A. R. & M. D. COOPER. 1974. Modification of B lymphocyte differentiation by anti-immunoglobulins. In Contemporary Topics in Immunobiology. M. D. Cooper & N. L. Warner, Eds.: 193-225. Plenum Publishing Co. New York, N.Y.

3. NOSSAL, G. J. V. & B. L. PIKE. 1975. Evidence for the clonal abortion theory of B-lymphocyte tolerance. J. Exp. Med. **141:** 904-917.

4. METCALF, E. S., A. S. SCHRATER & N. KLINMAN. 1979. Murine model of tolerance induction in developing and mature B cells. Immunol. Rev. **43:** 141-183.

5. OSMOND, D. G., M. FAHLMAN, G. M. FULOP & M. D. RAHAL. 1981. Lymphocyte differentiation in the bone marrow: Localisation and regulation of bone marrow lymphocyte production. In CIBA Foundation Symposium No. 84, Microenvironments in Hemopoietic and Lymphoid Differentiation. R. Porter & J. Whelan, Eds.: 68-82. Pitman. London, England.

6. LANDRETH, K. S., C. ROSSE & J. CLAGETT. 1981. Myelogenous production and maturation of B lymphocytes in the mouse. J. Immunol. **127**(5): 2027-2034.

7. DE FREITAS, A. A. & A. COUTINHO. 1981. Very rapid decay of mature B lymphocytes in the spleen. J. Exp. Med. **154:** 994-999.

8. KEARNEY, J. F., M. D. COOPER, J. KLEIN, E. R. ABNEY, R. M. E. PARKHOUSE & A. R. LAWTON. 1977. Ontogeny of Ia and IgD on IgM-bearing B lymphocytes in mice. J. Exp. Med. **146:** 297-301.

9. MOND, J. J., S. KESSLER, F. D. FINKELMAN, W. E. PAUL & I. SCHER. 1980. Heterogeneity of Ia expression on normal B cells, neonatal B cells, and on cells from B-cell defective CBA/N mice. J. Immunol. **124**: 1675–1682.

10. LALA, P. K., G. R. JOHNSON, F. L. BATTYE & G. J. V. NOSSAL. 1979. Maturation of B lymphocytes. I. Concurrent appearance of increasing Ig, Ia and mitogen responsiveness. J. Immunol. **122**: 334–341.

11. KINCADE, P. W., G. LEE, T. WATANABE, L. SUN & M. P. SCHEID. 1981. Antigens displayed on murine B-lymphocyte precursors. J. Immunol. **127**: 2262–2268.

12. KINCADE, P. W., L. FLAHERTY, G. LEE, T. WATANABE & J. MICHAELSON. 1980. Qa antigen expression on functional lymphoid, myeloid, and stem cells in adult mice. J. Immunol. **124**: 2879–2885.

13. SCHER, I., A. K. BERNING, S. KESSLER & F. D. FINKELMAN. 1980. Development of B lymphocytes in the mouse: Studies of the frequency and distribution of surface IgM and IgD in normal and immune-defective CBA/N F$_1$ mice. J. Immunol. **125**(4): 1686–1693.

14. OSMOND, D. G. & G. J. V. NOSSAL. 1974. Differentiation of lymphocytes in mouse bone marrow. I. Quantitative radioautographic studies of antiglobulin-binding by lymphocytes in bone marrow and lymphoid tissue. Cell. Immunol. **13**: 117–131.

15. SIECKMANN, D. G., I. SCHER, R. ASOFSKY, D. E. MOSIER & W. E. PAUL. 1978. Activation of mouse lymphocytes by anti-immunoglobulin. II. A thymus-independent response by a mature subset of B lymphocytes. J. Exp. Med. **148**: 1628–1643.

16. MOND, J. J. 1982. Use of the T lymphocyte regulated type 2 antigens for the analysis of responsiveness of Lyb5$^+$ and Lyb5$^-$ B Lymphocytes to T lymphocyte derived factors. Immunol. Rev. **64**: 99–115.

17. SIGAL, N. H. & N. R. KLINMAN. 1978. The B-cell clonotype repertoire. Adv. Immunol. **26**: 255–337.

18. KINCADE, P. W., G. LEE, M. P. SCHEID & M. D. BLUM. 1980. Characterization of murine colony-forming B cells. II. Limits to *in vitro* maturation, Lyb-2 expression, resolution of IgD$^+$ subsets and further population analysis. J. Immunol. **124**(2): 947–953.

19. OI, V. T., P. P. JONES, J. W. GODING, L. A. HERZENBERG & L. A. HERZENBERG. 1978. Properties of monoclonal antibodies to mouse Ig allotypes, H-2, and Ia antigens. Curr. Top. Microbiol. Immunol. **81**: 115.

20. KINCADE, P. W., G. LEE, C. J. PAIGE & M. P. SCHEID. 1981. Cellular interactions affecting the maturation of murine B lymphocyte precursors *in vitro*. J. Immunol. **127**(1): 255–260.

21. KINCADE, P. W. 1981. Formation of B lymphocytes in fetal and adult life. Adv. Immunol. **31**: 177–245.

22. BLACK, S. J., W. VAN DER LOO, M. R. LOKEN & L. A. HERZENBERG. 1978. Expression of IgD by murine lymphocytes. Loss of surface IgD indicates maturation of memory B cells. J. Exp. Med. **147**: 984–996.

23. SITIA, R., J. ABBOTT & U. HAMMERLING. 1979. The Ontogeny of B Lymphocytes. V. Lipopolysaccharide-induced changes of IgD expression on murine B lymphocytes. Eur. J. Immunol. **9**(11): 859–864.

24. ABBOTT, J. & K. NGIAM. 1981. Sequential expression of B lymphocyte surface antigens *in vitro*. Eur. J. Immunol. **11**: 411–417.

25. PAIGE, C. J., P. W. KINCADE, L. A. SHINEFELD & V. L. SATO. 1981. Precursors of murine B lymphocytes. Physical and functional characterization and distinctions from myeloid stem cells. J. Exp. Med. **153**: 154–165.

26. PAIGE, C. J., P. W. KINCADE, M. A. S. MOORE & G. LEE. 1979. The fate of fetal and adult B-cell progenitors grafted into immunodeficient CBA/N mice. J. Exp. Med. **150**: 548–563.

27. LANDRETH, K. S., P. W. KINCADE & G. LEE. 1981. Relationship between phenotypically and functionally defined precursors of B lymphocytes. Fed. Proc. **40**: 4990.

E. S. VITETTA: Does LPS in the cloning system create a problem with detecting or keeping IgD on the cells?

P. W. KINCADE: Would IgD be lost?

VITETTA: Yes, I mean why doesn't it disappear?

KINCADE: We can't know that. All we know is that the right sub-set, the half that is δ^+ and anti-δ sensitive, is sensitive to 50 nanograms of anti-δ. That would completely stop their proliferation. We can't know if they lose it or if the other half manages to survive anti-δ because they quickly lose it. That's one possible explanation.

VITETTA: And they are sensitive to intact molecule anti-delta, as well as F(ab')$_2$.

KINCADE: Yes, that's correct. F(ab')$_2$ works in our hands just as well as the intact molecule. Monomers, where we have used them, have no effect.

F. R. BLATTNER: The dogma now as far as the DNA level is concerned is that you make a variable region by a basically completely random process in which the V, D and J segments in the case of heavy chain, and in the case of light chains V and J are rearranged. Eventually you get a gene for a V segment, then the next thing is the cytoplasmic μ. I would like to know more about that cytoplasmic μ. I don't think any information about the structure of the constant region is known, but the point is, you still can't decide whether you can tolerize that cell, even if it has gotten to making cytoplasmic μ, because you still don't know what it's going to bind to. And this whole idea of deleting a clone or removing it from the population seems impossible to do at any of those early stages.

KINCADE: The best guess is that the cell is resistant to tolerization or anti-μ treatment because it doesn't express an intact surface IgM molecule. The experiments that best speak to that are those where, after the anti-μ suppression the numbers of cells in bone marrow that have cytoplasmic μ chains is not changed. The ones that are surface negative and have cytoplasmic μ chains are not changed by anti-μ suppression from birth. Furthermore, Owen and his colleagues have found that the rate of B-cell formation in a mouse, which is in the order of 10^8 μ^+ cells in the bone marrow every day, is not changed by depleting everything from surface Ig positive onwards by anti-μ treatment. So in that sense it says that there's no feedback. The population size doesn't control the rate at which B-cells are formed. So that's the best guess about that.

Whether or not immunoglobulin molecules get out of those pre-B cells has been a controversial issue and you probably know that there is evidence for and against that from Cooper's lab with different individuals working with human and mouse pre-B like cell lines. One seems to release μ chains and one does not. In the literature dealing with surface μ expression, using radio-iodination or rosetting procedures, some people have claimed to find μ chains on cells in very early embryos, whereas by fluorescence one don't see it.

LEN HERZENBERG: But is there really solid evidence that the pre-B cell is a precursor of the B-cell rather than just dying off?

KINCADE: It's solid circumstantial evidence. We have, for instance, a pre-B cell line that Chris Page developed in my lab that has pre-B characteristics. On exposure to LPS, they are induced to express intact surface Ig molecules. That was one example. There are also the very careful cell kinetics studies by my colleague, Ken Landreth. It seemed that once cells made cytoplasmic immunoglobulin (μ chains) they had the option of dividing maybe just once in the bone marrow before giving rise to two daughters, which, over a period of two days, would acquire surface immunoglobulin and at some random point along that pathway could escape to the periphery.

LEN HERZENBERG: So where is the wastage? The Tonagawa model and Weigert say you have wastage.

KINCADE: That's right. There could be wastage in the cells that we pull out as bearing a surface marker associated with the B-lineage. You pull the positive cells out from the bone marrow and half of them aren't making μ chains. Now we don't know what the other half are, maybe they are erroneously rearranged.

You must also consider the half life of cells that are made. One recent set of experiments by Coutinho suggested the cells that leave the bone marrow and go to the spleen have, on average, a very short half life. Within one day, half of the splenic population is gone. So there is this enormous production of cells, enormous migration of cells to peripheral tissues, and enormous death in those sites as well. We have an exception that I think is going to tell us a lot about regulation. By the time the NZB mouse, is 15 weeks old, this precursor population just disappears and perhaps they aren't making any more B-cells from that time on. Then we would expect that perhaps their repertoire might get simplified with time and all the consequences that would come about from that.

EFFECTS OF ALLOTYPE SPECIFIC ANTI-IgD ON THE IMMUNE RESPONSES OF HOMOZYGOUS MICE*

G. J. Thorbecke,† Y. Baine,† B. Xue,† Y.-W. Chen,‡ B. Pernis,§
G. W. Siskind,‡ and E. B. Jacobson¶

†Department of Pathology
New York University Medical Center
New York, New York 10016

‡Department of Medicine
Cornell University Medical Center
New York, New York 10021

§Department of Microbiology
Columbia University College of Physicians and Surgeons
New York, New York 10032

¶Department of Immunology
Merck Institute for Therapeutic Research
Rahway, New Jersey 07065

In previous studies[1] on mice treated with anti-IgD from birth we found no suppression of primary or secondary responses to trinitrophenylated B. abortus (TNP-BA) injected intravenously (i.v.). This was considered surprising in view of the low numbers of Ig-bearing cells present in the spleens of such anti-IgD treated mice. Primary responses to other antigens including TNP-hemocyanin (TNP-KLH) or TNP-ficoll were also found to be, if anything, enhanced rather than suppressed in spite of the virtual absence of IgD⁺ B-cells (TABLE 1). The presence of normal immune responses to TNP-ficoll, a response usually attributed to Lyb5⁺ cells,[2] prompted us to determine, in collaboration with R. Skelly and A. Ahmed (Merck Institute, Rahway, N.J.), whether Lyb5⁺ cells were present among the approximately 2–10% Ig⁺ cells found in the spleen of anti-IgD treated mice. A relatively high percentage of Lyb5⁺ cells was found.[3] In addition, histological observations of the lymphoid tissues of the anti-IgD treated mice showed the presence of germinal centers which had a normal mitotic rate, blast cell content, and affinity for peanut agglutinin,[1,4,5] even though the dense lymphocyte coronas, normally present next to each germinal center, were lacking. IgD⁺ cells could be detected in the coronas of normal mice by immunoperoxidase (PAP) staining,[1,4,5] but were absent in the suppressed mice. Similar findings have been reported by others.[5-7] It was concluded that the deficiency in recirculating IgD⁺ B-cells did not affect responses to intravenously injected antigens, and that the difference in B-cell maturation and/or proliferation between normal and anti-IgD suppressed mice was primarily quantitative, possibly because the deficiency in IgD⁺ B-cells, at least in the spleen, was compensated for by enhanced representation of IgM⁺ IgD⁻ B-cells.

Compensation for a B-cell defect with enhanced IgM⁺, IgD⁻ cell production would require time and could not occur in mice given antigen immediately after a

*This work was supported by research grants from the National Institutes of Health, U.S.P.H.S.: AI-03076, CA-20075 and AI-14398.

TABLE 1

PRIMARY RESPONSES IN BALB/C MICE TREATED WITH ANTI-Ig-5A FROM BIRTH

Antigen On Day 0‡	Anti-Ig-5a* Treatment	Geom. Mean ($\overset{\times}{\div}$ SE) of Anti-† TNP-PFC/Spleen on Day 4		Mean Percentage (± SE)§ of Spleen Cells Bearings	
		19S	7S	IgD	Ig
				%	%
TNP-Ficoll	−	269,200 (1.4)	251,200 (1.4)	19.0 (2.1)	24.6 (3.1)
TNP-Ficoll	+	457,100 (2.0)	489,800 (1.8)	0.8 (0.5)	8.2 (0.7)
TNP-KLH	−	10,200 (1.5)	7,200 (1.2)	17.1 (3.4)	18.1 (2.6)
TNP-KLH	+	30,900 (1.1)	15,500 (1.3)	0	8.0 (0.8)

*3×/week i.p. injections of 4.22 anti-Ig-5a:5 μg/inj. first 10 days, 10 μg/inj. next 10 days, and 50 μg/inj. thereafter.

†PFC = Plaque forming cells; Indirect PFC were developed by anti-Ig with goat anti-μ added to agar, n = 5−6.

‡10 μg TNP-ficoll or 100 μg TNP-KLH injected i.v.

§Determined by immunofluorescence, expressed as arithmetic mean ± S.E.

single injection of a large dose of anti-IgD. Therefore, additional experiments were performed in which the effect of a single iv injection of anti-Ig-5a(100 μg) was studied in BALB/c mice given an i.v. injection of either TNP-ficoll (10 μg) or TNP-KLH (100 μg). The results in TABLE 2 show that a significant inhibition of the response to TNP-ficoll was obtained both in normal and in athymic mice, while no significant effect was seen when a control protein of the same murine Ig class (IgG2a) was injected. The effect on the response to TNP-KLH was less marked but in the same direction. This result is in agreement with the possibility that cells with a high density of surface IgD are normally important for the response to TNP-ficoll, and are inhibited from responding by anti-IgD.

Other investigators have found enhancement rather than inhibition of the

TABLE 2

SUPPRESSIVE EFFECT OF ANTI-IgD ON PRIMARY PFC RESPONSE TO TNP-FICOLL OR TNP-HEMOCYANIN

Mice	Antigen	Injected With	Geom. Mean PFC/Spleen $\times 10^{-3}$ ($\overset{\times}{\div}$ SE)†	
			19S	7S
BALB/c	TNP-KLH*	None	23.4 (1.13)	5.6 (1.17)
		Anti-Ig-5a§	16.3 (1.14)	3.2 (1.58)
BALB/c	TNP-F‡	None	100.9 (1.16)	63.5 (1.13)
		LPC-1¶	89.1 (1.58)	56.2 (1.55)
		Anti-Ig-5a	37.9 (1.20)	22.0 (1.24)
Nu/Nu	TNP-F	None	269.1 (1.15)	93.3 (1.38)
BALB/c		LPC-1	204.2 (1.78)	120.2 (1.26)
		Anti-Ig-5a	55.0 (1.45)	28.2 (1.38)

*100 μg, i.v., on day 0.

†PFC determined on day 4, n = 5−15.

‡10 μg, i.v. on day 0.

§100 μg, i.v., monoclonal antibody 4.22, on the day before antigen.

¶100 μg, i.v., LPC-1.8.1.9, on the day before antigen.

TABLE 3

EFFECT OF ANTI-IgD ON PRIMARY RESPONSE TO TWO DIFFERENT
PREPARATIONS OF TNP-FICOLL

TNP-Ficoll* Preparation	Anti-Ig-5a (100 μg) On Day-1	Geom. Mean PFC/Spleen ×10⁻³ (× SE)	
		19S	7S
A	None	58.9 (1.05)	39.8 (1.16)
	+	66.1 (1.12)	56.2 (1.19)
B	None	38.9 (1.29)	28.2 (1.19)
	+	15.1 (1.17)	8.3 (1.23)

*10 μg TNP-Ficoll injected i.v. on Day 0. Preparations A and B were prepared from two different lots of ficoll.
†PFC determined on Day 4, n = 5.

response to TNP-ficoll after a single injection of anti-IgD, both in mice[7] and in rats.[8] Since the immunological properties of different preparations of TNP-ficoll can vary considerably, as we have demonstrated in other studies in our laboratory,[9] we studied the effect of anti-IgD on the response to two different preparations of this antigen (TABLE 3). The results showed that anti-IgD had no effect on the response to preparation A, while it significantly inhibited the response to preparation B. Different preparations of TNP-ficoll might vary in their ability to stimulate lymphokine production, thereby influencing the effect of anti-IgD. Therefore we included lymphokine injections in the experimental design of the next series of experiments (TABLES 4–6). The lymphokines used ("SN") were obtained from culture supernatants of SJL/J lymph node cells and syngeneic γ-irradiated (7500R) lymphoma cells ("γ-RCS"). It was shown previously that such supernatants contain large amounts of IL-2[10] and have a strong enhancing effect on antibody production by murine spleen cells in vitro.[11] The content of IL-2 was titrated by its effect on proliferation of IL-2 dependent T-cells (kindly donated by Dr. M. A. Palladino, Sloan-Kettering Institute for Cancer Research) using the probit analysis.[10,12] Clearly, SN contains a number of lymphokines in addition to IL-2, and furthermore, IL-2 is not necessarily relevant to the effect seen in the present studies, but its content is readily quantitated and provides some basis for comparison of different SN preparations. Usually 0.5 ml (200 U/ml IL-2) were injected i.v. at the same time as the antigen. The results in TABLE 4 show that SN alone caused a two to threefold enhancement of the response to

TABLE 4

ENHANCEMENT OF PRIMARY RESPONSE TO TNP-FICOLL* IN BALB/C MICE BY ANTI-IgD
AND LYMPHOKINES (SN)

Injected On		Geom. Mean PFC/Spleen ×10⁻³ (× SE)‡	
Day-1	Day 0	19S	7S
None	None	117.5 (1.15)	61.7 (1.20)
Anti-Ig-5a†	None	60.3 (1.20)	47.9 (1.26)
None	SN	223.9 (1.10)	190.6 (1.10)
Anti-Ig-5a	SN	316.2 (1.10)	251.2 (1.15)

*10 μg of TNP-Ficoll (preparation B) injected i.v. on Day 0.
†Anti-Ig-5a 100 μg injected i.v. on day before antigen.
‡ PFC determined on Day 4, n = 5.

TABLE 5

ANTI-TNP MEMORY CHALLENGE, 4 DAYS AFTER PRIMING,* BY INJECTION
OF ANTI-IgD AND LYMPHOKINES (SN)

Additional Treatment (Day)	PFC/Spleen on Day 8† Geom. Mean ($\overset{\times}{\div}$ SE)	
	19S	7S
None	4,756 (1.06)	2,690 (1.11)
Antigen (D4)‡	7,787 (1.18)	23,990 (1.14)
Anti-Ig-5a (D4)§	2,884 (1.38)	4,169 (1.20)
SN (D4, 5)¶	7,079 (1.15)	9,120 (1.14)
Anti-Ig-5a (D4) + SN (D4, 5)	28,840 (1.12)	27,542 (1.15)

*Primary TNP-KLH injection (100 μg, i.v.) on Day 0.
†PFC determined on Day 8, n = 5–15.
‡Second injection of antigen also 100 μg i.v.
§Anti-IgD, 100 μg, i.v. (monoclonal ab. 4.22).
¶SN = supernatant medium of SJL/J lymph node cells and γ-irradiated RCS after 48 hrs of culture.

TNP-ficoll. In combination with anti-IgD the enhancement was even greater, although the injection of anti-IgD alone caused an inhibition of the response to TNP-ficoll (preparation B). Thus, there appeared to be synergism between anti-IgD and SN in the enhancement of the antibody response induced.

We next studied whether simultaneous injection of anti-IgD and SN, injected without antigen several days after priming, could induce the primed B-cells to make a secondary response. It was considered possible that, in the presence of lymphokines, anti-IgD might take the place of antigen in triggering B-cells into

TABLE 6

SYNERGISM BETWEEN ANTI-IgD AND LYMPHOKINES (SN) IN THE ENHANCEMENT OF THE
SECONDARY* IMMUNE RESPONSE TO TNP-KLH

Experiment	Additional Treatment (Day)	PFC/Spleen on Day 8† Percentage of Control	
		19S	7S
		100%	100%
1	None	(9,636)	(24,460)
	SN (D4)‡	98	266
	Anti-Ig-5a (D4)§	32	79
	Anti-Ig-5a (D4) + SN (D4)	212	391
		100%	100%
2	None	(8,709)	(33,113)
	SN (D4, 5, 6)	380	178
	Anti-Ig-5a (D4)	112	129
	Anti-Ig-5a (D4) + SN (D4, 5, 6)	417	251

*Primary and secondary injections of 100 μg TNP-KLH i.v. on Day 0 and 4.
†Values in parenthesis represent geom. mean PFC/spleen in control mice. PFC determined on Day 8, n = 4–5.
‡SN = supernatant medium of SJL/J lymph node cells and γ-irradiated RCS after 48 hrs of culture.
§Anti-IgD, 100 μg, i.v. (monoclonal ab. 4.22).

antibody production. The results in TABLE 5 are consistent with this possibility. The injection of anti-IgD was given four days after priming, at a time when most antigen primed B-cells have not yet lost their surface IgD.[13] Boosting with antigen on day 4 elicited a marked secondary response, predominantly of 7S PFC, on day 8 after the primary injection. Injection of either anti-IgD or SN alone caused a slight increase in 7S PFC on day 8. Injection of both anti-IgD and SN simultaneously caused a marked increase in both 19S and 7S PFC responses, which was more than additive and similar in magnitude to that elicited with antigen. Since the 7S responses were enumerated with anti-μ antibody in the agar at a concentration which caused complete inhibition of IgM plaque formation,[14] the indirect PFC were truly 7S antibody secreting cells.

The synergy between anti-IgD and SN again suggested that anti-IgD was, in effect, replacing antigen in the triggering of B-cells, which it could not do in the absence of lymphokine as a second signal. In order to examine this possibility further, the effect of injecting additional antigen on day 4 was determined. It seemed likely that the synergy between anti-IgD and SN would be reduced in the presence of antigen. In the experiments shown in TABLE 6, all mice received two injections of TNP-KLH, on day 0 and 4. Additional injections on day 4 consisted of anti-IgD alone, SN alone, or both anti-IgD and SN. It can be seen that anti-IgD alone did not enhance the response to antigen significantly, and even inhibited the response slightly in experiment 1 (TABLE 6). Lymphokine alone enhanced the response to TNP-KLH, but the combination of anti-IgD and SN was still synergistic in causing enhancement of antibody production. This raises the possibility that additional B-cell activating effects can be seen with these agents. Such effects are explored further in studies by Jacobson et al.[15] employing allotype heterozygous mice. Thus, we conclude that lymphokine production can markedly modify the effects of a single injection of anti-IgD in vivo and that this could explain apparent inconsistencies between results of various investigators studying the effect of anti-IgD.

REFERENCES

1. JACOBSON, E. B., Y. BAINE, Y.-W. CHEN, T. FLOTTE, M. O'NEIL, B. PERNIS, G. W. SISKIND, G. J. THORBECKE & P. TONDA. 1981. J. Exp. Med. **154:** 318–332.
2. MOSIER, D. E., I. M. ZITRON, J. J. MOND, A. AHMED, I. SCHER, & W. E. PAUL. 1977. Immunol. Rev. **37:** 89–104.
3. SKELLY, R. R., Y. BAINE, A. AHMED, B. XUE & G. J. THORBECKE. J. Immunol. In press.
4. THORBECKE, G. J., T. FLOTTE, & Y. BAINE. 1982. Maturity of precursor cells for germinal centers. In In Vivo Immunology: Histophysiology of the Lymphoid System. P. Nieuwenhuis, A. A. van der Broek, & M. G. Hanna, Eds. Plenum. New York, N.Y. In press.
5. FINKELMAN, F., I. SCHER, J. J. MOND, S. WILBURN, K. CHAPMAN, & E. S. METCALF. 1981. Developments in Immunology **15:** 201–210.
6. BAZIN, H., & I. C. M. MACLENNAN. 1982. This volume.
7. FINKELMAN, F. D., V. L. WOODS, S. B. WILBURN, J. J. MOND, K. E. STEIN, A. BERNING & I. SCHER. 1980. J. Exp. Med. **152:** 493–506.
8. CUCHENS, M. A., K. L. BOST, M. L. HOOVER & G. A. LESLIE. 1981. Cell. Immunol. **63:** 293–299.
9. BHOGAL, B. S., E. A. GOIDL, G. W. SISKIND & G. J. THORBECKE. 1982. Fed. Proc. **41:** 290.
10. PONZIO, N. M., T. HAYAMA, C. NAGLER, I. R. KATZ, M. HOFFMANN, C. GILBERT, J. VILCEK, & G. J. THORBECKE. Manuscript in preparation.

11. HAYAMA, T., C. NAGLER, D. T. UMETSU, J. CHAPMAN-ALEXANDER & G. J. THORBECKE. Eur. J. Immun. In press.
12. GILLIS, S., N. A. UNION, P. E. BAKER & K. A. SMITH. 1978. J. Exp. Med. **149:** 1460–1476.
13. KANOWITH-KLEIN, S., E. S. VITETTA, E. L. KORN & R. F. ASHMAN. 1979. J. Immunol. **122:** 2349–2355.
14. GOIDL, E. A., T. J. ROMANO, G. W. SISKIND & G. J. THORBECKE. 1978. Cell. Immunol. **35:** 231–241.
15. JACOBSON, E. B., Y. BAINE, Y.-W. CHEN, B. PERNIS, G. W. SISKIND & G. J. THORBECKE. 1982. This volume.

DISCUSSION OF THIS PAPER BEGINS ON PAGE 314.

EFFECT OF ALLOTYPE SPECIFIC ANTI-IgD ON THE IMMUNE RESPONSES OF HETEROZYGOUS MICE

E. B. Jacobson,* Y. Baine,† Y. Wu-Chen,‡
B. Pernis,§ G. W. Siskind,‡ and G. J. Thorbecke†

*Department of Immunology
Merck Institute for Therapeutic Research
Rahway, New Jersey 07065

†Department of Pathology
New York University School of Medicine
New York, New York 10016

‡Department of Allergy and Immunology
Cornell University Medical Center
New York, New York 10021

§Department of Microbiology
Columbia University Medical Center
New York, New York 10032

With the use of allotype-specific antibody to IgD, some of the effects observed in homozygous mice can be characterized more definitively in allotype heterozygotes, since these mice serve, in a sense, as their own control with respect to the untreated allotype.

In our initial studies, we examined the effect of chronic exposure to anti-IgD on the secondary immune response to sheep erythrocytes (SRBC). The experimental procedure has been previously described.[1] Briefly, the mice were treated from birth to 11 weeks of age with weekly injections of anti-IgD. All of the mice were injected with antigen on week 6 and were boosted on week 11, in each case one day after an anti-IgD injection. PFC assays were done six days after boosting and one week after the last anti-IgD injection. As shown in TABLE 1, control mice, given two injections of antigen, made a 7S PFC response that was essentially equivalent with respect to allotype distribution. In mice injected with anti-5a or anti-5b, the IgG PFC response linked to the relevant IgD allotype was markedly reduced, while, in each case, a moderate compensatory increase was seen in the alternate allotype. However, if the mice were injected with both anti-5a and anti-5b, using the same injection schedule and the same amounts of each antibody, there was no suppression of the IgG response of either allotype. In fact, there was a slight increase over control levels. The latter results were in complete agreement with those obtained in homozygous BALB/c mice injected from birth with anti-5a.

We concluded from these results, since the mice were able to make a normal immune response in the absence of δ^+ cells, that an alternate pathway exists in which IgD⁺ cells are not required for a secondary in vivo response. A similar conclusion has been reported by Metcalf et al. using heterologous anti-IgD (this volume). However, in heterozygous mice treated with antibody directed against one allotype, the alternate pathway is not used, and a profound suppression of the linked IgG allotype is seen. Cells producing IgG of the untreated allotype respond well, suggesting that if IgD⁺ cells are present, they may be preferentially used.

0077-8923/82/0399-0310$01.75/0 © 1982, NYAS

TABLE 1

SECONDARY RESPONSE TO SRBC* IN ALLOTYPE-HETEROZYGOUS MICE
TREATED FROM BIRTH WITH ALLOTYPE-SPECIFIC ANTI-IgD

Antibody Injected	PFC/Spleen Percentage of Control Response	
	Allotype a	Allotype b
	%	%
None	100.0	100.0
	(79,600)	(70,700)
Anti-5a†	19.3	170.0
Anti-5b	193.0	16.3
Anti-5a + Anti-5b	154.4	134.4

*4 × 10⁸ SRBC injected i.v. on Day 42 and on Day 77 after birth (one day after an anti-delta injection), assayed six days after boost, developed with specific anti-allotype sera, 19S PFC subtracted.

†One i.p. injection per week of anti-5a (4.22) and/or anti-5b (H6/31 HL). 10 μg from birth to week 3 and 2 μg/g BW from week 4 to week 11.

However, quantitative aspects of B-cell representation will obviously influence which B-cells are activated.

An additional set of experiments was done to determine whether a single high dose of anti-5a or anti-5b, administered one day prior to antigen injection to six week old heterozygous mice, could replace the previous regimen of weekly injections given from birth to six weeks of age. It is clear from the results shown in TABLE 2 that a similar pattern of suppression was obtained, regardless of whether the treatment was continued through week 11 or not. Thus, unlike the effect seen

TABLE 2

SECONDARY RESPONSE TO SRBC* IN ALLOTYPE-HETEROZYGOUS MICE
TREATED AT SIX WEEKS OF AGE WITH ALLOTYPE-SPECIFIC ANTI-IgD

Antibody Injected	PFC/Spleen Percentage of Control Response	
	Allotype a	Allotype b
None	100.0	100.0
	(48,440)	(45,210)
Anti-5a†	23.0	141.4
None	100.0	100.0
	(163,000)	(168,110)
Anti-5b†	142.4	41.0
Anti-5b‡	147.4	29.6

*4 × 10⁸ SRBC injected i.v. on day 42 and on day 77 after birth, assayed six days after boost, developed with specific anti-allotype sera, 19S PFC subtracted.

†One injection of 100–200 μg of anti-5a (4.22) or anti-5b (H6/31HL) injected on day 41.

‡One injection of 100–200 4mg of anti-5a (4.22) or anti-5b (H6/31HL) injected on day 41 followed by one injection per week of 2 μg/g BW to day 76 (one day before antigen challenge).

TABLE 3

EFFECT OF TREATMENT WITH ANTI-Igh-5A AND/OR LYMPHOKINES (SN)
ON THE SECONDARY IMMUNE RESPONSE TO TNP-KLH IN (BALB × SJL)F₁ MICE*

Treatment	PFC/Spleen† Percentage of Control Response		
		7S	
	19S	Allotype a	Allotype b
	%	%	%
None	100	100	100
	(27,600)	(18,520)	(7,320)
Anti-5a (day 4)	276	94	263
SN (days 4, 5)	201	176	270
Anti-5a (day 4) and SN (days 4, 5)	594	130	516

*Primary and secondary injections of 100 μg TNP-KLH i.v. on days 0 and 4.
†PFC response assayed day 8. 7S PFC developed with allotype specific antisera, with anti-μ incorporated in the agar.

in homozygous mice, the result of chronic suppression in heterozygous mice treated with anti-IgD directed against one allotype and the result obtained with a single high dose, administered one day prior to antigen injection, is similar.

It was observed in homozygous mice that a suppressive effect of anti-IgD could be converted to an augmenting effect by the simultaneous injection of lymphokines (Thorbecke *et al.,* this volume). To further delineate the mechanism of this synergistic effect between anti-IgD and lymphokine, the secondary response of heterozygous mice was studied in a similar manner. TNP-KLH was injected on day 0 and day 4 and allotype specific anti-IgD was injected on day 4, either alone or together with the lymphokine preparation (SN), described by Dr. Thorbecke (this volume). The PFC response was determined on day 8. In some experiments, treatment with anti-5a alone had little effect on the 7S response of cells producing Ig^a antibody but augmented the Ig^b PFC response (TABLE 3). In other experiments, represented in TABLE 4, it had no effect on the response of either allotype. Injection of lymphokine alone resulted in an augmentation of the

TABLE 4

EFFECT OF TREATMENT WITH ANTI Igh-5A AND/OR LYMPHOKINES (SN)
ON THE SECONDARY IMMUNE RESPONSE TO TNP-KLH IN (BALB × SJL)F₁ MICE*

Treatment	PFC/Spleen† Percentage of Control Response		
		7S	
	19S	Allotype a	Allotype b
	%	%	%
None	100	100	100
	(4,540)	(5,990)	(2,620)
Anti-5a (day 4)	154	104	123
SN (days 4, 5)	400	376	466
Anti-5a (day 4) and SN (days 4, 5)	527	376	1,027

*Primary and secondary injections of 100 μg TNP-KLH i.v. on days 0 and 4.
†PFC response assayed day 8. 7S PFC developed with allotype specific antisera, with anti-μ incorporated in the agar.

response of both allotypes (TABLES 3 and 4). However, when anti-5a was injected together with lymphokine a marked increase (additive or super-additive) was seen in the Ig^b PFC response, although the Ig^a PFC response was not increased over that obtained with SN alone. Thus, the major augmenting effect, in which anti-IgD and lymphokine synergize, was on cells producing the allotype which the anti-IgD could not interact with directly. Comparable trans-stimulatory results were obtained using anti-IgD specific for the b allotype. From these data, we concluded that the mechanism of the augmenting effect of anti-IgD must be an indirect activation of B-cells.

The ability of anti-IgD to augment immune responses was first noted by Pernis[2] and has been observed by several workers since that time.[3-6] It is not clear, however, from these studies, whether this augmentation is due to a direct interaction between the antibody and the IgD bearing cells. Studies by Mond *et al.*[7] have clearly demonstrated an increase in sIA density on the surface of B-cells after treatment with anti-IgD, both *in vivo* and *in vitro*. This increase occurs early (3-9 hours) and is T-cell independent, suggesting a direct effect on IgD bearing cells. However, the later effect, represented by the production of IgG_1 antibody, is T-cell dependent.[6,7] This later effect might therefore be, at least partially, an indirect action of anti-IgD comparable to that which we have presented here.

Several possible mechanisms for this indirect effect of anti-IgD should be considered. First, it is possible that B-lymphocytes, following their interaction with anti-IgD, are induced to produce lymphokines. The production of MIF by B-cells[8] serves as a classical precedent for such a possibility. If such a B-cell lymphokine had an action synergistic with that of the lymphokine preparation injected in these experiments, it could account for the observed results. Second, the interaction of anti-IgD with at least certain B-cells can result in the shedding of immune complexes (Pernis, this volume). These immune complexes might have idiotype-specific augmenting effects on other B-cells, either directly or by activation of idiotype-specific helper cells.

The enhanced expression of Ia antigens by B-cells treated with anti-Ig suggests a third possibility. Such cells may be enhanced stimulators of autologous mixed lymphocyte reactions, as are LPS stimulated B-blast cells (Ponzio and Thorbecke, unpublished observation). The occurrence of an autologous MLR *in vivo* could lead to endogenous lymphokine production, resulting in a nonspecific augmentation of the immune response. It has been shown that *in vitro* the autologous MLR is accompanied by the elaboration of lymphokines into the medium,[9] (Hayama, *et al.*, unpublished). The allotype nonspecificity of augmentation which we have observed would thus be due to a nonspecific effect of lymphokine production. The failure to see augmentation of the allotype linked to the specificity of the anti-IgD injected could be explained as the result of competing suppression (direct effect of anti-IgD) and augmentation (indirect effect).

References

1. JACOBSON, E. B., Y. BAINE, Y. W. CHEN, T. FLOTTE, M. J. O'NEIL, B. PERNIS, G. W. SISKIND & P. TONDA. 1981. J. Exp. Med. **154**: 318–332.
2. PERNIS, B. 1975. *In* Membrane Receptors of Lymphocytes. M. Seligman, J. L. Preud'homme, and F. M. Dovrilsky, Eds.: 25–26. North Holland. Amsterdam.
3. MARTIN, L. N. & G. A. LESLIE. 1979. Immunology **37**: 253–262.
4. FINKELMAN, F. D. & P. E. LIPSKY. 1979. Immunological Rev. **45**: 117–139.
5. CUCHENS, M. A., L. N. MARTIN & G. A. LESLIE. 1978. J. Immunol. **121**: 2257–2262.

6. FINKELMAN, F. D., J. J. MOND, V. L. WOODS, S. B. WILBURN, A. BERNING, E. SEHGAL & I. SCHER. 1980. Immunological Rev. **52:** 55–74.
7. MOND, J. J., E. SEHGAL & F. FINKELMAN. 1981. *In* B Lymphocytes in the Immune Response: Functional, Developmental and Interactive Properties. N. KLINMAN, D. E. MOSIER, I. SCHER & E. S. VITETTA, Eds.: 177–184. Elsevier/North Holland.
8. ROCKLIN, R. E., R. P. MACDERMOTT, L. CHESS, S. F. SCHLOSSMAN & J. R. DAVID. 1974. J. Exp. Med. **140:** 1303–1316.
9. LATTIME, E. C., S. GILLIS, C. DAVID & O. STUTTMAN. 1981. Eur. J. Immunol. **11:** 67–69.

DISCUSSION OF THE TWO PRECEDING PAPERS

J. J. MOND: You've shown that anti-δ plus supernatant can, in fact, replace the need for antigen. Have you ever tried priming a nude mouse with a T-dependent antigen and then coming back with anti-δ and lymphokine to see, in fact, if you did have priming of B-cells in the absence of T-cells, and could now boost such a response by anti-δ and supernatant?

G. J. THORBECKE: We have tried supernatants along with antigen in nude mice to promote the priming of B-cells, but we have always challenged with T-independent antigens and found no memory at all. In a preliminary experiment in which we tried anti-δ along with lymphokine we have not obtained any effect.

D. W. SCOTT: What was the epitope density of the two preparations of TNP-Ficoll?

G. J. THORBECKE: Both were in the range of 40 to 50 TNP groups per 10^5 daltons.

F. R. BLATTNER: Is there any way that anyone can distinguish between the action of the antibody on the membrane form and the secreted form of IgD?

F. FINKELMAN: I think if you look at what happens when you give a very low dose of anti-δ, which could remove presumably all the circulating IgD but not all of the cell surface IgD, you can look at it that way.

J. W. GODING: I think the possibility does exist of making specific antibodies against the C-terminal extension portion, which lies between the end of the secretory form and the membrane. That segment is probably an open sort of conformation and I think antibodies might be made. It would be perhaps a worthwhile exercise for someone to attempt to make them and address this point.

H. BAZIN: Have you found the normal number of germinal centers in your anti-δ suppressed mice? In rats we actually think we have fewer germinal centers.

THORBECKE: We have not made an extensive search through all the tissues to quantitate this, but I think the germinal centers in Peyer's patches were relatively normal. The germinal centers in the lymph nodes were on the small side and there probably were fewer than in normal animals, but we did not actually count the germinal centers.

BAZIN: I believe that the maturity of the immune response is about normal in anti-δ suppressed animals, except, as Dr. Ovary showed in his poster, the IgE response is completely suppressed.

THORBECKE: In those experiments, in order to get IgE in the immune response we had to immunize in a special way. If you immunize that way in an anti-δ suppressed animal you get neither γ1, nor γ2 or IgE. In other words, the inhibition is not specific for ϵ. It is specific for the method of immunization. If, therefore, in serum, ϵ may be suppressed more than γ; it still does not reflect an effect on ϵ per se. It may mean that the route of immunization, leading ultimately to ϵ, is more sensitive to suppression by anti-δ. One has to distinguish that from a specific effect on the switch to ϵ.

BAZIN: I'm not absolutely sure because we use an interperitoneal route and a very common technique to obtain such a response.

THORBECKE: But you need a very low dose of antigen, and that may be exactly the clue why the whole response is inhibited because, as I said, in our hands the $\gamma 1$, the $\gamma 2$, and ϵ responses are inhibited when we immunize that way in an anti-δ suppressed animal. I think Dr. Vitetta would like very much this type of result, as she suggested that in the absence of δ a low dose of antigen might not fire and switch the cells properly because the cells have fewer receptors. We would like to know whether with a higher dose of antigen or with a different route of immunization we will still get the inhibition of IgE. Dr. Ovary and I are in the process of trying that.

BAZIN: I don't agree completely, because the level of IgE in the serum and also of IgG 2A are much lower in anti-δ suppressed, while all the other classes are normal. And curiously, IgE and IgG 2A are the most thymus dependent.

THORBECKE: You may be right, maybe there is an interaction with thymus dependency, but I just wanted to point out that it's not class specific in the sense that B-cells from anti-δ suppressed mice are not able to switch to one specific class.

STIMULATION OF THE MURINE IMMUNE SYSTEM BY ANTI-IgD ANTIBODIES: A POLYCLONAL MODEL OF B-LYMPHOCYTE ACTIVATION BY A THYMUS DEPENDENT ANTIGEN*

Fred D. Finkelman, Linda M. Muul, Lyn Yaffe, Irwin Scher,
James J. Mond, Steven W. Kessler, John Ryan, John T. Kung, and
Eleanor S. Metcalf

*Departments of Medicine, Microbiology and Biochemistry
Uniformed Services University of the Health Sciences
Bethesda, Maryland 20014
and
Divisions of Immunology and Pathology
Naval Medical Research Institute
Bethesda, Maryland 20814
and
Laboratory of Immunology
National Institutes of Health
Bethesda, Maryland 20205*

INTRODUCTION

Injection of a mouse with an immunogenic molecule will stimulate the production of antibodies specific for that molecule. If a haptenic determinant is conjugated to the same molecule, that molecule will act as a carrier, so that anti-hapten as well as anti-carrier antibodies will be produced. The roles of the haptenic determinant on the hapten-carrier conjugate in the stimulation of anti-hapten antibody production have been postulated to include direct stimulation of hapten specific B-lymphocytes by cross-linking of their surface (s) Ig as well as focusing of carrier specific helper cells or helper factors onto hapten specific B-cells.[1-2] In either case, injection of a mouse with a hapten-carrier conjugate, the haptenic determinants of which would bind to the sIg of all or nearly all B-lymphocytes, might be expected to stimulate polyclonal B-cell activation. Since the great majority of lymphocytes in a mature mouse bear sIgD[3-4] and since goat Ig is immunogenic for this species, a goat antibody to IgD (GaMδ) might be considered to represent such a "universal hapten" bound to an immunogenic carrier. GaMδ differs, however, from the standard hapten-carrier conjugate in that, with the exception of goat Ig specific B-cells, it is incapable of binding to B-cell sIgM or sIgG, and in that it binds to the constant rather than the variable region of sIgD. Previous studies, in which antibodies reactive with monkey,[5-7] mouse,[8-9] or rat[10-11] IgD had an adjuvant affect on antibody production to simultaneously injected antigens in these species but failed to induce polyclonal B-cell activation, raised the possibilities that a ligand-sIg V region interaction or the binding of ligand to sIgM might be obligatory for B-cell activation. The data that are presented in this paper provide evidence that

*Supported by USUHS research protocol Nos. RO8308, RO8315, CO7305, CO8310 and CO8327 and Naval Medical Research and Development Command Research Task No. M0095-PN.001-1030.

0077-8923/82/0399-0316$01.75/0 © 1982, NYAS

injection of mice with a sufficient quantity of heterologous or even homologous anti-δ antibody does indeed lead to polyclonal B-cell activation and, therefore, strongly suggests that the hapten's role in B-cell activation can be met by the crosslinking of sIgD in the absence of crosslinking of sIgM and that the sIgD V region need not be the site of such crosslinking.

EARLY EFFECTS OF GaMδ

In most of the studies presented here, 8–12 wk old BALB/c mice were injected i.v. with 800μg of affinity purified GaMδ or normal goat IgG and their sera and lymphoid cells were studied at various times thereafter. Multiple changes had occurred in splenic and lymph node B-cells by 24 hr after GaMδ injection at which time nearly all sIgD had been modulated from the B-cell surface. These changes included modifications in the B-cells' surface receptors as well as increases in B-cell size and DNA synthesis. While the percentage of sIa$^+$ cells in spleen was not changed, the quantity of sIa per B-cell had increased two-threefold.[12] Recent studies indicate that this is the result of an increase in Ia synthesis (J. Mond *et al.*, unpublished data). In addition, as is discussed by Yaffe in this volume, spleen cells from a mouse injected with GaMδ 24 hr prior to sacrifice had a 100–1,000 fold greater ability than control spleen cells to absorb the T-cell replacing activity from a T-cell replacing factor (TRF)[13] containing culture supernatant of concanavalin A stimulated spleen cells. Furthermore, Ryan has shown that there is an approximately tenfold increase in the ability of spleen cells from mice injected 24 hr previously with GaMδ to stimulate T-cell proliferation in an Mls-defined mixed lymphocyte reaction.[14] All of these features may increase the capacity of B-lymphocytes to interact with T-lymphocytes and macrophages as well as the lymphokines that these cells produce. GaMδ also has a rapid effect on B-cell size and DNA synthesis. Twenty-four hr after GaMδ injection a very substantial increase in the mean volume of spleen cells is seen as well as a more than twofold increase in the percentage of cells in the S, M, or G$_2$ phase of the cell cycle. Studies in which spleen cells were sorted into sIa$^+$ and sIa$^-$ populations with a fluorescence activated cell sorter (FACS) 48 hr after GaMδ injection indicated that a majority of splenic sIa$^+$ (B) lymphocytes had greatly increased in size and that splenic B-cell DNA synthesis, as measured by *in vivo* thymidine incorporation, had increased more than eightfold.[15] T-cell size and DNA synthesis were not measurably increased at this time.[15]

Activation of T-Lymphocytes

This lack of detectable T-lymphocyte participation in the GaMδ stimulated system ended three–four days after GaMδ injection. FACS purified Thy 1.2$^+$ lymphocytes from mice injected three or four days before sacrifice with GaMδ and 24 hr prior to sacrifice with ^{3}H-thymidine had incorporated respectively 1.7 and 3.1 times as much ^{3}H-thymidine as equal numbers of Thy 1.2$^+$ cells from control mice. The stimulation indices for Thy 1.2$^-$ spleen cells from the same mice were 9.4 and 8.0, respectively.

Activation of an sIgM to sIgG Switch and Ig Secretion

Further evidence of GaMδ induced B-lymphocyte activation was seen six days after GaMδ injection, when a sixfold increase in the percentage of spleen cells

TABLE 1

LATE EFFECTS OF GaMδ ON SPLEEN CELL NUMBER AND PERCENTAGES OF sIgG⁺ AND cIG⁺ CELLS

Day	Antibody Injected	Cells/Spleen × 10⁻⁶	Percent of Spleen Cells with sIgG	cIgM	cIgG
3	G IgG	79 (1.06)*	3.6		
	GaMδ	119 (1.10)	2.8		
5	G IgG	85 (1.17)	3.9	0.9 (1.45)	<0.2
	GaMδ	187 (1.27)	6.2	2.2 (1.53)	0.4 (2.03)
6	G IgG	77 (1.14)	2.0	0.3 (2.07)	0.5 (1.50)
	GaMδ	308 (1.18)	12.3	4.9 (1.04)	3.1 (1.57)
7	G IgG	76 (1.17)	4.6	0.4 (1.09)	0.5 (2.14)
	GaMδ	352 (1.22)	23.8	2.5 (1.67)	15.7 (1.28)

*Geometric means (geometric standard deviation)

with sIgG, and 16 and sixfold increases in the percentages of spleen cells that stained brightly for intracytoplasmic (c) IgM or IgG respectively were seen. By seven days after GaMδ injection the percentages of spleen cells with surface and intracytoplasmic IgG were respectively 20-35% and 12-18%.[16] The increases in the absolute numbers of sIgG⁺ and cIgG⁺ spleen cells were considerably greater than the percentage increases, since spleens from GaMδ treated mice contained, at day seven, three-six times as many cells as control spleens (TABLE 1).[15] Two lines of evidence suggested that much of the sIgG found on 20-35% of spleen cells at this time was intrinsic rather than cytophilic. sIgM⁺ and sIgG⁺ cells were found to be mostly nonoverlapping populations, i.e.; most sIgM⁺ cells were sIgG⁻ and vice versa (TABLE 2). In addition, greater than 90% of cIgG⁺ cells were found within the sIgG⁺ population while greater than 90% of cIgM⁺ cells were sIgG.⁻[16] Furthermore, sodium dodecyl sulphate-polyacrylamide gel electrophoretic analysis of ¹²⁵I-labeled sIg from spleen cells of day seven GaMδ treated mice indicated the presence of considerable amounts of IgG with a γ chain characteristic of cell membrane IgG,[16] which has an apparent molecular weight 10 kd greater than that of secreted IgG and which is barely detectable on lymphoid cells from control mice.[17-18]

Other experiments indicated that the IgG response induced by GaMδ was

TABLE 2

sIGM⁺ AND sIGG⁺ SPLEEN CELLS ARE MOSTLY NONOVERLAPPING POPULATIONS

Day	Antibody Injected	sIgM⁺	Percent of Spleen Cells* sIgG⁺	sIgM⁺ or sIgG⁺
7	G IgG	48.0	3.9	50.9
	GaMδ	42.5	21.7	59.3
13	G IgG	56.7	4.1	59.1
	GaMδ	40.0	13.9	53.2

*Pools of spleen cells from three mice injected with normal goal IgG or GaMδ seven or 13 days before sacrifice were stained with FITC-labeled antibodies specific for mouse μ or δ chain, or with a mixture of both antibodies. Percentages of specifically stained cells were determined with a FACS.

polyclonal rather than specific for constituents of goat serum. While 10–20% of spleen cells from mice injected seven days earlier with GaMδ exhibited bright intracytoplasmic fluorescence after staining with fluorescein isothiocyanate (FITC) labeled anti-mouse γ, less than 0.1% of the same cells were stained by FITC-goat IgG, and IgG levels in sera from the same mice were not decreased by absorption with goat IgG or goat serum.[16] Furthermore, absorption of small amounts of ^{3}H-labeled Ig secreted by cultured cells from the same mice with large quantities of goat serum immobilized on Sepharose suggested that no more than 20% of this Ig could have even low avidity for constituents of goat serum.[16]

Differentiation of T-Independent from T-Dependent Effects of GaMδ

Two lines of experimental evidence suggest that the B-cell activating effects observed one–two days after GaMδ injection result directly from sIgD crosslinking, while the effects seen six–seven days after injection require the production of T-cell helper factors. First, B-lymphocyte activation in congenitally athymic

TABLE 3

ROLES OF T-LYMPHOCYTES AND CARRIER DETERMINANTS IN ANTI-δ INDUCED IMMUNE ACTIVATION

Mice	Day	Antibody Injected	>429μ³	>2C DNA	sIgG⁺	cIgM⁺	cIgG⁺
BALB/c	3	G IgG	3	5.5	3.6		
		GaMδ	12	12.5	2.8		
	7	G IgG	2	5.5	4.6	0.4	0.5
		GaMδ	24	12.1	23.8	2.5	15.7
BALB/c nu/nu	2	G IgG	5	7.0	8.6		
		GaMδ	15	13.4	6.1		
	7	G IgG	5	7.6	6.6	2.6	0.8
		GaMδ	7	8.6	11.2	1.7	1.2
BALB/c Tolerized to G IgD	2	G IgG	3	5.8			
		GaMδ	15	15.4			
	7	G IgG	2	5.2	5.6	0.5	0.6
		GaMδ	5	5.2	5.7	1.2	1.5

(nude) mice injected two days previously with GaMδ resembles that of normal mice with respect to increases in B-cell sIa, size, and DNA synthesis. However, seven days after GaMδ injection no increases in spleen cell number or percent of cells with intracytoplasmic Ig and only a small and variable increase in the percentage of sIgG⁺ spleen cells were seen.[15-16] Second, similar findings were seen in mice made tolerant to goat IgG prior to injection of GaMδ. B-cell activation in these mice was similar to that seen in goat IgG reactive mice two days after GaMδ injection. However, B-cells from goat IgG tolerant mice failed to differentiate into cells with sIgG or cIgG seven days after GaMδ injection (TABLE 3).[15-16] Similar results were also found in experiments in which BALB/c and (BALB/c × C57BL/6)F₁ (BCF₁) mice were injected with 10-4.22, a monoclonal mouse IgG₂ₐ of the b allotype with specificity for IgD of the a allotype[19] or with a control monoclonal IgG₂ₐ of the b allotype, CBPC-101. 10-4.22, which reacts with all sIgD⁺ BALB/c lymphocytes and 50% of sIgD⁺ BCF₁ lymphocytes[20] and which is seen as foreign by the inbred but not by the hybrid mice, increased B-cell sIa density and B-cell size in both the BALB/c and F_1 mice two days after injection, but, seven days after injection, only increased spleen cell DNA synthesis and the percentages of sIgG$^+$ and cIg$^+$ cells in the BALB/c mice (TABLE 4).[15-16] We interpret these data to indicate that the crosslinking of sIgD by antibodies with anti-δ specificity leads to the presentation of those antibodies to T-lymphocytes and, in the presence of T-cells specific for those antibodies, leads to the production of helper factors that are required in our system for B-cells to acquire sIgG and to secrete Ig.

RELATIONSHIP OF EARLY AND LATE B-CELL ACTIVATING EVENTS

While it might be expected that anti-δ induction of polyclonal antibody production is totally dependent upon the early B-cell activating effects of anti-δ, examination of the ontogeny of responses to anti-δ injection suggests that this is not the case. Increases in B-cell sIa, size and proliferation were not seen in

TABLE 4

ROLE OF CARRIER DETERMINANTS IN ANTI-δ INDUCED IMMUNE ACTIVATION

Mice	Day	Antibody Injected	>429μ³	Percent of Spleen Cells				
				>2C DNA	sIa$^+$	sIgG$^+$	cIgM$^+$	cIgG$^+$
BALB/c	2	CBPC-101	2.5	5.4	39 (123)*			
		10-4.22	4.8	6.0	32 (249)			
BCF$_1$	2	CBPC-101	1.7	4.5	46 (121)			
		10-4.22	3.0	5.2	42 (193)			
BALB/c	7	CBPC-101	1.9	5.3		5.2	1.1	0.3
		10-4.22	14.	11.0		12.9	5.0	6.4
BCF$_1$	7	CBPC-101	1.2	6.0		3.6	0.9	0.3
		10-4.22	1.7	2.6		4.0	0.7	0.4

*(Median Fluorescence Intensity) of specifically stained cells. Note that all BALB/c sIgD$^+$ cells will be bound by 10-4.22, but that only 50% of BCF$_1$ sIgD$^+$ cells will be bound by this antibody.

16-day-old mice that had been injected two days earlier with GaMδ. However, 13–15-day-old mice that had been injected seven days earlier with GaMδ showed definite increases in spleen cell sIa, size, proliferation and antibody production seven days after GaMδ injection. Thus; the late effects of GaMδ injection are seen in mice too immature to experience the early effects. Despite this finding, the early events stimulated by GaMδ may contribute to the magnitude of the day seven antibody response, since the percentage of cIgG$^+$ spleen cells seen seven days after GaMδ injection of eight-day-old mice is only 10–20% of that seen in similarly treated adult mice (L. Muul et al., unpublished data). As is discussed by Muul et al. in this volume, experiments with mice with the CBA/N X-linked immune defect reinforce this conclusion.

Studies of the effects of different doses of GaMδ or GaMδ plus normal goat IgG (G IgG) also provided information about the relationship between the early and late phases of anti-δ stimulated B-cell activation. Injection of mice with 200 or 800 μg of GaMδ had qualitatively similar effects both two and seven days after injection, although the lower dose stimulated less lymphocyte proliferation and less of an increase in spleen cell number than the higher dose. In contrast, injection of 50μg of GaMδ induced a substantial increase in B-cell sIa two days after injection, but little or no increase in lymphocyte proliferation or differentiation into antibody secreting cells, and injection of 12.5μg of GaMδ had no effects on B-cell sIa, DNA synthesis, or antibody production, even though it caused B-cells to lose most of their sIgD. Supplementing the quantity of GaMδ injected with enough G IgG to keep the total dose of goat IgG injected constant at 800μg had little effect on B-cell sIa, proliferation, or total spleen cell numbers, but had important effects on the differentiation of B-cells into IgG secreting cells. Ten to fifteen percent of spleen cells from mice injected seven days earlier with 50μg of GaMδ plus 750μg of G IgG contained intracytoplasmic IgG, while the percentage of $cIgG^+$ spleen cells in mice injected with 200μg of GaMδ plus 600μg of G IgG (30–40%) was two–threefold above that seen in mice given 800μg of GaMδ. These data provided evidence that the proliferative and differentiative events induced by GaMδ were under separate controls and that, under some circumstances (low GaMδ concentration) an increase in B-cell sIa might be required for the events leading to the generation of Ig secreting cells to transpire. In addition, these data suggested that the T-cell stimulating (carrier) roles of injected GaMδ could be divided into at least 2 components; 1) the initial presentation of goat IgG by GaMδ stimulated B-cells to goat IgG specific T-cells and 2) the stimulation of activated goat IgG specific T-cells to secrete helper factors. While both components would be required to induce B-cells to differentiate into antibody secreting cells, the first component would be inducible by GaMδ but not by G IgG, while the latter component would be inducible by either. This concept was supported by studies in which mice were first injected with 200μg of GaM^δ plus 600μg of G IgG, then injected one, two, three, or five days later with 1 mg of TEPC-1017 $(IgDκ)$[21] in order to neutralize the injected GaMδ, and sacrificed seven days after the initial injection. Seven days after injection of 200μg of GaMδ plus 600μg of G IgG an average of 30% of spleen cells were $cIgG_1^+$. Injection of 1 mg of TEPC-1017 one or two days after GaMδ injection inhibited the percentage of splenic $cIgG_1^+$ cells by 88% or 71% respectively, but neutralization of GaMδ three or more days after injection did not inhibit the generation of $cIgG_1^+$ spleen cells. Thus, it is only for the first three days after GaMδ injection (the period required for initiation of T cell proliferation) that the effects of GaMδ necessary for stimulation of polyclonal antibody production cannot be duplicated by G IgG.

Suppressive Effects of Anti-δ on B-Cell Differentiation

The observation that 200μg of GaMδ plus 600μg of G IgG is a stronger stimulus of IgG_1 secretion than 800μg of GaMδ suggested that the binding of GaMδ to B-cell sIgD might, in addition, to its stimulatory effects, have a suppressive effect on the differentiation of B-cells into IgG secreting cells, as has been described *in vitro*.[9,22–24]

Further evidence for this was obtained from experiments in which mice were injected with immune complexes of goat anti-rabbit Ig and rabbit anti-goat Ig, then injected four days later with 800μg of G IgG or GaMδ and sacrificed four days after that. The mice injected with immune complexes followed by G IgG showed only 1.3-fold and 1.5-fold increases respectively in spleen cell number and the percent of spleen cells with greater than 2C DNA as compared to controls, but demonstrated a greater than 50-fold increase in the percent of spleen cells with intracytoplasmic IgG_1. Similar evidence for *in vivo* polyclonal activation of antibody production by rabbit IgG immune complexes has been reported by Rosenberg.[25-26] In contrast, the number and percentage of greater than 2C DNA containing spleen cells from the mice injected with immune complexes followed by GaMδ were increased 2.6- and 3.3-fold respectively while the percentage of $cIgG_1^+$ spleen cells in these mice was only 17% of that found in the mice treated with immune complexes followed by G IgG.

Specificity of GaMδ Induced Polyclonal Activation

While the experiments presented here strongly suggest that sIgD crosslinking could play a major role in B-cell activation, it was possible that the crosslinking of any cell surface molecule would induce similar effects. To test this possibility, mice were injected with 800μg of a monoclonal antibody specific for the ThB determinant,[15] which is present on B-lymphocytes and a population of thymus cells.[27] Unlike anti-δ antibodies, this antibody induced no increase in B-cell sIa, size, DNA synthesis, or differentiation into antibody secreting cells either two or seven days after injection, even though it modulated ThB from splenic B-cells

TABLE 5

FAILURE OF AN ANTIBODY TO ThB TO DUPLICATE THE ACTIVATING EFFECTS OF ANTI-δ

Day	Antibody Injected	Cells/Spleen × 10^{-6}	>429μ^3	Percent of Spleen Cells			
				>2C DNA	$sIgG^+$	$cIgM^+$	$cIgG^+$
2	RaDNP	76	3.	3.8			
	RaThB	54	3.	3.5			
	GaMδ	92	18.	17.6			
7	RaDNP	128	5.	9.0	2.2	1.3	1.1
	RaThB	96	3.	6.0	2.1	0.5	0.5
	GaMδ	419	19.	14.4	23.0	3.6	16.7

(TABLE 5). Thus, the effects of anti-δ antibodies on B-cell activation do not result simply from the binding of a foreign Ig to the B-cell surface and probably involve the transmission of specific signals via sIgD.

Collapse of the Activated Immune System

As described above, seven days after injection of 800μg of GaMδ the number of spleen cells had increased three–sixfold and the percentages of spleen cells with surface and intracytoplasmic IgG had increased 10–20 fold and 25–100 fold, respectively. However, 10 days after GaMδ injection the number of spleen cells had decreased to less than two times the control value and, by 14 days after injection, it was no longer elevated above control. Furthermore, by day 14 the percentages of $sIgG^+$ and $cIgG^+$ spleen cells had also decreased to control values. The disappearance of activated lymphoid cells from lymphoid organs probably resulted from death *in situ* rather than from migration to other organs, since histologic studies of spleen and lymph nodes removed from mice 10 days after GaMδ injection demonstrated large numbers of pyknotic and smudge cells.[15] The reasons for collapse of the activated immune system are not clear. Since activated helper T-cells have been shown to induce suppressor T-cell activation,[28] it seems likely that suppressor cells may have a role in the retrenchment of the immune system. This possibility is supported by preliminary in vitro studies that indicate that spleen cells removed from mice seven days after GaMδ injection can suppress the LPS induced proliferative response of normal spleen cells, while spleen cells from mice injected with GaMδ one day before sacrifice lack this suppressive effect (J. Mond and F. Finkelman, unpublished data).

Another reason for the death of activated B-lymphocytes may be the disappearance of helper factors. Melchers et al. have shown that proliferation and antibody production by activated B-cells can be maintained in vitro by B-cell maturation and replication factors that are produced by antigen specific T-lymphocytes only so long as they are simulated with antigen.[29] Mice injected with GaMδ produce considerable quantities of antibody to goat Ig, with the result that this molecule is rapidly catabolized. Once injected goat IgG has been fully catabolized, activated goat Ig specific T-cells may no longer be stimulated to secrete the factors that may be required for the survival of activated B-lymphocytes. Indeed, the collapse of the activated immune system can be prevented to a considerable extent by giving mice multiple injections of G IgG after an initial injection of GaMδ. (F. Finkelman et al., unpublished data).

A third possible reason for the immunological retrenchment may be that B-cells activated by GaMδ and T/macrophage helper factors to acquire sIgG probably lose sIgD (as they lose sIgM) and thus; can no longer be directly stimulated by anti-δ antibody. This represents a major difference between antigen induced and GaMδ induced B-cell activation, since antigen specific B-cells will continue to have the capacity to interact directly with antigen or antigen-associated helper factors after undergoing an sIgM/sIgD to sIgG shift. Since we have so far been unable to demonstrate that GaMδ induces the polyclonal appearance of large numbers of cells with the functional characteristics of memory B-lymphocytes, it is tempting to speculate that such sIgG mediated interactions may be important for the generation and/or survival of memory B-cells. Preliminary observations that spleen cells that have sIgG but not cIgG and that, like memory B-cells, bind peanut agglutinin (Dr. T. Flotte and Dr. J. Thorbecke, personal communication) are seen in the spleen between days seven and 13 but disappear by day 14 after GaMδ injection, favor the possibility that sIgG mediated interactions may have more of a role in memory B-cell maintenance and stimulation than in memory B-cell generation.

CONCLUDING DISCUSSION

The potential of a B-lymphocyte is realized only when it is stimulated to become a clone of antibody secreting cells. The experiments discussed in this paper indicate that the sIg-ligand interaction has several roles in this process, which can include the direct initiation of B-cell proliferation, the presentation of antigen to T-lymphocytes and the induction of changes in the B-cell's compliment of surface receptors that make it more capable of interacting with T-cell and macrophage-generated lymphokines. Other data, not presented in this paper, suggest that in addition to having a direct stimulatory effect on B-cell proliferation and an indirect stimulatory effect on the differentiation of B-cells into antibody secreting cells, relatively weak crosslinking of sIg, that by itself is incapable of inducing B-cell proliferation, can act synergistically with helper lymphokines to induce proliferation. Similar observations have been described *in vitro.*[30] The complexity of surface immunoglobulin's role in B-cell activation is underlined by the findings that sIgD crosslinking can have both a stimulatory and an inhibitory effect on B-cell differentiation and that the anti-δ induced changes in B-cell surface receptors, DNA synthesis and antibody production can occur independently of each other. This complexity is magnified by the existence of several different carrier specific and non-specific lymphokines that affect B-cell proliferation and differentiation, the B-cell receptors for most of which have not yet been defined as constitutive or inducible.[13,29,31-41] The data that are currently available lead us to believe that there is considerable redundancy in the pathways that can lead to B-cell clonal expansion and antibody production and that any one pathway may become crucial only when other pathways are blocked by an inherited defect,[42] when an antigen is incapable of activating B-lymphocytes via one or more pathways,[43] or when the speed and magnitude of antibody production are essential for the survival of an organism.[44-45]

While our experiments with anti-δ antibodies have helped to elucidate the roles of sIg by allowing us to crosslink the sIgD of the great majority of B-cells rather than just those B-cells specific for a given antigen, it must be considered that our system may distort some of the effects produced when antigen crosslinks the sIg of a more limited number of cells. As we have already mentioned, anti-δ loses its ability to interact directly with B-cells when their DNA is rearranged to allow the production of sIgG but not sIgD, while antigen can continue to interact with sIgG$^+$ antigen specific B-cells. Furthermore, the polyclonal nature of the anti-δ induced response may itself distort the nature of the response. In particular, the low concentration of antigen specific B- and T-cells may make B-cell antigen presentation to T-cells physiologically much less important than antigen presentation by accessory cells. On the other hand, the architectural localization of a clone of B-cells that has expanded as a result of a direct ligand-sIg interaction may have an antigen presenting function if the circulatory patterns of T-lymphocytes can increase the likelihood that antigen specific T-cells and antigen stimulated B-cells will be brought into close proximity. Such events would not be expected to be observed in *in vitro* studies, in which normal architectural and circulatory patterns are destroyed.

The polyclonal nature of GaMδ-induced immune activation may also distort the normal humoral immune responses by stimulating suppressive influences on B-cell differentiation that are greatly in excess of those induced by a normal T-dependent antigen. Such suppressive influences may have a role in the collapse of the anti-δ activated immune state that greatly exaggerates their roles in the regulation of the humoral immune response to a conventional antigen. Finally, GaMδ, unlike a conventional antigen, fails to interact with the sIgM on the B-cells that it stimulates. While our data indicate that an sIgM-ligand interaction is unnecessary for B-cell activation, *in vitro* studies of B-cell activation by anti-μ antibodies[46] and *in vivo* studies of antigen induced antibody production in mice suppressed from birth with anti-δ antibodies suggest that the roles of sIgM and sIgD in B-cell activation are very similar.[47-48] Furthermore, recent studies of the nucleic acid sequences of the terminal exons for the cell surface forms of μ and δ chains suggest that sμ and sδ share the identical sequence of amino acids that penetrate into the interior of the cell, and thus reinforce the likelihood that sIgM and sIgD may link to the same internal structures and transmit the same signals.[49] *In vitro* studies, however, indicate that anti-μ antibodies are more suppressive of antigen induced antibody responses than are anti-δ antibodies. Some, but not all, of this increased suppressive effect may result from an association under physiological conditions of sIgM (but not sIgD) with the FcIgG receptor,[50-51] since triggering of the FcIgG receptor may suppress B-cell differentiation. In addition, recent experiments performed by Dr. B. Pernis (personal communication) and by us indicate that the ligand-sIgM complexes produced by continous culture of B-cells with anti-μ antibody may remain associated with the B-cell for a longer period of time than the ligand-sIgD complexes produced by culturing B-cells with anti-δ antibody. This relative persistence may provide a mechanism by which the suppressive effects of a ligand-sIgD interaction can be amplified by a ligand-sIgM interaction. Since sIgM is the predominant sIg of newly generated B-lymphocytes, while more mature B-cells are sIgD predominant,[9,52] the association of a greater suppressive effect with sIgM may have a role in the clonal abortion or suppression of auto-reactive B-cells.[53-56]

Summary

The injection of mice with affinity purified GaMδ leads to polyclonal activation of the murine immune system. Within 24 hr after injection B-cells have increased in size and DNA content and have acquired increased quantities of sIa and receptor(s) for T-helper factors. These changes appear to be T-independent. Within three-four days after GaMδ injection the activated B-cells have induced goat Ig specific T-cells to proliferate and to generate lymphokines that, by six-seven days after GaMδ injection, induce up to 50% of splenic B-cells to proliferate further, to acquire sIgG and to secrete Ig. Antibodies to a non-Ig B-cell determinant lack any *in vivo* B-cell activating effect. Ontogeny experiments suggest that the early, direct, T-independent effects of GaMδ amplify, but are not required for, the late, indirect, T-dependent effects such as antibody production. Injection of mice with greater than optimal quantities of GaMδ appears to have suppressive effects on antibody production, but stimulatory effects on spleen cell proliferation.

By 14 days after GaMδ injection the number of spleen cells, which at day seven had increased to 3-6 times baseline, has returned to baseline, as have the percentages of sIgG$^+$ and Ig secreting cells. The development of suppression, the termination of the generation of T-help, and the lack of ability of anti-δ to react with the sIgG on activated B-cells may have roles in this collapse of the activated immune system, which involves the death of activated B- and T-cells. Comparison of sIgD and sIgM function suggests that the crosslinking of either receptor can activate B-cells, but that ligand-sIgM interactions may have a more suppressive effect on B-cell differentiation than do sIgD-ligand interactions. A possible explanation for this increased suppressive effect may be provided by preliminary experiments that suggest that sIgM-ligand complexes may remain in association with B-cells longer than do sIgD-ligand complexes.

Acknowledgments

We thank Mr. N. Belcher and Drs. P. Fox, J. Kappler, P. Marrack, K. Ozato, J. Paslay, M. Potter, D. Sachs, and E. Vitetta for their gifts of reagents; Drs. R. Ashman, A. DeFranco, T. Flotte, M. Fultz, L. A. Herzenberg, E. Jacobson, D. Parker, W. Paul, B. Pernis, J. Thorbecke, and I. Zitron for their helpful conversations; and Mrs. J. Smith, Mr. P. Acala, and Mr. E. Daco for their expert technical assistance.

REFERENCES

1. MOLLER, G. 1975. Transplant. Rev. **23**: 126.
2. BRETSCHER, P. A. & M. COHN. 1970. Science **169**: 1042.
3. PARKHOUSE, R. M. E. & M. D. COOPER. 1977. Immunol. Rev. **37**: 105.
4. SCHER, I., A. K. BERNING, S. KESSLER & F. D. FINKELMAN. 1980. J. Immunol. **125**: 1686.
5. PERNIS, B. 1977. Immunol. Rev. **37**: 210.
6. FINKELMAN, F. D. & P. E. LIPSKY. 1979. Immunol. Rev. **45**: 117.
7. MARTIN, L. M. & G. A. LESLIE. 1979. Immunology. **37**: 253.
8. FINKELMAN, F. D., V. L. WOODS, S. B. WILBURN, J. J. MOND, K. E. STEIN, A. BERNING & I. SCHER. 1980. J. Exp. Med. **152**: 493.
9. FINKELMAN, F. D., J. J. MOND, V. L. WOODS, S. B. WILBURN, A. BERNING, E. SEHGAL & I. SCHER. 1980. Rev. **52**: 38.
10. CUCHENS, M. A., L. N. MARTIN & G. A. LESLIE. 1978. J. Immunol. **121**: 2257.
11. CUCHENS, M. A., K. L. BOST, M. L. HOOVER & G. A. LESLIE. 1981. Cellular Immunol. **63**: 293.
12. MOND, J. J., E. SEHGAL, J. KUNG & F. D. FINKELMAN. 1981. J. Immunol. **127**: 881.
13. WATSON, J., L. AARDEN & I. LEFKOVITS. 1979. J. Immunol. **122**: 209.
14. RYAN, J. J., J. J. MOND, F. D. FINKELMAN & I. SCHER. 1981. In B Lymphocytes in the Immune Response. N. Klinman, D. Mosier, I. Scher & Vitetta, Eds. **2**: 185. Elsevier/ North Holland.
15. FINKELMAN, F. D., I. SCHER, J. J. MOND, J. T. KUNG & E. S. METCALF. 1982. J. Immunol. **129**: 629.
16. FINKELMAN, F. D., I. SCHER, J. J. MOND, S. KESSLER, J. T. KUNG & E. S. METCALF. 1982. J. Immunol. **129**: 638.
17. OI, V. T., V. M. BRYAN, L. A. HERZENBERG & L. A. HERZENBERG. 1980. J. Exp. Med. **151**: 1260.
18. WORD, C. J. & W. M. KUEHL. 1981. Mol. Immunol. **18**: 311.
19. OI, V. T., P. P. JONES, J. W. GODING, L. A. HERZENBERG & L. A. HERZENBERG. 1978. In Current Topics in Microbiology & Immunology. F. Melchers, M. Potter & N. L. Warner, Eds: **81**: 115–129. Springer-Verlag. New York, N.Y.
20. VITETTA, E. & K. KROLICK. 1980. J. Immunol. **124**: 2988.
21. FINKELMAN, F. D., S. W. KESSLER, J. F. MUSHINSKI & M. POTTER. 1981. J. Immunol. **126**: 680.
22. ZITRON, I. M., D. E. MOSIER & W. E. PAUL. 1977. J. Exp. Med. **146**: 1707.
23. CAMBIER, J. C., F. S. LIGLER, J. W. UHR, J. R. KETTMAN & E. S. VITETTA. 1978. Proc. Natl. Acad. Sci. USA. **75**: 432.
24. PURÉ, E. & E. S. VITETTA. 1980. J. Immunol. **125**: 420.
25. ROSENBERG, Y. J. & J. M. CHILLER. 1979. J. Exp. Med. **150**: 517.
26. ROSENBERG, Y. J. 1981. Cell. Immunol. **61**: 416.
27. LEDBETTER, J. A. & L. A. HERZENBERG. 1979. Immunol. Rev. **47**: 362.
28. L'AGE-STEHR, J., H. TEICHMANN, R. K. GERSHON & H. CANTOR. 1980. Eur. J. Immunol. **10**: 21
29. ANDERSSON, J., M. H. SCHREIER & F. MELCHERS. 1980. Proc. Natl. Acad. Sci. USA. **77**: 1612.
30. PARKER, D. C. 1980. Immunol. Rev. **52**: 115.
31. APTE, R. N., I. LOWY, P. DEBAESTSELIER & E. MOXES. 1981. J. Immunol. **127**: 25.
32. SCHIMPL, A. & E. WECKER. 1972. Nature. **237**: 15.
33. DUTTON, R. W. 1975. Transplant. Rev. **23**: 66.
34. MIZEL, S. B., J. J. OPPENHEIM & D. L. ROSENSTREICH. 1978. J. Immunol. **120**: 1504.
35. HOFFMANN, M. K., S. KOENIG, R. S. MITTLER, A. F. OTTGEN, P. RALPH & U. HAMMERLING. 1978. J. Immunol. **122**: 497.
36. FARRAR, J. J., J. FULLER-FARRAR, P. L. SIMON, M. L. HILFIKER, B. M. STADIER & W. L. FARRAR. 1980. J. Immunol. **125**: 2555.
37. TAKATSU, K., K. TANAKA, A. TOMINAGA, Y. KUHMAHARA & T. HAMAOKA. 1980. J. Immunol. **125**: 2646.

38. HARWELL, L., B. SKIDMORE, P. MARRACK & J. KAPPLER. 1980. J. Exp. Med. **152:** 893.
39. BASHAM, T.Y., S. TOYOSHIMA, F. FINKELMAN & M. J. WAXDAL. 1981. Cell. Immunol. **63:** 118.
40. GILLIS, S. & S. B. MIZEL. 1981. Proc. Natl. Acad. Sci. USA. **78:** 1133.
41. PURE, E., P. C. ISAKSON, K. TAKATSU, T. HAMAOKA, S. L. SWAIN, R. W. DUTTON, G. DENNERT, J. W. UHR & E. S. VITETTA. 1981. J. Immunol. **127:** 1953.
42. MOND, J. J., I. SCHER, J. COSSMAN, S. KESSLER, K. A. MONGINI, C. HANSEN, F. D. FINKELMAN & W. E. PAUL. 1982. J. Exp. Med. **155:** 924.
43. AMBSAUGH, D. F., C. T. HANSEN, B. PRESCOTT, P. W. STASHAK, D. R. BARTHOLD & P. J. BAKER. 1972. J. Exp. Med. **136:** 931.
44. HUNTER, K. W., JR., G. T. FINKELMAN, G. T. STRICKLAND, P. T. SAYLES & I. SCHER. 1979. J. Immunol. **123:** 133.
45. O'BRIEN, A. D., I. SCHER, G. H. CAMPBELL, R. P. MacDERMOTT & S. B. FORMAL, 1979. J. Immunol. **123:** 720.
46. PARKER, D. C., J. J. FOTHERGILL & D. C. WADSWORTH. 1979. J. Immunol. **123:** 931.
47. METCALF, E. S., I. SCHER, J. J. MOND, S. WILBURN, K. CHAPMAN & F. D. FINKELMAN. 1981. *In* B Lymphocytes in the Immune Response: Functional, Developmental & Interactive Properties. N. Klinman, D. E. Mosier, I. Scher & E. S. Vitetta, Eds.: 221. Elsevier/North-Holland.
48. JACOBSON, E. B., Y. BAINE. Y. W. CHEN, T. FLOTTE, M. J. O'NEIL, B. PERNIS, G. W. SISKIND, G. J. THORBECKE & P. TONDA. 1981. J. Exp. Med. **154:** 318.
49. CHENG, H. L., F. R. BLATTNER, L. FITZMAURICE, J. F. MUSHINSKI & P. W. TUCKER. Submitted for publication.
50. FORNI, L. & B. PERNIS. 1975. *In* Membrane Receptors of Lymphocytes. M. Seligman, J. L. Preud'homme & F. M. Kourilsky, Eds.: 193. American Elsevier. New York, N.Y.
51. DICKLER, H. B., M. T. KUBICEK & F. D. FINKELMAN. 1982. J. Immunol. **128:** 1271.
52. VITETTA, E. S., U. MELCHER, M. McWILLIAMS, J. PHILLIPS-QUAGLIATA, M. LAMM & J. W. UHR. 1975. J. Exp. Med. **141:** 206.
53. VITETTA, E. S., J. C. CAMBIER, F. S. LIGLER, J. R. KETTMAN & J. W. UHR. 1977. J. Exp. Med. **146:** 1804.
54. CAMBIER, J. C., E. S. VITETTA, J. R. KETTMAN, G. WETZEL & J. W. UHR. 1977. J. Exp. Med. **146:** 107.
55. SCOTT, D. W., J. E. LAYTON & G. J. V. NOSSAL. 1977. J. Exp. Med. **146:** 1473.
56. VITETTA, E. S. & J. W. UHR. 1977. Immunol. Rev. **37:** 50.

—◆—

DISCUSSION OF THE PAPER

J. W. GODING: I suppose we normally think of Ia these days as being an antigen presenting molecule, but do you think that there's any possibility that you see the increase in TRF receptors and Ia at the same time because they actually are the same thing?

F. D. FINKELMAN: I would certainly think that Ia may very well have a role as a helper factor receptor. On the other hand, we can only see about a two to threefold increase in surface Ia and we see 100- to 1000-fold increase in ability to absorb out "TRF," so unless there's a change in the quality of the Ia as well as in its quantity I don't think one would totally explain the other. I think that there's probably a fairly global modification of B-cell surface receptors and we're just beginning to scratch the surface of this phenomenon.

B. G. PERNIS: I agree with your interpretation. As a matter of fact that's what we thought years ago looking at the effect in the monkey, that it did involve a so called polyclonal T help. The reason we thought of that was that it took two weeks to take effect and we thought that was the time necessary for priming of the T-cells with the foreign gammaglobulin. Not only two weeks but it took also, as in your case, very large amounts of anti-δ, much beyond what was necessary to wipe out the serum δ and also all the membrane δ. We thought we needed that much because we need the anti-δ there to bridge to the T-help two weeks after the injection. Since it decays in these two weeks, you have to give a large shot to start with. This is probably true in your case as well.

Another point is that of the antibody nature of the extra immunoglobulin. In our case we could adsorb out about one-third of the extra immunoglobulin with a total rabbit serum or goat serum, depending on what we used. So this is still much more than just a random representation of the anti-goat or anti-rabbit specificity that might be present in the precursor B-cells. So this indicates that there is not only a polyclonal effect by the anti-δ but also an adjuvant effect.

FINKELMAN: In some studies we injected IgD after injection of a combination of anti-δ and normal goat IgG so as to neutralize the anti-δ but not remove the normal goat IgG. These studies show that if you neutralize the anti-δ one or two days after you inject it you very substantially suppress the polyclonal response. However, if you neutralize it three days or longer after you inject it, you no longer affect the polyclonal antibody response. This three day period is precisely the time it seems to take T-cells to become activated, at least as judged by proliferation and cell size increase, and it may also be the time in which the B-cells stop reexpressing IgD and start switching to other isotypes. We can say from these data that this polyclonal activation does not result from the removal of serum IgD, because an amount of anti-δ which is quite capable of removing serum IgD for the duration of the experiment doesn't induce polyclonal activation.

BLATTNER: Obviously, the rapid effects are going to be as a result of the anti-δ serving as a mimicker of antigen, as you state, and those certainly have to be separated from any effect of serum IgD removal by some reasonably sophisticated experiments. I think Goding's idea to try to make an antibody specific for the serum of cell surface IgD is a very good one that has occurred to us as well.

FINKELMAN: We have tried and Mike Parkhouse was kind enough to send me some of the anti-serum that he made against membrane IgD preps. Unfortunately we find we can absorb it all with the TEPC-1017 protein.

BLATTNER: Unfortunately, there's membrane material in that, too.

THE ENHANCING EFFECTS OF ANTI-IgD ON B-LYMPHOCYTE FUNCTIONS IN RATS*

Marvin A. Cuchens,† Marie L. Hoover,† Kenneth L. Bost,† and Gerrie A. Leslie‡

†Department of Microbiology
University of Mississippi Medical Center
Jackson, Mississippi 39216
and
‡Department of Microbiology and Immunology
Oregon Health Sciences University
Portland, Oregon 97201

INTRODUCTION

The disproportionately high expression of IgD on B-cell surfaces as compared to low serum concentrations of IgD has led to the hypothesis that IgD may function primarily as a B-cell antigen receptor.[1] However, the coexpression of IgD with IgM on the majority of normal, resting B-lymphocytes suggests that the function of membrane IgD (and IgM) may be more intricate than merely to serve as an antigen focusing receptor. Along these lines murine studies suggest that antigen interactions with membrane IgD (mIgD) may be necessary for B-cell triggering, whereas membrane IgM interactions may elicit tolerogenic or suppressive signals.[2-5] However, antibodies directed against IgD or IgM induce ^{3}H-thymidine incorporation in vitro,[6-9] suggesting that both IgD and IgM membrane receptors elicit proliferative events in the B-cell population. It remains to be determined whether these coexpressed receptors have different[10] or complementary[11] functions.

One approach employed to examine the functional role of mIgD has been to determine the effects of anti-δ specific antisera on B-cell responses. Due to the low concentrations of serum IgD, in vivo studies with anti-δ have been feasible. One of the most dramatic responses involving mIgD interactions yet described has been the hypergammaglobulinemia elicited in anti-δ injected monkeys and rats.[12-16] The hypergammaglobulinemia observed in these studies has been attributed to an adjuvant effect of the anti-δ:mIgD interactions on antibody responses to the heterologous serum proteins in the antisera employed rather than a polyclonal differentiation of the B-cell population. More recent studies in our laboratory with rats[17] and by Finkelman et al.[18] with mice have also demonstrated enhanced antibody responses to more defined antigens in anti-δ treated animals. However, different effects on the B-cell populations have been noted, possibly due to the different species, protocols, or reagents employed. Thus, the cellular events involved in the anti-δ augmentation of immune responses are yet to be defined. Furthermore, contradictory results from several in vitro studies demonstrating anti-δ induced suppression rather than enhancement of antigen stimulated cultures have been reported.[19-23]

In the present report we have further examined the effects of mIgD interac-

*This investigation was supported by grants from the National Institutes of Health (7R23 CA28046) and the National Institute of Child Health and Human Development (HD 12381).

0077-8923/82/0399-0329$01.75/0 © 1982, NYAS

tions on B-lymphocytes in rats and have developed *in vitro* correlates in order to better understand the apparent enhancing effects of anti-δ in immune responses in this species.

Anti-δ Induced B-Cell Proliferation

Our laboratories have conducted studies to determine if anti-δ:mIgD interactions alter the normal expression of the B-lymphocyte membrane immunoglobulins and whether changes in the number of B-cells occur in anti-δ injected rats, which may be indicative of proliferative and/or differentiation events. In a previous study, a rapid decrease, followed by a twofold increase in the percentages of $\mu^+\delta^+$ lymphocytes was observed in rabbit anti-rat membrane δ (R anti-δ) treated rats.[12] The transient decrease in circulating B-cells subsequent to the *in vivo* administration of anti-δ was not merely due to mIgD modulation since mIgM was also not detected. Furthermore, direct fluorescent antibody stains with fluorochrome conjugated sheep anti-rabbit Ig were negative, suggesting that the B-cells were not negative for mIg because they were coated with the *in vivo* administered R anti-δ such that *in vitro* binding of the anti-rat μ or anti-rat Ig was sterically blocked.

Transient decreases in the number of peripheral blood B-cells have also been reported in anti-δ injected monkeys.[8,14] However, increased numbers of B-lymphocytes, indicative of B-cell proliferation induced by the anti-δ, were not observed. Since a temporary sequestering of B-lymphocytes followed by a recirculation back in the blood could explain the results obtained in the rat, the effects of anti-δ injections on the number and metabolic activity of the B-cell populations in the peripheral lymphoid organs of rats were examined. Inbred August rats were injected with γ-globulin fractions of either R anti-δ, prepared as previously described,[12] or normal rabbit serum (NRS) adjusted to an equivalent protein concentration. Our rationale for using IgG enriched fractions as opposed to whole serum for these studies was to minimize the immune responses to the numerous heterologous proteins in order to more directly examine the effects of anti-δ on the B-cells. Three rats in each treatment group were sacrificed at the times indicated in Figure 1 and Table 1, and cell suspensions of the excised spleens and lymph nodes (a pool of the popliteal, inguinal and submaxillary lymph nodes) examined with membrane immunofluorescence stains. The reagents and staining procedures employed have been described.[24] Increased percentages of B-lymphocytes in the spleen and lymph nodes were detected as early as 24 hr after the anti-δ injection. As previously reported,[12] circulating $\mu^+\delta^+$ lymphocytes were not detected at this time (data not shown), possibly suggesting that peripheral blood B-cells "home" to the spleen and lymph nodes as a result of anti-δ interactions with the mIgD receptors. However, the subsequent increase in the number of B-lymphocytes in the spleen and lymph nodes concomitant with either normal or increased percentages of circulating B-cells indicates that anti-δ induced B-cell proliferation in the rat. Although dual fluorescent antibody stains were not done, the similar percentages of cells positively stained with the anti-δ, anti-μ and anti-polyvalent immunoglobulin (anti-Ig) reagents indicates that $\mu^+\delta^+$ B-cells were actively dividing. However, at this time we have not ruled out the possibility that a third immunoglobulin isotype is also coexpressed with mIgD and mIgM.

In addition to the fluorescence microscopy studies, the splenic and lymph node cell isolates were cultured without any further *in vitro* stimulation, immedi-

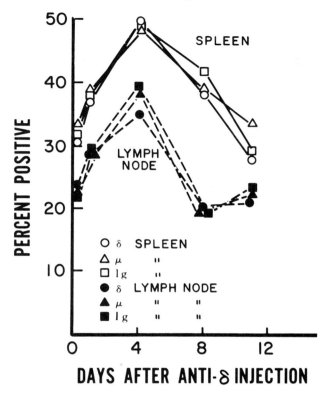

DAYS AFTER ANTI-δ INJECTION

FIGURE 1. The effect of an injection of anti-δ on δ⁺, μ⁺ and Ig⁺ lymphocytes in the spleen and lymph nodes. Membrane immunofluorescent stains and procedures have been described.[24] Results are compiled from duplicate determinations (>200 cells/determination) of three rats per day. Day 0 values represent preinjection percentages.

TABLE 1

³H-THYMIDINE INCORPORATION IN UNSTIMULATED CULTURES OF SPLENIC AND LYMPH NODE CELLS FROM ANTI-δ TREATED RATS

Day of Sacrifice	Spleen CPM*	Spleen Fold Increase†	Lymph Node CPM*	Lymph Node Fold Increase†
1	304 ± 40	0.9	214 ± 71	1.2
4	912 ± 51	2.7	351 ± 120	2.0
8	2,945 ± 461	8.7	1,051 ± 253	5.9
11	2,218 ± 311	6.6	888 ± 158	4.9

*Mean ± standard deviation of the means of triplicate cultures from each of three sacrificed rats. Microtiter (96 well) cultures containing 5 × 10⁵ cells/well in 0.2 ml of RPMI 1640 with 5% fetal calf serum were pulsed with ³H-thymidine (0.5 μCi/culture), incubated for 24 hr at 37°C in 5% CO₂, humidified air and harvested for liquid scintillation counting.

†Fold increase of the mean CPM over the mean CPM of unstimulated control cultures of noninjected rats. CPM of control splenic and lymph node cultures were 338 ± 25 and 180 ± 29, respectively.

ately pulsed with ³H-thymidine upon initiation of the cultures and harvested 24 hr later to assess the radioactivity incorporated into cellular DNA. Cultures of cell isolates from noninjected control rats incorporated low levels of ³H-thymidine (see TABLE 1). Similarly, no significant thymidine incorporation was observed in the cell isolates from NRS γ-globulin injected rats (maximum percent increases in the CPM over the control responses in the splenic and lymph node cultures were 1.8% and 1.5%, respectively). In contrast, significantly increased metabolic activity as judged by DNA synthesis was observed in the splenic and lymph node cultures from anti-δ injected rats. Interestingly increased ³H-thymidine incorporation in cells isolated 24 hr after the injection of anti-δ and cultured for an additional 24 hr was not detected. Thus, the lack of metabolic activity in conjunction with the respective decreased and increased percentages of circulating and peripheral lymphoid B-cells supports the hypothesis that anti-δ:mIgD interactions induce changes in the peripheral blood B-cells. These changes then appear to result in the migration or homing of these cells to the peripheral lymphoid organs. However, the elevated ³H-thymidine incorporation in cultures without *in vitro* stimulation that was observed by day 4 post anti-δ injection suggests that the splenic and lymph node cells were prestimulated *in vivo*. Furthermore, the increase in the metabolic activity may be correlated with the anti-δ induced B-cell proliferative event. It should also be pointed out that similar responses have also been observed with sheep anti-rat membrane δ.

Anti-δ Enhancement of Immune Response

The enhancing effects of anti-δ on primary *in vivo* immune responses in rats have been well documented.[12,17] In our earlier studies, augmented antibody responses to the heterologous serum proteins of the antiserum were detected in R anti-δ injected animals.[12] More recently we have employed a sheep anti-rat membrane δ (S anti-δ) antiserum[17] to examine the effects of anti-δ on antibody responses to more defined antigens. The switch to a sheep reagent was dictated by the requirement for larger quantities of antisera, as well as the variabilities in antibody titer and specificity, which are inherent problems in the polyclonal antibody responses of multiple immunized outbred rabbits. The preparation and specificity of the S anti-δ have been described.[17,25]

A secondary type of antibody response was observed in rats treated with the S anti-δ (γ-globulin preparation) in conjunction with a primary SRBC injection; i.e., responsiveness to lower antigen doses, increased antibody production, earlier antibody production, a rapid shift to 2ME-resistant low-molecular weight antibodies and prolonged antibody production. Similar results were obtained with DNP-Ficoll (a presumed T-independent antigen), with the exception that only IgM anti-DNP hemagglutinins were detected. Antibody responses to either SRBC or DNP were not observed in rats injected with only S anti-δ, suggesting that at least two events, i.e., one involving anti-δ and the other involving an antigenic challenge, are necessary to elicit enhanced B-cell responses. Furthermore, this data argues against polyclonal B-cell differentiation induced by the anti-δ:mIgD interactions as being the sole factor involved.[17]

The secondary nature of the enhanced primary antibody responses in S anti-δ plus antigen treated rats led us to examine whether memory or secondary antibody responses were elevated upon subsequent rechallenge with the antigen. Rats treated with S anti-δ plus SRBC, as previously described,[17] were rested for one month after the hemagglutinin serum antibody titers had dropped to preimmune levels and then rechallenged with only SRBC. No significant differences

TABLE 2

SECONDARY ANTI-SRBC RESPONSES OF RATS PREVIOUSLY
INJECTED WITH ANTI-IgD AND ANTIGEN

| Original Treatment* | Pre | HA Titer (Log $_2$) | | |
		3 day	6 day	9 day
Ag Only	0	6.0	8.3	7.0
Anti-IgD −3 days	0	5.0	7.3	5.7
Anti-IgD plus Ag	0	6.0	7.0	7.3
Anti-IgD +3 days	0	7.3	7.3	5.7

*All rats were rested for a month after preimmune antibody titers were obtained following the original treatment. All rats were then challenged with 1 ml 0.1% SRBC.

between the hemagglutinin titers of the S anti-δ plus antigen treated rats and the rats primed only with antigen were observed when the rats were boosted with the antigen (TABLE 2). Similarly, enhanced secondary responses were not detected in rats immunized with SRBC, rested as above and then treated with S anti-δ upon rechallenge with the antigen (TABLE 3). Thus, at least with the *in vivo* protocols used in these studies, S anti-δ treatments in conjunction with either a primary or secondary antigenic stimulus does not enhance the secondary antibody responses that are observed without anti-δ.

Further studies employing our *in vivo* rat model to examine the cellular mechanisms involved in the anti-δ enhanced responses were limited by difficulties in assessing the role of the T-cell population, presentation of defined concentrations of anti-δ to the B-cells, and possible interactions of anti-δ with serum IgD (albeit in low concentrations). Furthermore, studies in mice have suggested that anti-δ may have a suppressive effect on *in vitro* immune responses.[19-23] Therefore, in order to establish whether a suitable *in vitro* immune response correlate in the rat could be established, our initial studies have employed a combination of *in vivo* anti-δ or antigen treatments with *in vitro* antigen and/or anti-δ stimulation. Such an approach should also address the questions of whether 1) *in vivo* and/or *in vitro* treatments can modulate the generation of antibody producing cells *in vitro* and 2) anti-δ or antigen prestimulation in an *in vivo* environment is a prerequisite for enhanced *in vitro* responses.

Lymph node cell suspensions, isolated from rats subcutaneously injected with

TABLE 3

EFFECT OF ANTI-IgD ON SECONDARY ANTI-SRBC RESPONSES AFTER
ANTIGEN PRIMING

| Treatment* | Pre | HA Titer (Log$_2$) | | |
		4 day	7 day	11 day
SRBC Only	1	7.0	8.7	7.0
Anti-IgD 3 days before SRBC	0	6.0	8.7	8.0
Anti-IgD plus SRBC	0	7.3	7.7	7.7
Anti-IgD 3 days after SRBC	0	7.3	8.0	7.0

*Rats were immunized with 1 ml 0.1% SRBC, rested for one month after the primary antibody titers dropped to preimmune levels, then boosted with 1 ml 0.1% SRBC, with or without anti-IgD.

S anti-δ three days previously, were used to examine the effects of *in vivo* anti-δ pretreatments on the generation of antibody producing cells in antigen stimulated cultures. Low numbers of plaque forming cells (PFC) to SRBC, indicative of a primary *in vitro* response, were detected in antigen stimulated control cultures of lymph node cells from NSS γ-globulin injected rats (TABLE 4). These responses represented significant increases over the low numbers of PFC which were detected prior to culture or after five days *in vitro* without antigenic stimulation of either the NSS or S anti-δ pretreated lymph node cell suspensions. In contrast to the relatively low PFC responses in the NSS pretreated control cultures, *in vivo* anti-δ prestimulation resulted in enhanced PFC responses in SRBC stimulated cultures. Thus it appears that anti-δ prestimulation *in vivo* "staged" the B-cells in such a way to enhance the generation of PFC upon subsequent antigenic stimulation. Furthermore, the addition of S anti-δ to these antigen stimulated cultures markedly altered the generation of antibody producing cells. A high concentration of anti-δ was completely inhibitory whereas lower concentrations induced even greater PFC responses. Therefore anti-δ prestimulation may not be an absolute prerequisite in these enhanced PFC responses since additional *in vitro* stimulation with the appropriate dose of anti-δ further enhanced the *in vitro* PFC responses.

We have also examined the effects of anti-δ on the generation of antibody producing cells in antigen stimulated cultures of lymph node cells which were antigen primed *in vivo*. For these studies rats were sacrificed eight days after a

TABLE 4

EFFECTS OF ANTI-δ ON *IN VITRO* PFC RESPONSES TO SRBC

In Vivo Treatment	In Vitro Treatment	PFC/Culture*					
		Experiment 1			Experiment 2		
		0.01%	0.1%	1.0%‡	0.01%	0.1%	1.0%
NSS γ-globulin†	—	0¶	30	30	40	80	180
S anti-δ	—	1,210	1,220	710	2,050	3,020	3,410
S anti-δ	S anti-δ (150 μg/culture)§	0	0	0	—	—	—
S anti-δ	S anti-δ (15 μg/culture)	580	1,100	3,860	2,600	1,950	6,370
S anti-δ	S anti-δ (1.5 μg/culture)	280	2,880	780	2,730	5,130	3,440
S anti-δ	S anti-δ (0.15 μg/culture)	1,180	5,520	900	—	—	—

*Lymph node cells were cultured in 24 well Linbro plates (1×10^7 cells/well) in Click's modified Mishell-Dutton media[26] without 2-mercaptoethanol and with 5% fetal calf serum. Cultures were incubated at 37°C in humidified, 5% CO_2, and harvested after five days. The number of plaque forming cells (PFC) per culture was assessed by a slide modification of the Jerne hemolytic plaque assay.

†NSS and S anti-δ were twice precipitated with 40% saturated NH_4Cl, dialyzed versus phosphate buffered saline and filter sterilized (0.45 μ Millipore). Three rats per group were subcutaneously injected as previously described with 1.5 ml of equivalent protein concentrations (22.5 mg/rat) of either γ-globulin NSS or S anti-δ.

‡Cultures were stimulated with 0.1 ml per culture of SRBC at the concentrations indicated.

§Protein concentration of the γ-globulin preparation of S anti-δ incorporated in the culture.

¶Background subtracted PFC per culture.

TABLE 5

IN VITRO EFFECTS OF ANTI-δ AFTER IN VITO SRBC
STIMULATION

Culture	PFC/Culture†		
Treatment*	0.01%	0.1%	1.0%
Control	240	240	3,480
Anti-δ (150 μg/culture)	0	0	0
Anti-δ (15 μg/culture)	1,890	2,370	24,590
Anti-δ (1.5 μg/culture)	810	990	5,780

*Cell suspensions were prepared from a pool of the lymph
nodes excised from three rats sacrificed eight days after
subcutaneous immunization with 1.5 ml of 0.1% SRBC.
Antigenic stimulation, anti-δ treatments and culture conditions are described in TABLE 4.

†Background subtracted PFC/culture after five days *in
vitro*.

subcutaneous immunization with SRBC. Lymph node cell suspensions were
prepared and cultured as above. Prior to culture 150–300 PFC/10^7 lymph node
cells were detected. After five days in culture low numbers of PFCs (<50 PFC/
culture) were detected in cells which were either not antigen stimulated or were
treated only with anti-δ. The addition of SRBC to such cultures stimulated an
increased number of PFCs over the PFC response in the control cultures,
although the PFC responses in the 0.01% and 0.1% SRBC stimulated cultures do
not represent an increase over the precultured numbers of antibody producing
cells (see TABLE 5). Again, as observed above, the inclusion of anti-δ into the
antigen stimulated cultures either suppressed (with a high concentration of anti-δ)
or significantly enhanced (with lower concentrations of anti-δ) the differentiation
of PFCs to SRBC. These results suggest that anti-δ:mIgD interactions do not
induce B-cell differentiation events in an antigen primed population of cells
without further antigenic stimulation. Thus, antigenic stimulation of anti-δ pretreated B-cells induces differentiation of a greater number of antibody producing
cells, whereas anti-δ stimulation of antigen prestimulated B-cell populations does
not initiate differentiation events.

DISCUSSION

The data presented indicate that mIgD interactions with anti-rat membrane δ
specific antisera induce changes in the percentages of B-cells in the peripheral
blood and peripheral lymphoid organs. Anti-δ elicited a rapid decrease (within 24
hr) in the circulating B-cell population, concomitant with an increased number
of B-cells, which were not metabolically active in the assay employed, in the
spleen and lymph nodes. One possible explanation for these early events may be
an anti-δ plus complement mediated cytolysis of only the circulating B-cells,
possibly due to differences in the density of mIgD expressed on circulating versus
peripheral lymphoid organ B-cells or nonuniform distribution of the anti-δ in the
blood versus the lymphoid organs. However, if a preferential cytolysis of the
peripheral blood B-cells occurred, the increased number of B-cells in the spleen
and lymph nodes must be due to proliferation of the B-cell population already

present in these lymphoid organs. This would imply that our *in vitro* assay to assess DNA synthesis was insensitive to the early proliferative events. A more likely possibility is that the anti-δ interactions with the circulating B-cells initially induce a "homing" of these cells to the peripheral lymphoid organs. This could be due to an increase in the size of the B-cells, resulting in trapping of the peripheral blood B-cells in the spleen and lymph nodes in conjunction with an immobilization of the B-cells already present. An increase in splenic B-cell size, as well as DNA synthesis, has been observed in anti-δ injected mice (Finkelman and coworkers, personal communication) and may in part support this hypothesis. Further studies using flow cytofluorometry methods are underway to determine if there are differential effects of anti-δ interactions on the circulating versus lymphoid organ B-cell populations in the rat.

Following the apparent localization of the circulating B-cells in the spleen and lymph nodes 24 hr after the anti-δ injection, increased numbers of circulating B-cells, as well as further increases in the percentages of splenic and lymph node B-cell populations, were detected. In addition, increased DNA synthesis was measured in unstimulated cultures of lymphoid cell isolates from the anti-δ treated rats. Collectively these data suggest that anti-δ stimulated B-cell proliferation. It should be pointed out that other metabolically active cells, such as antigen stimulated T-cells, may have contributed to the increased DNA synthesis observed, since previous studies have shown active immune responses to the heterologous proteins in R anti-δ treated rats.[12] However, *in vitro* studies have demonstrated increased ³H-thymidine incorporation in anti-δ stimulated mouse and human lymphocyte cultures,[6-9] as well as in rats wherein stimulation indices of 5–10 are observed with anti-δ stimulated splenic cultures (unpublished observations). Thus it seems likely that the metabolic activity observed in the cells isolated from anti-δ injected rats was in part, if not *in toto*, due to the proliferation of anti-δ stimulated B-cells.

In light of the apparent polyclonal expansion of B-cells stimulated by anti-δ:mIgD interactions, one interpretation of the previously reported enhancing effects of anti-δ on *in vivo* primary immune responses[17] is simply an increase in the number of antigen specific B-cells. However, one would expect an increase in the number of PFC to be proportional to the increased number of B-cells, i.e., a maximum increase of approximately twofold based on the percentages of B-cells in anti-δ injected rats (see FIGURE 1). Surprisingly, much greater than anticipated PFC response were detected in 1) the anti-δ plus antigen injected animals as compared to the responses in the antigen immunized control animals[17] or 2) the antigen stimulated cultures of lymph node cells isolated three days after anti-δ treatments *in vivo* (see TABLE 4). These data indicate that there is either a clonal expansion of antigen specific B-cells or a greater recruitment of the antigen specific B-cells already present. Therefore, B-cell and/or T-cell events, rather than simply a polyclonal B-cell expansion, may be involved in the cellular processes leading to enhanced antibody production initiated by anti-δ.

Based on several lines of evidence polyclonal differentiation of anti-δ stimulated B-cells is unlikely. Firstly, in the *in vitro* experiments presented above PFC responses were not detected in anti-δ treated cultures unless the cultures were costimulated with antigen. Furthermore, enhanced PFC responses were observed in antigen stimulated cultures of anti-δ prestimulated lymph node cells but not in anti-δ stimulated cultures (without antigen) of antigen prestimulated cells. This suggests that anti-δ:mIgD interactions do not signal B-cell differentiation either with or without prestimulation with antigen, but that anti-δ interactions may partially activate the B-cells so that differentiation events are enhanced after an antigenic stimulus. Secondly, polyclonal B-cell differentiation was not observed in anti-δ stimulated mouse splenic cultures without the addition of concanavilin A stimulated T-cell supernatant factors.[16] And thirdly, antibody responses were not detected in rats and mice injected only with anti-δ, whereas enhanced immune responses were elicited in anti-δ plus antigen treated animals.[17,18,27] In our rat studies optimal responses were observed in rats injected with anti-δ three days before immunization, again suggesting that anti-δ prestimulation of the B-cells may facilitate enhanced B-cell differentiation after an antigenic stimulus. Collectively these data support the hypothesis that B-cells are activated via anti-δ:mIgD interactions and that terminal differentiation is initiated only in conjunction with a second stimulus or signal. Along these lines, the studies of Parker[6] suggest that T-cells or T-cell factors may provide the second stimulus. Extrapolating to the enhanced immune responses observed *in vivo* and *in vitro*, antigen stimulated T-cells or their products may also be necessary in order to signal clonal differentiation of the antigen specific B-cells in a polyclonally activated B-cell population. The T:B cell interactions which ensue may be augmented by an increased density of Ia antigens on the activated B-cells, as indicated by the studies of Finkelman *et al.*[18,27] However, it should be pointed out that antibody responses to presumed T-independent antigens can be enhanced with anti-δ stimulation of the B-cells.[17,18] Therefore at this time we cannot rule out the possibility that anti-δ:mIgD interactions activate the B-cells such that with subsequent antigenic stimulation the generation of antibody producing cells is T-independent.

The presented data suggests that different concentrations of anti-δ may have different effects on the *in vitro* PFC responses in antigen stimulated cultures, i.e., suppression or enhancement. Since mIgD interactions may stimulate polyclonal proliferation, as well as polyclonal activation, of the B-cells a basic question is whether these events represent dependent versus independent cellular processes. Preliminary studies in our laboratories indicate that concentrations of anti-δ which optimally stimulate DNA synthesis suppress the PFC responses in SRBC immunized cultures whereas lower concentrations of anti-δ which optimally enhance *in vitro* antibody responses do not stimulate *in vitro* B-cell proliferation. These studies may indicate that B-cell proliferation is not a prerequisite to the activation processes. It should also be pointed out that differential effects of high vs low concentrations of anti-δ on the PFC responses in LPS stimulated cultures have also been reported.[28] It is unclear at this time whether different B-cell subpopulations or the same B-cell population are preferentially stimulated by different concentrations of anti-δ to either proliferate or to be activated. However, an important point from these studies is that much lower ligand to mIgD ratios may be necessary to elicit the B-cell activation events than are required to stimulate B-cell proliferation, which may explain the apparent suppressive effects of anti-δ on *in vitro* immune responses previously reported.[19-23]

As a final point, anti-δ may have different effects on virgin versus memory B-cells. Anti-δ injections had no significant effect on the secondary antibody responses *in vivo*, nor were the secondary responses enhanced in rats which were initially injected with anti-δ plus antigen. Based on these results, one interpretation of the enhancing effects of anti-δ on cultures of lymph node cells isolated from antigen primed rats (see TABLE 5) is that the anti-δ enhanced an ongoing primary immune response rather than a secondary response. Also preliminary studies have indicated that enhanced secondary PFC responses are not induced in anti-δ plus antigen stimulated cultures of cells from rats which were rested for one month prior to sacrifice. These results may imply that virgin versus memory B cells either express different membrane immunoglobulin isotypes or respond differently to anti-δ:mIgD interactions (assuming that both cell types express mIgD). However, further studies are needed to examine the possible effects of antigen and/or anti-δ concentrations, as well as the regulatory influences of T-cells in these responses.

REFERENCES

1. ROWE, D. S., K. HUG, L. FORNI & B. PERNIS. 1973. J. Exp. Med. **138:** 965–972.
2. CAMBIER, J. C., E. S. VITETTA, J. R. KETTMAN, G. WETZEL & J. W. UHR. 1977. J. Exp. Med. **146:** 107–117.
3. VITETTA, E. S., J. C. CAMBIER, F. S. LIGLER, J. R. KETTMAN & J. W. UHR. 1977. J. Exp. Med. **146:** 1804–1808.
4. SCOTT, D. W., J. E. LAYTON & G. J. V. NOSSAL. 1977. J. Exp. Med. **146:** 1473–1483.
5. DOSCH, H., S. KWONG, F. TSUI, B. ZIMMERMAN & E. W. GELFAND. 1979. J. Immunol. **123:** 557–560.
6. PARKER, D. C. 1980. Immunol. Rev. **52:** 115–137.
7. PURÉ, E. & E. S. VITETTA. 1980. J. Immunol. **125:** 1240–1242.
8. LESLIE, G. A. & L. N. MARTIN. 1978. Contemp. Top. Mol. Immunol. **7:** 1–49.
9. SIECKMANN, D. G. 1980. Immunol. Rev. **52:** 181–210.
10. VITETTA, E. S. & J. W. UHR. 1975. Science **189:** 964–969.
11. FINKELMAN, F. D. & P. E. LIPSKY. 1978. J. Immunol. **120:** 1465–1472.
12. CUCHENS, M. A., L. N. MARTIN & G. A. LESLIE. 1978. J. Immunol. **121:** 2257–2262.
13. CUCHENS, M. A. & G. A. LESLIE. 1977. *In* Developmental Immunobiology. J. B. SOLOMON & J. D. HORTON, Eds.: 197–204. Elsevier/North Holland Biomedical Press. Amsterdam, the Netherlands.
14. FINKELMAN, F. D. & P. E. LIPSKY. 1979. Immunol. Rev. **45:** 117–139.
15. MARTIN, L. N. & G. A. LESLIE. 1979. Immunol. **37:** 253–262.
16. PERNIS, B. 1975. *In* Membrane Receptors of Lymphocytes. M. SELIGMANN, J. L. PREUD'HOMME & F. M. KOURILSKY, Eds.: 25–26. North Holland Publishing Co. Amsterdam, the Netherlands.
17. CUCHENS, M. A., K. L. BOST, M. L. HOOVER & G. A. LESLIE. 1981. Cell Immunol. **63:** 293–299.
18. FINKELMAN, F. D., V. L. WOODS, S. B. WILBURN, J. J. MOND, K. E. STEIN, A. BERNING & I. SCHER. 1980. J. Exp. Med. **152:** 493–506.
19. PIERCE, C. W., S. M. HOLLIDAY & R. ASOFSKY. 1972. J. Exp. Med. **135:** 675–697.
20. ANDERSON, J., W. W. BULLOCK, & F. MELCHERS. 1974. Eur. J. Immunol. **4:** 715–722.
21. ZITRON, I. M., D. E. MOSIER & W. E. PAUL. 1977. J. Exp. Med. **146:** 1707–1718.
22. CAMBIER, J. C., F. S. LIGLER, J. W. UHR, J. R. KETTMAN & E. S. VITETTA. 1978. Proc. Natl. Acad. Sci. USA **75:** 432–435.
23. PURÉ E. & E. S. VITETTA. 1980. J. Immunol. **125:** 420–427.
24. LESLIE, G. A. & M. A. CUCHENS, 1982. Ann. N.Y. Acad. Sci. This volume.
25. GOLDING, H., M. A. CUCHENS, G. A. LESLIE & M. B. RITTENBERG. 1979. J. Immunol. **123:** 2751–2755.
26. CLICK, R. E., L. BENCK & B. J. ALTER. 1972. Cell. Immunol. **3:** 264–276.
27. FINKELMAN, F. D., J. J. MOND, V. L. WOODS, S. B. WILBURN, A. BERNING, E. SEHGAL & I. SCHER. 1980. Immunol. Rev. **52:** 55–74.
28. BERNADE, R. & A. C. MARTINEZ. 1980. Basel Institute for Immunology Annual Report. 54.

DISCUSSION OF THE PAPER

F. D. FINKELMAN: I think the whole idea of B-cells as antigen presenters to T-cells, whether this is merely an artifact of a situation in which B-cells are polyclonally stimulated or whether this is a true physiological activity of B-cells is something that really should be explored a great deal more. I think if you just activate T-cells there are pathways by which the activated T-cells can activate B-cells, probably without the B-cells having their surface immunoglobulin triggered at all. I think that the systems of B-cell activation must be tremendously redundant.

LEN HERZENBERG: A very good way to make anti-allotype antibodies, we found years ago, is by using a little bit of anti-H2 antibody of the right allotypes directed against the recipient H-2. It's a very good way to immunize against the allotype of the injected antibody. You can use .1 to 1 μg and it works extremely well. Possibly this involves a similar mechanism as is being discussed here. Therefore, when you inject anti-δ of one allotype into another allotype animal you should be making antibodies against the allotype of the injected antibody. Since anti-δ antibody is not the easiest to make, it might be worthwhile to look in the injected mice for antibody against the other allotype.

FUNCTIONAL ASPECTS OF
IMMUNOGLOBULIN D (IgD)

R. M. E. Parkhouse, Ann Chayen, and S. Marshall-Clarke

National Institute for Medical Research
London, NW7 1AA United Kingdom

INTRODUCTION

Although the original discovery of IgD is almost twenty years old,[1] nonetheless a distinct functional role for this immunoglobulin class remains an enigma. This deficiency in our knowledge is all the more surprising in view of the availability of a mouse model for the last ten years.[2,3] The most striking aspect of IgD is its distribution; present in normal serum in very low quantities and yet found on the surface of most B-lymphocytes as a membrane Ig (mIg), usually in association with another immunoglobulin class sharing the same $V_H V_L$ pair.[4] Early ideas, not surprisingly therefore, focused on the possibility that IgD might be a specialized antigen receptor for B-cells, the other Ig classes serving their defined roles as secreted molecules. A wealth of evidence now suggests that all immunoglobulin classes can be found on B-cells,[5] where they are thought to function as antigen receptors.[6,7] Thus IgD is not the sole immunoglobulin serving receptor function. In fact, in some,[8] but not all[9,10] studies there was a failure to demonstrate IgD on antigen-sensitive memory cells. Thus it is clear that the possession of mIgD is not a mandatory feature of memory cells. Furthermore, immature B-lymphocytes, lacking in all isotypes other than IgM, can be stimulated by LPS to differentiate into cells secreting IgM, IgA or IgG.[11] During this mitogen-independent differentiation sequence there is no transitory expression of IgD and thus synthesis of serum immunoglobulin can apparently occur in the absence of IgD expression at any stage in the process of differentiation of those plasma cells. Similarly, IgD is not an intermediate in the expression of IgM, IgG or IgA at the level of the lymphocyte surface.[5] Perhaps significantly, IgD is rapidly lost from the surface of lymphocytes as a result of antigenic or mitogenic stimulation.[5,12,13] These observations and their implications for B-cell differentiation have been discussed.[5] In essence, the suggestion, based on the evidence was that independent cell lines with commitment for production of the major heavy chain isotypes (IgD, IgA, IgE and IgM) are seeded from IgM-positive B-lymphocytes bearing a selected $V_H V_L$ pair. Their commitment is indicated by the expression of the appropriate mIg in addition to IgM. Next, IgD is added to these various sublines and so the precursors of IgA-, IgG- and IgE- secreting cells simultaneously bear three different Ig classes, all sharing the same $V_H V_L$ pair originally expressed by the mIgM-positive precursor cell. Since each class is functionally distinct, the system is consequently designed so that a selected combining site can be expressed in association with all possible Ig effector mechanisms. Following interaction with antigen, there is a preferential loss of mIgD and later mIgM. In agreement with this, anti-IgD is found to inhibit primary, but not secondary, responses of all Ig classes to a thymus-independent antigen.[14] To generalize, virgin B-lymphocytes are IgD positive, whereas memory B-cells are often not.

In the work to be described, the role of IgD as a receptor in immune responses has been examined in two ways. First, by extending our investigation into the

340

0077-8923/82/0399-0340$01.75/0 © 1982, NYAS

effects of anti-IgD upon immune responses, and second, by determining the IgD status of subpopulations of B-cells separated using monoclonal antibodies.

MATERIALS AND METHODS

Animal and Immunization Protocols

CBA × BALB/c, CBA and CBA/b20 strains of mice raised under specific pathogen free conditions were used at 8–12 weeks of age.

Anti-IgD Reagents

Rabbit anti-IgD was prepared against isolated normal mIgD[15] or a purified myeloma IgD protein, TEPC 1033,[16] and then converted to the F(ab)$_2$ derivative by

TABLE 1

TISSUE DISTRIBUTION OF MONOCLONAL ANTIBODIES NIM-R2 AND NIM-R3*

Antibody	% of Cells Fluorescent in Tissue				
	Spleen	Thymus	Lymph Node	Peyer's Patches	Bone Marrow
Goat anti-MIg	50.1	0	14.7	41.8	6.7
NIM-R1 (anti-Thy-1)	39.5	97.0	80.2	25.8	2.7
NIM-R2	25.4	35.0	6.5	14.3	63.8
NIM-R3	7.9	0	2.4	1.4	33.2

*Adult CBA × BALB/c mice were killed and cell suspensions prepared from the organs indicated were stained. Staining for sIg and Thy-1 was direct using FITC-GaMIg and FITC-NIM-R1, respectively. For NIM-R2 and NIM-R3, staining was indirect using ascitic fluids at a dilution of 1/100 followed by FITC-OX-12. Samples were analyzed in the FACS and the numbers reported are with the control samples set at zero. Controls used were; FITC-GaRGG for GaMIg and NIM-R1 staining and normal rat serum, diluted 1/100, followed by FITC-OX-12 for NIM-R2 and NIM-R3. All fluorochromes were used at 200 μg/ml.

pepsin digestion. Mouse monoclonal allo-antibodies 10-4.22 and 11-6.3[17] directed to IgD of the Ig-5a and Ig-5b alleles respectively were purified by affinity chromatography on protein A from culture supernatants (10-4.22) or by preparative isoelectric focusing from ascitic fluid (11-6.3). Mice used expressing IgD of the Ig-5a and Ig-5b alleles were CBA (Ig-5a) and CBA/b20 (Ig-5b).

Derivation of Monoclonal Anti-B-Cell Antibodies

Two monoclonal antibodies reactive with subpopulations of murine B-lymphocytes were prepared from rat X rat fusions. (Chayen and Parkhouse, submitted to *European Journal of Immunology*.) Their reactivities with cells from a variety of lymphoid organs is given in TABLE 1. The antibody NIM-R2 stains most B-cells providing a sufficient degree of amplification (e.g., hapten-linked indirect fluorescence) is used (FIGURE 1). Under these conditions the FACS fluorescence intensity profile may be arbitrarily divided into four numerically equal fractions, A, B, C and D (see FIGURE 1), and the resultant subpopulations examined for immune reactivity. When this is done,[18] the majority of cells responsible for mounting a primary response to both T-independent and T-dependent antigens are found in the groups with a relatively high degree of fluorescence (76–94% of the recovered direct plaque forming cells [PFC] in fractions C and D). Conversely, 83% of the PFC from secondary responses were found in fractions A and B. Thus cells that stain weakly with NIM-R2 are enriched for memory cells, while those that stain strongly are enriched for virgin

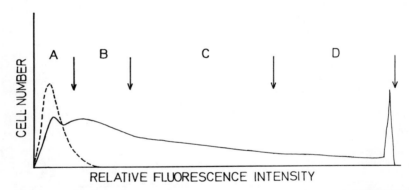

FIGURE 1. FACS profile of the fluorescence given by Ars-NIM-R2 and FITC-GᾱArs on spleen cells showing the fractions separated for the biological experiments. CBA × BALB/c strain spleen cells, depleted of T-cells by treatment with NIM-R1 and complement, were incubated (10[8] cells/ml) with Ars-NIM-R2 (300 μg/ml) followed by FITC-GᾱArs (200 μg/ml). The fluorescence profile (———) shows a gradation of intensity. For sorting, the profile was divided into four numerically equally sized fractions, from weak (A) through to D, strongly stained cells. The arrows indicate the positions of the "gates" used in the sorting. The profile (----) was given by FITC-GᾱArs (200 μg/ml) alone.

cells. The antibody NIM-R3, on the other hand, reacts strongly with B-cells, staining very weakly, if at all, with NIM-R2, and preliminary experiments indicate that this population includes memory cells.

Depletion of T-Cells

Spleen cells were depleted of T-cells by treatment with monoclonal rat anti-mouse Thy-1 antibody, NIM-R1[19] and guinea pig complement. After this treatment, the cell suspensions contained <3% Thy-1 positive and 90–95% mIg-positive cells.

Fluorescent Staining

Lymphocytes (10^8/ml) in phosphate-buffered saline containing bovine serum albumin (1 mg/ml) and sodium azide (2 mg/ml) (PBS-B-A) were incubated in antibody at 0.1–0.3 mg/ml for 30 min on ice. After washing they were examined or, when appropriate, similarly treated with another antibody. Stained cells were processed on the fluorescence-activated cell sorter (FACS II, Becton Dickinson).

Generation of Primary Responses In Vitro

B-lymphocytes (5×10^5) were cultured in RPMI 1640 medium supplemented with 5% (v/v) foetal calf serum, 2 mM glutamine, 50 U/ml penicillin, 50 μg/ml streptomycin, 5×10^{-5} M mercaptoethanol and 5 mM HEPES (0.2 ml). Cultures were stimulated by: dinitrophenylated lipopolysaccharide (DNP-LPS) (20 ng/culture), trinitrophenyl-Ficoll (TNP-Ficoll) (2 ng/culture) or TNP-sheep red cells (TNP SRC) (5×10^5/culture). For the T-independent responses (DNP-LPS and TNP-Ficoll), the cultures were supplemented with syngeneic thymocytes (10^6/culture), and for the T-dependent responses (TNP-SRC) carrier-primed cells were added (10^6 SRC primed spleen cells, irradiated by 1500 R per culture).

Plaque Assay

PFC were assayed[20] on day 4 (T-independent responses) or day 5 (T-dependent responses), using TNP-SRC (T-independent responses) or TNP-horse RBC and SRC (T-dependent responses) as indicators.

Antibodies

Antibodies were purified and derivatized with haptens and fluorochromes as previously described.[19] OX-12, a mouse monoclonal anti-rat K chain, was given to us by Dr. A. Williams (Sir William Dunn School of Pathology, University of Oxford, England), coupled with fluorescein and used for revealing rat monoclonal antibodies (NIM-R1, NIM-R2 and NIM-R3) in a two-step staining procedure.

RESULTS

Effect of Anti-IgD on Primary Responses

Addition of purified monoclonal anti-IgD allo-antibody to cultures of appropriate splenic B-cells markedly reduced T-dependent primary responses, but was without effect upon T-independent type I (DNP-LPS) and type II (TNP-Ficoll) responses. Thus addition of as little as 0–1 μg/ml 11-6.3 antibody to cultures of splenic CBA/b20, B-cells caused 50% inhibition of the PFC response to TNP-SRC. More antibody (10–100 μg/ml) resulted in 75–80% inhibition of the anti-TNP-SRC response in the CBA/b20 mouse, but was without effect upon the same

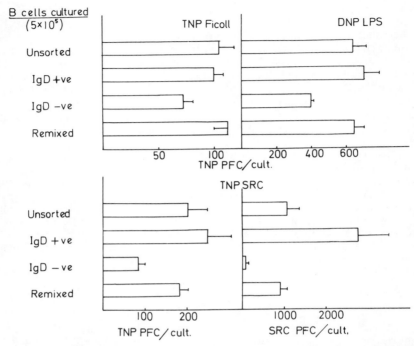

FIGURE 2. *In vitro* responses of FACS separated B-cells stimulated with T-independent and T-dependent antigens. Splenic B-cells from CBA mice sorted into IgD-positive and -negative populations were cultured *in vitro* with the antigens indicated and then PFC were measured. Details in the MATERIALS AND METHODS and RESULTS sections.

response in the CBA mouse. The observed inhibition is thus the consequence of the anti-IgD activity of the alloantibody. There was no inhibition of the PFC response to DNP-LPS or TNP-Ficoll. Using the reverse monoclonal anti-IgD (10-4.22) similar results were obtained, but here, of course, the inhibition was noted in CBA and not CBA/b20 mice.

One explanation for the failure of anti-IgD to inhibit T-independent responses could be that these are the property of cells with a relatively low concentration of mIgD. To test for this, T-depleted splenic B-cells from CBA mice were stained with rabbit F(ab)$_2$ anti-IgD-FITC-Gα-rabbit Ig, and then sorted into the brightest 60% (IgD + ve) and dullest 30% (IgD − ve). By reference to an FITC-Gα-rabbit Ig negative control about 70% of the cells were positive for IgD. Both negative and positive fractions were tested for responsiveness *in vitro* (FIGURE 2), using in addition unsorted and remixed (positives plus negatives) cells as controls. As is apparent in FIGURE 2, T-independent responses were recovered to a similar degree in both IgD-positive and -negative populations, whereas the T-dependent responses were enriched in the IgD-positive subpopulation. All of these responses were then tested for sensitivity to inhibition by monoclonal anti-IgD. As expected, the T-dependent response given by the IgD-positive was inhibited. Interestingly, however, the T-independent responses given by IgD-positive B-cells were not inhibited by anti-IgD.

Expression of mIgD on B-Lymphocyte Subpopulations

Splenic B-cells were separated using monoclonal rat antibody NIM-R2-FITC-OX12 into the four subpopulations A, B, C, D indicated in FIGURE 1, and then counterstained with rhodamine labelled (TRITC) anti-MIg (absorbed on rat Ig-Sepharose), anti-mouse μ chain (absorbed on NIM-R2-Sepharose) and anti-mouse δ chain. Some of the sorted cells were cultured overnight to allow for loss of the surface-bound immune complexes; the cells were then restained with FITC GαMIg (absorbed on rat Ig-Sepharose) or FITC-peanut lectin (PNA) (Vector Labs., California). The frequencies observed, visually for TRITC-reagents and using the cell sorter for the FITC-reagents, are reported in TABLE 2.

All four B-cell subpopulations, A-D, exhibited identical fluorescence intensity FACS profiles when stained with FITC GαMIg. However, those in group A (which includes the memory cells) had a higher percentage of IgD-bearing cells compared to those in group D (primary cells). Conversely, group D had a higher percentage of IgM-bearing cells than group A.

About 60% of lymphocytes in all subpopulations, A-D, reacted with PNA. This lectin has been reported to react preferentially with memory cells.[21] The only difference in profile was that population A (which includes the memory B-cells, contained 6.4% arbitrarily defined very bright cells, whereas population D (containing primary cells) contained only 1.8% of these very bright cells.

As an alternative approach to the same question, splenic B-cells were stained for mIgD (rabbit F(ab)$_2$ anti-IgD-FITC Gα-rabbit Ig) and then the profile was divided into two numerically equal sized fractions, designated IgD-weak and IgD-strong. There were cultured overnight to allow for loss of surface-bound antibodies and then restained with NIM-R2 and NIM-R3 (TABLE 3) in combination with FITC-OX-12. As can be seen, NIM-R2, which preferentially stains primary cells, is found enriched in the IgD-weak subpopulation. Conversely, NIM-R3 which preferentially stains the alternative subpopulation is enriched in the IgD-strong subpopulation.

TABLE 2

ANALYSIS OF SURFACE IMMUNOGLOBULIN ISOTYPE AND PEANUT AGGLUTININ BINDING CHARACTERISTICS OF POPULATIONS OF SPLEEN CELLS DEFINED BY NIM-R2*

Population	% sIg Positive TRITC-GαMIg	% of sIg Positive Cells Stained With		% of Total Cells Stained With FITC-Peanut Lectin
		TRITC-GαMμ	TRITC-RαIgD	
Unsorted	82	90	78	62
A	85	91	97	60
B	91	94	86	66
C	88	94	76	65
D	85	102	66	67

*The fractions of spleen cells defined by NIM-R2 were sorted as described in Materials and Methods with fraction A representing the weakest stained cells and fraction D, the strongest stained. All sIg analyses were measured visually by counter staining with the TRITC-coupled reagents indicated. The percentage of cells positive with FITC-peanut lectin on modulated cells was measured using the FACS. (NIM-R2 stained and sorted cells were modulated to remove surface stain by overnight culture). All the fluorochromes were used at 200 μg/ml.

DISCUSSION

In agreement with earlier work done *in vivo*,[14] anti-IgD was found to inhibit primary T-dependent immune responses *in vitro*. Using the cell sorter, it was possible to show that these responses were enriched in the IgD-positive fraction of splenic B-cells. This finding contrasts with a previous report using the T-dependent splenic focus assay of Klinman,[22] where equal numbers of anti-DNP precursor frequencies were found in IgD-positive and -negative populations. No explanation for this discrepancy, other than the different assay systems employed, is immediately apparent.

Also in agreement with earlier work is the finding that the Type I T-independent response (DNP-LPS) can not be inhibited by anti-IgD.[23,24] This is also the case *in vivo* when anti-IgD is given to mice subsequently infected with LPS. Here, the enormous increase in splenic "reverse" PFC (total IgM-secreting cells) is unaffected by administration of anti-IgD under conditions which greatly inhibit a primary response to SRC (A. Popham, D. W. Dresser, and R. M. E. Parkhouse, unpublished work).

Type II, T-independent responses *in vitro* are also unaffected by anti-IgD, although previously work has suggested that they may be susceptible.[23] In this

TABLE 3

REACTIVITY OF IgD-POSITIVE CELLS WITH NIM-R2 AND NIM-R3*

	IgD-weak	IgD-strong
NIM-R2	63.7	33.1
NIM-R3	18.6	29.0

*Splenic B-cells were stained with affinity purified rabbit F(ab)₂ anti-mouse IgD and FITC goat anti-rabbit Ig. Positive cells divided into two numerically equal sized fractions: "weak" and "strong" and cultured overnight for modulation of reagents. Cells were then stained with rat antibodies and FITC-OX-12.

case the discrepancy might be the presence of unsuspected antibody specificities in the alloantisera used by the previous investigators. A similar lack of influence of anti-IgD upon responses to TNP-ficoll *in vivo* has also been seen (A. Popham, D. W. Dresser, and R. M. E. Parkhouse, unpublished work).

The most interesting aspect of the work was the finding that T-independent responses are not only represented in IgD-positive and negative populations,[25,26] but even the selected IgD-positive B-cells will respond normally to Type I and II T-independent antigens in the presence of anti-sIgD. This must indicate an as yet undefined difference in triggering requirements for these T-independent responses as opposed to the T-dependent variety.

The study correlating the presence or absence of mIgD on B-cells defined by the monoclonal antibodies NIM-R2 and NIM-R3 does not offer an immediately attractive pattern. Whilst NIM-R2 and NIM-R3 appear to preferentially react with virgin and antigen-experienced B-cells, respectively, it was surprising to note that the cells reacting most extensively with anti-IgD were enriched to some extent in the B-cell subpopulation containing memory cells. Similarly, the Ig strong population was relatively enriched for the NIM-R3 marker. In spite of the fact that some memory responses do appear to derive from IgD-negative cells,[14] there certainly are some IgD-positive memory cells[27]; so the main conclusion that can be drawn from this part of the study is that further work is required in order to fit the presence and absence of mIgD into a differentiation scheme for B-cells.

As to the function of IgD, it is still elusive. It probably does not define susceptibility to tolerance, nor does it distinguish T-independent from T-dependent responses. Its presence is clearly not mandatory for expression of the other Ig classes. If it is simply a "filler" immunoglobulin adjusting Ig receptor density up to a certain critical level,[14] then this will be hard to test experimentally. Perhaps it is time that we tried to design experiments to test the hypothesis that IgD acts *off* the cell, rather than *on* the cell. As previously suggested,[28] it is still possible that IgD, lost from B-cells as a consequence of antigen stimulation, serves to elicit a regulatory anti-idiotype response. Since all of the progeny of the original B-cell will bear the same idiotype as the original activated B-cell, then the resulting clone would be susceptible to regulation by the anti-idiotype antibody. In this way IgD would contribute a loop in the idiotype network hypothesis of Jerne. To say this, however, is far from proving it.

ACKNOWLEDGMENTS

We thank Keith Keeler for operating the cell sorter and Graham Preece for considerable technical assistance. We are grateful to Dr. F. D. Finkelman for the gift of the purified IgD myeloma protein TEPC 1033.

[**Note Added in Proof:** Since the submission of this paper we have noted a great variation in the number of cells reactive with NIM-R3, particularly weakly stained cells measured with the FACS. By binding studies we have shown that the antibodies NIM-R3 also reacts with granulocytes, and assume that this reactivity is a cause of variability, since the number of non-B, non-T cells in spleens is widely disparate depending disparate upon the biological history of the mouse. At the same time cells positively selected by NIM-R3 have been shown to transfer antibody responses and so the reactivity of NIM-R3 with cells of the B-lineage is confirmed, although the number of such cells is normally a low percentage of spleens from mice kept under specific pathogen free conditions.]

REFERENCES

1. ROWE, D. S. & J. L. FAHEY. 1965. J. Exp. Med. **121:** 171–184.
2. ABNEY, E. R. & R. M. E. PARKHOUSE. 1974. Nature **252:** 600–602.
3. MELCHER, U., E. S. VITETTA, M. MCWILLIAMS, M. E. LAMM, J. M. PHILLIPS-QUAGLIATA & J. W. UHR. 1974. J. Exp. Med. **140:** 1427–1431.
4. PARKHOUSE, R. M. E. & M. D. COOPER. 1977. Immunological Rev. **37:** 105–126.
5. ABNEY, E. R., M. D. COPPER, J. F. KEARNEY, A. R. LAWTON & R. M. E. PARKHOUSE. 1978. J. Immunol. **120:** 2041–2049.
6. MASON, D. W. 1976. J. Exp. Med. **143:** 1122–1130.
7. OKOMURA, K., M. H. JULIUS, T. TSU, L. A. HERZENBERG & L. A. HERZENBERG. 1976. Eur. J. Immunol. **6:** 467–472.
8. ABNEY, E. R., K. D. KEELER, R. M. E. PARKHOUSE & H. N. A. WILLCOX. 1976. Eur. J. Immunol. **6:** 443–450.
9. COFFMAN, R. L. & M. COHN. 1977. J. Immunol. **118:** 1806–1815.
10. ZAN-BAR, I., S. STROBER & E. S. VITETTA. 1977. J. Exp. Med. **145:** 1188–1205.
11. KEARNEY, J. F., A. R. LAWTON & M. D. COOPER. 1977. *In* Immune System: Genetics and Regulation. ICN-UCLA Symposia on Molecular and Cellular Biology. E. Sercarz, L. A. Herzenberg & C. F. Fox, Eds. **6:** 313–320. Academic Press. New York, N.Y.

12. COOPER, M. D., J. F. KEARNEY, A. R. LAWTON, E. R. ABNEY, R. M. E. PARKHOUSE, J. L. PREUD'-HOMME & M. SELIGMAN. 1976. Ann. Immunol. (Inst. Pasteur) **127c:** 573–581.
13. BOURGOIS, A., K. KITAJIMA, I. R. HUNTER & B. A. ASKONAS. 1977. Eur. J. Immunol. **7:** 151–153.
14. DRESSER, D. W. & R. M. E. PARKHOUSE. 1978. Immunology **35:** 1027–1036.
15. ABNEY, E. R., I. R. HUNTER, R. M. E. PARKHOUSE. 1976. Nature **259:** 404–1406.
16. FINKELMAN, F. D., S. W. KESSLER, J. F. MUSHINSKI & M. POTTER. 1981. J. Immunol. **126:** 680–687.
17. OI, V. T., P. P. JONES, J. W. GODING, L. A. HERZENBERG & L. A. HERZENBERG. 1978. Curr. Top. Microbiol. Immunol. **81:** 115–129.
18. MARSHALL-CLARKE, S., A. CHAYEN & R. M. E. PARKHOUSE. 1981. *In* B Lymphocytes in the Immune Response: Functional, Developmental and Interactive Properties. N. R. Klinman, D. Mosier, I. Scher & E. S. Vitetta, Eds.: 95–101. Elsevier/North Holland.
19. CHAYEN, A. & R. M. E. PARKHOUSE. 1982. J. Imm. Meth. **49:** 17–23.
20. MARSHALL-CLARKE, S. & J. H. L. PLAYFAIR. 1975. Immunology **29:** 477–486.
21. ROSE, M. I. & F. MALCHIOLDI. 1981. Immunol. **42:** 583–591.
22. LAYTON, J. E., J. M. TEALE & G. J. V. NOSSAL. 1979. J. Immunol. **123:** 709–713.
23. ZITRON, I. M., D. E. MOSIER & W. E. PAUL. 1977. J. Exp. Med. **146:** 1707–1718.
24. KETTMAN, J. R., J. C. CAMBIER, J. W. UHR, F. S. LIGLER & E. S. VITETTA. 1979. Immunol. Rev. **43:** 69–95.
25. LAYTON, J. E., B. L. PIKE, F. L. BATTYE & G. J. V. NOSSAL. 1979. J. Immunol. **123:** 702–708.
26. BUCK, L. B., D. YUAN, & E. S. VITETTA. 1979. J. Exp. Med. **149:** 987–992.
27. BLACK, S. J., W. VAN DER LOO, M. R. LOKEN & L. A. HERZENBERG. 1978. J. Exp. Med., **147:** 984–995.
28. BOURGOIS, A., E. R. ABNEY & R. M. E. PARKHOUSE. 1977. Eur. J. Immunol. **7:** 210–213.

DISCUSSION OF THE PAPER

LEN HERZENBERG: Several years ago, Sam Black, Lee and others in the lab showed that IgG is present on early memory cells and is lost from later memory cells. There's a lot of other evidence that has been published from our lab on the association between IgD positive memory cells and low affinity versus IgD negative cells and high affinity IgG responses made by the decendents of those cells. So the notion was simply one of mass action, e.g., a cell which has a lot of receptors on the surface, and these would be μ and δ, will be able to bind antigen when it is present at low concentration even though the affinity of an individual FAB fragment may be relatively low. Because there are a lot of receptor molecules on the surface, in spite of low FAB fragment binding, you still get very good binding because of effectively high avidity of the cell as a whole.

When one gets less antigen, as we all expect happens during immune response, then what contributes to the competition for antigen which allows an IgG response to end up predominating? Well, obviously one component that leads to this is the increase in affinity, not avidity, of these IgG molecules. The cell that has a high affinity but smaller number of receptors, namely just IgG receptors, would finally actually win out. The only role of IgD, which is perhaps disappointing if that really is the final role, since it is nothing very specific but just quantitative, is that evolution has made use of the fact it exists there and keeps it because it serves a perfectly useful role in allowing the progression of immune responses from high avidity and low affinity to one with high avidity and high affinity, even though the cell has fewer receptors on it.

R. M. E. PARKHOUSE: I think that's a very reasonable thing and perhaps it would be nice to be able to correlate the appearance of IgD in evolution together with the appearance of well regulated affinity maturation in a variety of different animals.

E. VITETTA: I think it's fair to say that the ability of a cell lacking IgD, that is an IgM only cell, to respond to any kind of antigen is still very questionable because of the technicalities involved in the systems. I think when you sort for IgD you always have the risk of removing the receptor from the cell so when something comes out of the pot IgD negative it doesn't mean that it really is. Secondly, if you put a cell into a long term assay and it's IgM only to start with, it can certainly develop IgD before it responds. That leaves us with a lot of problems in terms of how to actually look at cells bearing only IgM. We have, in our lab, questioned what kind of system to use and finally gone to one where we actually do a panning in the cold with azide, or without it, and immediately take the cells up to the FACS to see how many IgD cells are left. And then we put the rest of the cells in a limiting dilution system and a rapid antibody forming assay for a few days only. In these experiments every time you deplete IgD positive cells you deplete response precursor cells. So even if you start with a neonatal population where half the cells bear only IgM, if you deplete the cells bearing IgD you completely eliminate the reactive precursor. So I'm not convinced that the cell lacking IgD can respond and I think it's still an open question we have to accept. We have to look at the fact that in these systems it is difficult to really know what's on that cell when one is getting a response. Most of the assays are reading down the road and that's the thing I don't like about them.

PARKHOUSE: But that's not the case in Ethel Jacobson's data, is it? I mean Ethel's mice are under this blockade of anti-δ and I would very much agree with what she said, that while normally one may very well produce immune responses from cells that do have IgD on them, the IgD itself is a sort of superimposed, optional extra which I would say was for some fine tuning role, because if one gets rid of it the cells can still go on and give their basic responses.

G. J. THORBECKE: I agree. The only reservation I think we should keep in the back of our mind is that we can never be completely sure that a hundred percent of all the cells were suppressed to the point where nobody had any δ on them at any time.

VITETTA: I understand that's the interpretation of those experiments. The reason we went to the very short term experiments with panning was precisely to get everything shortened down considerably and know really what number, three percent, is left. Is there a compensatory increase from the cells? One can't do precursor frequencies *in vivo*. It is very difficult and I don't know when I get a response whether it's coming from two percent of remaining cells or from 50 percent of the remaining cells.

THORBECKE: I think there can be a very big difference between those cells that respond *in vivo* or *in vitro* as, for instance, suggested by the result of Shortman *et al.*

VITETTA: Well, would you agree that in a neonate the cells bearing IgM only, let's say in the first three days after birth, are unresponsive B-cells?

PARKHOUSE: There are a large number of things going on in that developing B-cell other than acquisition of IgD. We charted in a particular series of experiments three markers, IgD, Ia and H2, and by the time we get more markers you'll see all sorts of things going on in those first two weeks.

J. J. MOND: Just to address what Vitetta had mentioned, in experiments that Marion Fultz is doing together with Irwin Scher, Fred Finkelman and me, we're suppressing mice from birth with anti-Ia. Presumably we don't affect their Ig receptor, but if you look at such mice four weeks after birth, after they have been chronically suppressed with anti-Ia, they have only IgM positive cells; they have no IgD positive cells and no Ia positive cells. They respond perfectly well to TNP Ficoll and TNP *Brucella abortus*. In addition, after we have looked at their responses, we kill the mice and we analyze their cells again and find that they stay IgD negative, Ia negative, and only surface IgM positive. So at least in that situation we can say we haven't fooled around with the Ig receptor until they've encountered antigen and, nevertheless, in the presence of μ positive only cells they respond very nicely to at least those two antigens.

PARKHOUSE: I think that's an absolutely fascinating observation, but you are still doing something to the cell surface.

MOND: We are doing something to the cell surface, but we also know that if we do a similar treatment with anti-Ia in the adult, we don't appear to modulate the response very much to anything.

PARKHOUSE: I'd certainly view that experiment with the same sort of spectacles as you. However, perhaps the most famous example of anti-cell surface antibody doing unlikely things is the old example of the sea urchin egg which can be turned into division and blastulation with antibodies, even with just a prick from a needle, so there's no question that cell surface related "scratching" can have indirect as well as direct effect.

J. W. GODING: In relation to one of the postulates, which was that cleavage of IgD may be important, one thing which perhaps hasn't been discussed sufficiently is the fact that IgM is a class that doesn't have a hinge while not only IgD but all of the other classes do. I suppose we tend to think of a hinge as being something which imparts flexibility for antigen binding of different spacing of epitopes. However, the hinge may have some other more subtle role, perhaps as a cleavage site in all of the immunoglobulins as part of the activation of cells in a receptor mechanism.

F. FINKELMAN: I wanted to clear up perhaps one possible point of misunderstanding about activation of B-cells by anti-immunoglobulins. We have some data which is entirely consistent with that of the Jacobson-Thorbecke group, which says that if one gives 4.22, the anti-δ allotype hybridoma, to adult B6XBALB/c F1 mice and just keep giving it over a period of weeks, one gets a situation very similar to what one sees when one gives 4.22 to the neonatal mice. One seems to totally ablate the B-cell population which has the IgA allotype lineage. This also makes me feel that when I give anti-δ to neonatal mice, or in any circumstance where I get T-cell tolerance to the anti-δ molecule, I am ablating rather than activating the B-cells involved. While one cannot be absolutely sure that there are not a few B-cells sneaking through to become γ positives I also feel, as does Dr. Thorbecke, that it is unlikely that the excellent immune responses we can see in the mice treated from birth with anti-δ could possibly all be coming from these few sneak through cells.

G. LESLIE: There is a group of patients who are dysgammaglobulinemic with a hyper-IgM. They have virtually only IgM and in very high concentration and are agammaglobulinemic with respect to the rest of the immunoglobulins. My question to Dr. Cooper is, I've never seen anything published on these patients insofar as what the B-cell picture is in these people. Do these people only have IgM on their B-cells and what is their immune response?

M. D. COOPER: Those boys have plenty of IgM plus IgD cells in their circulation. They also have an excess of blasts that have IgM only on their cell surface and some of them have cytoplasmic IgM. Interestingly, they also have elevated levels of serum IgD, but they don't seem to express the isotype switch even at a B-cell level. That is, they lack detectable γ and α B-cells as well as plasma cells.

B-CELL FUNCTION IN MICE TREATED WITH ANTI-IgD FROM BIRTH*

Eleanor S. Metcalf,† James J. Mond,‡ Irwin Scher,‡§
Moira A. LaVeck,† and Fred D. Finkelman‡

Departments of †Microbiology and ‡Medicine
Uniformed Services University of the Health Sciences
Bethesda, Maryland 20814
and
§The Naval Medical Research Institute
Bethesda, Maryland 20814

INTRODUCTION

The mechanism(s) by which B-cells are activated to differentiate into either memory cells or plasma cells remains obscure. Nevertheless, the initial step in B-cell activation is well characterized and involves the binding of antigen to the antigen-specific receptor on the surface of the B-cell. This receptor is cell surface immunoglobulin (sIg).[1] Two surface immunoglobulin isotypes, sIgM and sIgD, are coexpressed on the vast majority of B-cells from adult mice.[2] When these two sIg molecules are expressed on a single cell, they share identical idiotypic determinants[3,4] and antigen binding specificity.[5,6] The presence on a given B-cell of two isotypes with identical antigen binding specificity implies that these two isotypes may have different functions. However, several studies have shown that *both* sIgM and sIgD can independently cause activation of mature B-lymphocytes.[7-10] These observations suggest that either sIgM and sIgD is, by itself, sufficient to activate mature B-cells but is not *required* to activate these cells. Therefore, the significance of two discrete isotypes on the surface of mature B-cells remains unclear.

Several theories have been proposed which attempt to rationalize the apparent redundancy of two different activable sIg molecules on the B-cell surface.[11-17] Taken together, these studies indicate that the physiological role(s) of sIgD are still not well defined. It should be noted that the majority of the conclusions were derived from studies in which adult B-cells were manipulated. However, it is not clear whether a mature B-cell from which the sIgD has been removed is identical to a cell which has never expressed sIgD. If B-cells could be generated which had never expressed surface IgD, then analysis of these B-cells should provide a more physiologically relevant model with which to study the functional capabilities of sIgM$^+$sIa$^+$sIgD$^-$ B-cells.

One approach which obviates this criticism would be to raise mice in the absence of sIgD-bearing B-cells by treatment from birth with anti-IgD antibody. Previous studies by Lawton et al.,[18] Bazin et al.,[17] and Manning and Jutila[19] have demonstrated that this approach is feasible since they showed that chronic treatment of mice or rats from birth with goat anti-mouse (rat) IgM could abort all B-cell function. In the studies presented herein we use a similar model to study the role of sIgD in B-cell function.

*These studies were supported in part by Uniformed Services University of the Health Sciences protocol numbers C07305 and R08308.

351

MATERIALS AND METHODS

Neonatal Treatment of Mice with Anti-IgD

BALB/c or C3H/HeN mice were injected three times with 0.5 mg of either affinity purified rabbit anti-mouse IgD (RaMδ) or rabbit anti-keyhole limpet hemocyanin (RaKLH) during the first week of life: once within 24 hrs after birth, and two additional times thereafter for a total dose of 1.5 mg. This procedure tolerized the mice to rabbit immunoglobulin (Ig). After the first week, mice received 0.2 mg per week for the duration of the experiments.

Antibody Assays

At 8–12 wks, the mice were bled (for serum immunoglobulin level determinations) and were then injected either i.v. with 0.2 ml of a 10% TNP-SRBC suspension or i.p. with 100 μg of TNP-Ficoll. Serum samples were obtained five and seven days later and IgM and IgG anti-TNP antibody titers were determined by RIA or ELISA.[20] One month later those mice which had previously received TNP-SRBC were reimmunized with TNP-SRBC and the secondary anti-TNP antibody titers were assessed. The relative affinity of the anti-TNP antibodies was determined by a modification of the method of Herzenberg et al.[21] This technique utilizes the observation that the relative affinity of anti-TNP antibodies is proportional to the amount of binding of these antibodies to microtiter plate wells coated with a high epitope density TNP-BSA conjugate. In these experiments, $TNP_{6.3}$-BSA and TNP_{67}-BSA were the low and high epitope density conjugates utilized, respectively.

Enumeration of Plaque Forming Cells and Cell Culture

Spleen cells were cultured in modified Mishell-Dutton medium containing 10% endotoxin free fetal calf serum and 5×10^{-5} M 2-mercaptoethanol in flat bottom microtiter trays (Falcon no. 3040 Falcon Plastics, Div. of BioQuest, Oxnard, Ca.) at a density of 10^6 cells in 0.2 ml medium per well. Plates were incubated for three–four days in a humidified 5% CO_2, 95% air atmosphere. Cells were collected and IgM PFC were enumerated by a modification of Jerne and Nordin hemolysis in gel assay.[22]

Treatments with Goat Anti-Mouse IgM or IgD

One to 5×10^5 B-cells from suppressed or control mice were cultured in the presence or absence of 100 μg/ml goat anti-mouse IgM (GaMμ) in 0.2 ml modified Mishell-Dutton medium containing 5×10^{-5} M 2-mercaptoethanol and 1% glutamine[23] in a 5% CO_2 atmosphere. One μCi of ^{3}H-TdR (5 Ci/mmol, Amersham/Searle Corp., Arlington Heights, Ill.) was added at 48 hr. After an additional 16 hr of culture, incorporation of ^{3}H-TdR was measured by harvesting the cells onto glass fiber filters using a semi-automated harvester (Mash II, Microbiological Associates, Walkersville, Md.). These cells were also examined for an increase in the expression of surface Ia.

Control or neonatally treated RaMδ mice were injected with 800 μg of goat anti-mouse IgD (GaMδ) or goat anti-ferritin (GaF), as previously described.[24] Seven days thereafter, the spleens of these mice were removed, single cell suspensions were prepared and the size of the cells was determined by analysis on a Coulter Channelizer, as described elsewhere.[24] In addition, the cell surface phenotype of these mice was examined by fluorescence staining, as described below.

Quantitation of Immunoglobulin on Mouse Spleen Cells

Single cell suspensions were prepared from spleens (or other lymphoid organs) of the mice to be analyzed. The red cells were lysed with a NH_4Cl containing buffer and the remaining white cells were suspended in Hank's balanced salt solution which contained 10% newborn calf serum and 0.2% NaN_3 (HNA). Aliquots of 2×10^6 spleen cells in 100 μl of HNA were stained for 30 min. at 0°C with 100 μg of fluorescein-labeled (FITC-labeled) affinity purified $F(ab')_2$ fragments of RaMδ, RaMμ, RaMγ, RaKLH, or monoclonal FITC-anti-Thy 1.2, or

TABLE 1

EFFECT OF CHRONIC RaMδ TREATMENT ON CELL SURFACE PHENOTYPE

		Percentage of Cells Which Express:		
Organ	Treatment	sIgD	sIgM	sIa
Spleen	RaKLH	37.1 (1.19)*	39.0 (1.21)	38.3 (1.20)
	RaMδ	<1	11.7 (1.47)	11.0 (1.41)
Mesenteric	RaKLH	29.2	26.4	24.4
Lymph Node	RaMδ	<1	2.1	3.3
Peripheral	RaKLH	31.5	26.0	25.4
Lymph Node	RaMδ	<1	4.4	5.1
Bone Marrow	RaKLH	5.2	10.8	20.3
	RaMδ	<1	8.6	18.0

*Geometric mean (standard error)

monoclonal FITC-anti-Ia^k. The stained cells were subsequently washed and analyzed for surface fluorescence with a fluorescence activated cell sorter (FACS II, Becton-Dickenson FACS Systems, Mountain View, Ca.). In some cases the median fluorescence intensity (i.e., that channel above and below which 50% of the specifically stained cells are observed) was determined to provide a measure of the average fluorescence of the specifically stained cell population.

RESULTS AND DISCUSSION

Characterization of B-Cells from Neonatal Anti-IgD Treated Mice

When mice are treated with RaMδ from birth, the total number of B-cells in 8–12 week old mice is significantly reduced and their cell surface phenotype is changed. The results of the fluorescence activated cell sorter (FACS) analysis are shown in TABLE 1. Normal numbers of sIa$^+$sIgM$^+$sIgD$^+$ bearing cells were observed in the control RaKLH-treated mice; however, none of the cells in RaMδ treated animals expressed sIgD and the percentage of sIa⁺sIgM⁺ splenic cells was reduced by 60–80%. In addition, the number of sIa⁺sIgM⁺ cells was decreased by 80–90% in peripheral and mesenteric lymph nodes of these mice, but was relatively normal in their bone marrow. However, B-cells from anti-δ treated mice bore, on the average, about two times more sIgM and one and one half times more sIa than did B-cells from control mice. Finally, none of the lymphoid cells from anti-δ treated mice had detectable rabbit immunoglobulin bound to their surface.

We also carried out experiments to determine whether the absence of sIgD on B-cells from neonatal anti-IgD treated mice was a result of modulation of the sIgD. Both in vivo and in vitro regeneration experiments were completed and the results indicated that the vast majority of B-cells from chronically anti-IgD suppressed mice do not regenerate their surface IgD.[25] In addition, the median fluorescence intensity (a measurement of the density of sIgD after staining with fluorescein-conjugated anti-IgD) of B-cells which do reexpress their sIgD is much lower than that of normal B-cells. Nevertheless, we were concerned that neonatal anti-IgD treated mice did not have B-cells which were totally sIgD⁻. It was possible that these B-cells had very small amounts of sIgD, below the detectability of the FACS, and that the presence of this low quantity of sIgD made activation of these B-cells possible. To address this problem we took advantage of recent studies from this laboratory which demonstrated that the spleen cells from normal adult mice treated seven days earlier with 800 μg goat anti-mouse IgD (GaMδ) increased in number and percentage of cells with sIgG bearing cells, intracytoplasmic IgG₁, whereas control GaF-treated mice showed no effects.[24] We reasoned that if there were small quantities of sIgD on the B-cells from neonatal anti-IgD treated mice, then these B-cells could be stimulated with GaMδ. Therefore, neonatal anti-IgD treated or control mice were injected with 800 μg of GaMδ or 800 μg of GaF i.v. and the size, cell surface phenotype, and number of cytoplasmic Ig positive splenic B cells were determined seven days later. The results indicate that B-cells from neonatal anti-IgD treated mice were not increased in cell size or number, nor did they express greater than control levels of surface or intracytoplasmic IgG₁. Spleen cells from mice treated from birth with anti-IgD also did not show an increase in cytoplasmic IgG₁ after in vitro treatment with GaMδ (data not shown). These findings demonstrate that B-cells from chronically anti-IgD treated mice did not have sufficient levels of sIgD to be stimulated by GaMδ. Taken together with the earlier observations, these findings indicate that the B-cells from the RaMδ suppressed mice are sIgD⁻.

To further examine the characteristics of neonatal anti-δ treated mice, experimental and control mice were bled and their serum immunoglobulin levels

TABLE 2

SERUM IMMUNOGLOBULIN LEVELS OF MICE TREATED WITH RaMδ SINCE BIRTH

Exp. No.	Treatment	Serum Immunoglobulin Levels (mg/ml)			
		IgG₁	IgG₂ₐ&ᵦ	IgM	IgA
1	RaKLH	7.72	3.57	0.60	0.47
	RaMδ	7.47	2.24	1.06	0.59
2	RaKLH	5.86	1.64	0.49	0.40
	RaMδ	4.16	0.61	0.59	0.56

TABLE 3

EFFECT OF CHRONIC RaM TREATMENT ON THE PRIMARY ANTI-TNP
RESPONSES TO TNP-SRBC AND TNP-FICOLL

	Serum Titer*			
	RaKLH-Treated		RaMδ-Treated	
Antigen	IgM†	IgG	IgM	IgG
TNP-SRBC	43 (1.25)	97 (1.14)	186 (1.14)	131 (1.21)
TNP-Ficoll	62 (1.07)	232 (1.21)	88 (1.11)	99 (1.48)

*Geometric Mean (standard error)
†Sera obtained five and seven days after immunization were titered for IgM and IgG anti-TNP antibody levels, respectively.

determined. Surprisingly, the ranges for IgG_1, $IgG_{2a\&b}$, IgM, and IgA were similar in both RaMδ and RaKLH treated mice (TABLE 2). However, the total number of B-cells in RaMδ-treated mice was significantly reduced when compared to control mice. Therefore, these data suggested that the turnover rate of the B-cells from neonatal RaMδ-treated mice might be higher. In order to evaluate this hypothesis, control or experimental mice were either given saline or 5×10^8 SRBC i.p. on day 0, 200 μCi ^{3}HTdR on day 1 and their spleens removed on day 2. These labeled spleen cells were sorted into $sIgM^+$ and $sIgM^-$ pools and counts per minute per 2×10^6 cells were determined. The results showed there was very little difference in the turnover rate between RaKLH-treated control mice or the neonatal RaMδ-treated mice either in the presence or absence of SRBC. These data also support the notion that these B-cells are not activated. Finally, results of the cytoplasmic staining studies are consistent with the data which indicated that, even after treatment of neonatal RaMδ treated mice with GaMδ, no increase in cytoplasmic IgG_1 was detected. Taken together, these studies strongly suggest that the B-cells from neonatal RaMδ-treated mice are a phenotypically stable population of resting $sIgM^+sIa^+sIgD^-$ B-cells.

Immune Function of Neonatal RaMδ-Treated Mice after Antigenic Challenge

To evaluate the functional capabilities of B-cells from RaMδ-treated mice following antigenic challenge, we first examined in vivo antibody responses to thymus dependent (TD) and thymus independent (TI) type 2 antigens. In spite of the depletion of total B-cells, RaMδ-treated mice were able to produce both IgM and IgG primary serum anti-TNP antibody responses after immunization with either the TD antigens TNP-SRBC or the TI-2 antigen TNP-Ficoll. As shown in TABLE 3, these serum antibody responses did not differ significantly from those responses generated by the RaKLH-treated control mice. The capacity of $sIgD^-$ B-cells to generate in vitro primary antibody responses was subsequently examined. TABLE 4 shows that B-cells from neonatal anti-IgD treated mice can also respond to TI-1, TI-2 and TD antigens in vitro.

RaMδ-treated mice were also able to generate both IgG_1 and IgG_2 in vivo memory B-cell responses. The level of IgG_1 anti-SRBC antibody seven days after secondary immunization was greater than 100 times that seen at seven days after primary immunization with SRBC. The titers of these secondary serum antibody responses were similar to titers observed in sera from similarly immunized neonatal anti-KLH treated mice. Additional evidence for the development of B-memory cells was derived from antibody affinity studies of anti-TNP antibodies produced after primary and secondary immunization with TNP-SRBC. Results of these studies indicate that affinity maturation was observed in both IgG_1 and IgG_2 anti-TNP antibodies produced after primary immunization of both anti-δ and anti-KLH treated mice. These antibodies were of relatively low affinity (i.e. they bound to TNP_{67}-BSA but not to $TNP_{6.3}$-BSA). In contrast, IgG_1 anti-TNP antibodies produced after a second injection of TNP-SRBC were of high affinity (i.e., their binding to $TNP_{6.3}$-BSA was equal to or greater than their binding to TNP_{67}-BSA).

Although the serum antibody responses to TNP-KLH and TNP-Ficoll in neonatal anti-IgD treated mice appear to be relatively normal, these data do not indicate whether $sIgD^-$ B-cells can be activated by all antigens or even if the activation requirements for $sIgD^-$ B-cells are more stringent. The experiments described below were designed to approach to these questions. To determine whether $sIgD^-$ B-cells could respond to antigens other than TNP-carrier or SRBC, neonatal anti-IgD treated mice were immunized with phosphocholine (PC) conjugated to KLH in complete Freund's adjuvant. The mice were bled on day 7

TABLE 4

IN VITRO RESPONSE OF SPLEEN CELLS FROM
MICE TREATED WITH RaMδ SINCE BIRTH

Experimental Group	Antigen	Anti-TNP PFC/Culture*	
		RaKLH	RaMδ
1	—	54 (1.17)	40 (1.29)
	TNP-SRBC	280 (1.11)	298 (1.10)
	TNP-BA	520 (1.06)	234 (1.13)
2	—	10 (1.32)	42 (1.03)
	TNP-Ficoll	72 (1.64)	124 (1.15)

*Geometric mean of triplicate cultures (standard error)

and then reimmunized to induce secondary responses. Seven days after the second immunization, the mice were rebled. Both primary and secondary sera were analyzed for anti-PC antibodies and anti-TEPC-15 antibodies. The preliminary data indicate that the response of neonatal RaMδ-treated mice was similar to that of control mice treated from birth with rabbit anti-ferritin for both PC and TEPC-15. These studies suggest that the B-cell pool in neonatal anti-IgD-treated mice may be heterogeneous and moreover that PC-specific B-cells, which may have stringent activation requirements (E.S. Metcalf and J.J. Kenny, manuscript in preparation) are present in the $sIgD^-$ B-cell pool from these mice.

Recently Puré and Vitetta proposed that the roles of sIgM and sIgD could be distinguished in part by the nature of the antigen.[15] They demonstrated that, in their system, the requirement for sIgD was inversely proportional to the epitope density of the antigen. These findings suggested that B-cells from neonatal anti-IgD treated mice ($sIgD^-$ B-cells) should not respond to low epitope density hapten-carrier conjugates. To study this hypothesis, mice treated from birth with anti-IgD or anti-ferritin were immunized either with low epitope density conjugate TNP_4-KLH or with TNP_{51}-KLH which was the immunogenic conjugate used in the initial in vitro serum antibody response studies. The results of the initial studies indicate that RaMδ treated mice respond to TNP$_4$-KLH as well as control mice. These findings do not support the idea that sIgD is required for crosslinking both surface isotypes when the epitope density of the antigen is low.[15]

A second approach to the study of the functional capacity of sIgD⁻ B-cells is to ask whether or not these B-cells can respond to signals other than antigen. For example, previous studies have shown that normal adult, mature B-lymphocytes can be activated by such reagents as lipopolysaccharide (LPS)[26] and anti-immunoglobulin (anti-Ig).[27] In addition, B-cell subsets have been identified as a consequence of their capacity to respond to these reagents. Therefore, we reasoned that we could learn more about the role of sIgD or sIgD⁺ B-cells by determining whether or not sIgD⁻ B-cells can be activated by LPS or anti-Ig.

In the first series of experiments, 2.5×10^5 spleen cells from RaMδ or control treated mice were stimulated with 50 μg of E. coli 011B4 LPS. Proliferation was measured by the incorporation of ^{3}H-TdR as described in the MATERIALS AND METHODS section. The results indicated that sIgD⁻ B-cells could generate significant responses to LPS (data not shown). Although fewer counts per minutes of ^{3}H-TdR were incorporated into RaMδ-treated spleen cells, this reduction may be a consequence of the decreased number of B-cells in the RaMδ-treated mice. Studies in which equivalent numbers of purified B-cells from experimental and control animals are used in the LPS proliferation assay are currently underway.

The capacity of neonatal RaMδ-treated spleen cells to proliferate in response to goat anti-mouse IgD and goat anti-mouse IgM (GaMμ) was also analyzed. As expected, spleen cells from neonatal RaMδ treated mice did not respond to GaMδ. More importantly, however, these studies also demonstrated that spleen cells from neonatal anti-IgD treated mice did not proliferate in response to GaMμ whereas spleen cells from control mice responded to GaMμ, as previously reported.[24] Developmental immaturity could possibly explain the inability of the B-cells from neonatal RaMδ treated mice to respond to GaMμ. It has been previously shown that normal B-cells can not respond by proliferation to anti-IgM until approximately two weeks of age.[27] Therefore, it is conceivable that the B-cells in these RaMδ-suppressed mice have not matured beyond the late stages of normal neonatal development. In contrast, adult CBA/N mice do not possess the B-cell subset which responds to anti-IgM.[27] Thus, it is also possible that the inability of the sIgD⁻ B-cells to respond to GaMμ may be a result of the absence of this particular B-cell subset.

Finally, proliferation is not the only evidence for activation after interaction with these inducing agents. Recent studies have shown that adult, but not neonatal, B-cells significantly increase their sIa after incubation with anti-Ig.[28] Therefore, the capacity to activate sIgD⁻ B-cells was evaluated by determining the increase in their sIa after stimulation with GaMμ. The results demonstrate that B-cells from mice treated from birth with anti-IgD do not increase their sIa after stimulation with GaMμ (data not shown). These findings again suggest that the B-cell population in neonatal anti-IgD treated mice may be fixed at a neonatal level of differentiation since normal neonatal B-cells also do not increase their sIa in response to GaMμ stimulation until about two weeks after birth.[28]

Taken together, these observations suggest that the B-cells from mice which have been treated with RaMδ since birth represent a lineage which is distinct from the normal sIgM⁺sIgD⁺ major B-cell population, and that the expansion of the sIgM⁺sIgD⁻ subset may be a result of suppression of the normal sIgM⁺sIgD⁺ subset of RaMδ. The emergence in mice of a large population of B-cells which lack detectable sIgD and incorporate little or no IgD into their surface membranes provides a powerful tool for the investigation of the role of sIgD in the immune response. The results of the studies described herein clearly indicate that the sIgM⁺ sIgD⁻ B-cells from mice chronically suppressed with RaMδ can generate primary and secondary *in vivo* antibody responses as well as IgM and IgG *in vivo* and *in vitro* antibody responses to TI-1, TI-2, and TD antigens. However, not all B-cell functions are normal since these mice cannot proliferate in response to GaMμ and fail to show an increase in sIa after anti-Ig stimulation. Other functional differences probably exist between normal sIgM⁺ sIgD⁺ B-cells and the sIgM⁺ sIgD⁻ B-cells which are present in mice treated with RaMδ from birth. Preliminary studies indicate that C3H/HeN mice injected from birth with RaMδ die when infected i.p. with a dose of *Salmonella typhimurium* which is nonlethal for their control littermates. These studies suggest that the sIgD bearing B-cell has certain unique immunological capacities which may be required for an optimal immune response to natural pathogens, but the mechanisms of B-cell activation are sufficiently redundant to permit antibody production even in the absence of this cell type.

ACKNOWLEDGMENTS

We greatly appreciate the critical review of the manuscript by Drs. W.E. Biddison and S. Vogel. A special thank you to Ms. Rita Guimond for her preparation of the manuscript.

REFERENCES

1. WARNER, N. L. 1976. Adv. Immunol. **17:** 67.
2. GODING, J. W., D. W. SCOTT & J. E. LAYTON. 1977. Immunol. Rev. **37:** 152.
3. SALSANO, F., S. FROLAND, V. NATVIG & T. MICHAELSON. 1974. Scand. J. Immunol. **3:** 841.
4. FU, S. M., R. J. WINCHESTER & H. G. KUNKEL. 1975. J. Immunol. **114:** 250.
5. PERNIS, B., J. C. BROUET & M. SELIGMANN. 1974. Eur. J. Immunol. **4:** 776.
6. GODING, J. W. and J. E. LAYTON. 1976. J. Exp. Med. **144:** 852.
7. SIECKMANN, D. G. 1980. Immunol. Rev. **52:** 181.
8. PARKER, D. C. 1980. Immunol. Rev. **52:** 115.
9. FINKELMAN, F. D., J. J. MOND, V. L. WOODS, S. B. WILBURN, A. BERNING, E. SEHGAL & I. SCHER. 1980. Immunol. Rev. **52:** 55.
10. VITETTA, E. S. & J. W. UHR. 1977. Immunol. Rev. **37:** 50.
11. SCOTT, D. W. 1977. J. Exp. Med. **146:** 1473.
12. VITETTA, E. S., J. C. CAMBIER, F. S. LIGLER, J. R. KETTMAN & J. W. UHR. 1977. J. Exp. Med. **146:** 1804.
13. LAYTON, J. E., J. M. TEALE & G. J. V. NOSSAL. 1979. J. Immunol. **123:** 709.
14. FINKELMAN, F. D. & P. E. LIPSKY. 1978. J. Immunol. **120:** 1465.
15. PURÉ, E. & E. VITETTA. 1980. J. Immunol. **125:** 1240.
16. BOURGOIS, A., E. R. ABNEY & R. M. E. PARKHOUSE. 1977. Eur. J. Immunol. **7:** 210.
17. BAZIN, H., B. PLATTEAU, A. BECKERS & R. PAUWELS. 1978. J. Immunol. **121:** 2083.
18. LAWTON, A. R., R. ASOFSKY, M. B. HYLTON & M. D. COOPER. J. Exp. Med. **135:** 277.
19. MANNING, D. D. & J. W. JUTILA. 1972. J. Immunol. **108:** 282.
20. FINKELMAN, F. D., V. L. WOODS, S. B. WILBURN, J. J. MOND, K. E. STEIN, A. BERNING & I. SCHER. 1980. J. Exp. Med. **152:** 493.
21. HERZENBERG, L. A., S. J. BLACK, T. TOKUHISA & L. A. HERZENBERG. 1980. J. Exp. Med. **151:** 1071.
22. RITTENBERG, M. B. & K. L. PRATT. 1969. Proc. Soc. Exp. Biol. Med. **132:** 575.

23. MOND, J. D., E. SEHGAL & F. D. FINKELMAN. 1981. *In* B Lymphocytes in the Immune Response. N. R. Klinman, D. E. Mosier, I. Scher & E. S. Vitetta, Eds.:177. Elsevier-North Holland. New York, N.Y.

24. FINKELMAN, F. D., J. J. MOND, I. SCHER, S. W. KESSLER and E. S. METCALF. 1981. *In* B Lymphocytes in the Immune Response. N. R. Klinman, D. E. Mosier, I. Scher & E. S. Vitetta, Eds.:201. Elsevier-North Holland. New York, N.Y.

25. METCALF, E. S., I. SCHER, J. J. MOND, S. WILBURN, K. CHAPMAN & F. D. FINKELMAN. 1981. *In* B Lymphocytes in the Immune Response. N. R. Klinman, D. E. Mosier, I. Scher, and E. S. Vitetta, Eds.:211. Elsevier-North Holland. New York, N.Y.

26. ANDERSSON, J., A. COUTINHO & F. MELCHERS. 1977. J. Exp. Med. **145:** 1520.

27. SIECKMANN, D., I. SCHER, R. ASOFSKY, D. E. MOSIER & W. E. PAUL. 1978. J. Exp. Med. **148:** 1628.

28. MOND, J. J., E. SEHGAL, J. KUNG & F. D. FINKELMAN. 1980. J. Immunol. **127:** 881.

DISCUSSION OF THIS PAPER BEGINS ON PAGE 365.

CHRONIC SUPPRESSION IN MICE WITH ANTI-IgD: ROLE OF B-CELL NUMBERS*

Y. Baine,† Y.-W. Chen,† E. B. Jacobson,‡ B. Pernis,§
G. W. Siskind,¶ and G. J. Thorbecke*

†Department of Pathology
New York University Medical Center
New York, New York, 10016

¶Department of Medicine
Cornell University Medical College
New York, New York 10021

‡Department of Immunology
Merck Institute for Therapeutic Research
Rahway, New Jersey 07065

§Department of Microbiology
College of Physicians and Surgeons
Columbia University
New York, New York 10031

INTRODUCTION

Early studies on mice treated with anti-IgD from birth have suggested the presence of certain deficiencies in their immune response.[1,2] However, no detrimental effects on antibody production in the spleen were detected in two recent studies[3,4] in spite of the absence of detectable IgD⁺ B-cells and markedly reduced number of Ig⁺ cells. Since the spleen contains an IgM⁺ IgD⁻ B-cell population which is lacking in the lymph node,[5] it is possible that anti-IgD treatment more severely depletes the B-cell compartment of the lymph node than of the spleen. Therefore, in the present study a comparison was made of the effect of chronic suppression with anti-IgD from birth on the immune response in the spleen and lymph nodes. In addition, the ability of splenic B-cells from anti-IgD treated mice to transfer an immunologic response was studied.

MATERIALS AND METHODS

Animals and Immunizations

BALB/c mice, purchased from Charles River Laboratories, were bred in our facilities, and their progeny were suppressed with anti-IgD using hybridoma 4.22 anti-Ig-5a as described previously.[3] Control and treated mice were immunized with trinitrophenylated B. abortus (TNP-BA) intravenously (i.v.) or in the front footpads (see tables). Plaque forming cell (PFC) assays were performed four days after the last injection. Anti-IgD-treated and control mice used as donors in cell transfer studies were primed with 800 μg TNP-BA i.v. at four weeks, or at three

*This work was supported by research grants from the National Institutes of Health, U.S.P.H.S.: AI-03076, CA-20075 and AI-14398.

360

and five weeks of age, and were used three weeks after the last injection. Recipients received 250 mg/kg cyclophosphamide intraperitoneally (i.p.) on day 0, followed by TNP-BA primed spleen cells and 800 μg TNP-BA i.v. on day 1. The number of PFC/recipient spleen was determined on day 8.

Plaque-Forming Cell Assay

Anti-TNP PFC were assayed by a slide modification[6] of the Jerne technique[7] using TNP-coupled sheep erythrocytes.[8] Further, as antibody secreting PFC were determined by incorporating goat anti-μ into the agar (to inhibit IgM antibody secreting PFC) and developing with rabbit anti-Ig.

Assay of Surface Ig and IgD

The percentage of Ig^+ and IgD^+ cells in spleens and lymph nodes was determined by fluorescence microscopy using rhodamine labeled rabbit anti-mouse Ig and either fluorescein labeled 4.22 anti-5a or biotinylated 4.22 anti-5a followed by fluorescein labeled avidin, as described previously.[3]

Results

A comparison of the number of B-cells remaining in the axillary lymph node and spleen of IgD-suppressed mice is presented in FIGURE 1. There is an absence of IgD^+ cells in both lymphoid organs. However, while approximately 7% B-cells remain in the spleen, there are only 2-3% Ig^+ cells in the lymph node. As a result, the number of B-cells in the spleen is reduced approximately fourfold, whereas the number of B-cells in the lymph node is reduced approximately eightfold. Despite the effect of anti-IgD on the number of IgD^+ and Ig^+ cells in the spleen of suppressed mice, their secondary response to iv priming and challenge with TNP-BA is not significantly different from that of control littermates (TABLE 1, representative experiment No. 1). In contrast, the memory response obtained in the brachial lymph nodes of the suppressed mice, after subcutaneous priming and challenge in the footpad, was much lower than that of normal mice (TABLE 1, representative experiment No. 2). Since the mice treated with anti-IgD were still able to develop a secondary response to some degree, their diminished lymph node response may reflect the even more severe depletion of B-cells in their lymph nodes than in their spleen. It was, therefore, possible that the deficiency in the lymph node responses could be overcome by i.v. priming followed by challenge in the footpad, since, in such a situation, the cells primed in the spleen might migrate to the lymph node and establish a secondary response there. However, as seen in TABLE 1 (representative experiment No. 3) this immunization regimen also resulted in much lower responses in the lymph nodes of anti-IgD-suppressed than of control mice.

In view of the substantial reduction in the number of B-cells in the spleens of suppressed mice, it was surprising that the anti-IgD treatment did not affect the splenic memory response. An attempt was made to determine whether a decrease in immunologic memory would become apparent following adoptive transfer of graded numbers of spleen cells from primed suppressed mice. TABLE 2 shows the results of experiments in which various numbers of TNP-BA primed spleen cells

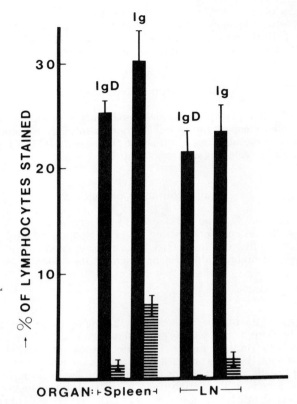

FIGURE 1. Percentage of IgD and Ig-bearing cells in spleens and lymph nodes of anti-IgD treated and normal BALB/c mice: IgD-suppressed mice were injected i.p. with 4.22 anti-Ig-5a three times per week in the following doses: 5 μg/injection from birth to day 10, 10 μg/injection from day 10 to day 20, and 50 μg/injection thereafter. The % of IgD$^+$ and Ig$^+$ cells in spleens and axillary lymph nodes (LN) was determined by immunofluorescence. ■ Normal mice (n = 9); ☰ anti-IgD suppressed mice (n = 12).

from anti-IgD-suppressed or control mice were compared with respect to their ability to transfer a memory response. The B-cells of suppressed mice had a reduced capacity to transfer a 7S memory response when low numbers of donor cells were used. Although it is not possible to precisely compare different pools of donor cells, it appears that the dminished ability of suppressed mice to transfer the 7S response was proportional to their reduction in B-cell number. However, with respect to the 19S memory response the spleen cells from primed anti-IgD treated mice were equivalent to (TABLE 2, Experiment 1) or only about 50% as effective (Experiment 2) as cells from control mice. The ratio of 19S to 7S PFC in spleens of recipients of cells from control primed mice was approximately 0.5 or less, whereas 19S/7S ratio in recipients of cells from suppressed donors was 1.0.

In other studies it was shown that transfer of memory B-cells into immunosuppressed recipients, which had been previously injected with antigen in the

TABLE 1

EFFECT OF ANTI-Ig-5A TREATMENT FROM BIRTH ON THE SECONDARY RESPONSE TO
TNP-BA INDUCED IN BALB/C MICE 10 DAYS AFTER PRIMING

| Expt. No. | Anti-Ig-5a* Treated | Route of† Immunization | Geometric Mean ($\overset{\times}{\div}$ SE) of Anti-TNP PFC/Organ‡ on Day 14 | | |
			19S	7S	Organ
1	−	Intravenous	269,153 (1.4)	891,251 (1.5)	
		Primary and			Spleen
	+	Secondary	213,796 (1.3)	478,630 (1.3)	N.S.
2	−	In Footpads	1,230 (2.3)	3,631 (1.5)	
		Primary and			Lymph Node
	+	Secondary	257 (1.4)	158 (1.5)	p < .01
3	−	Intravenous	14 (1.5)	1,148 (1.9)	
		Primary and			
		In Footpads			Lymph Node
	+	Secondary	41 (1.2)	71 (1.3)	p < .05

*3x/wk injections of 4.22 anti-Ig-5a: 5 μg/inj. first 10 days; 10 μg/inj. next 10 days, and 50 μg/inj. thereafter.

†Dose of TNP-BA in footpads: primary 0.8 μg and secondary 8 μg. Dose of TNP-BA iv: primary and secondary 800 μg.

‡n = 4–12.

TABLE 2

TRANSFER OF ANTI-TNP B-CELL MEMORY BY TNP-BA PRIMED IgD-SUPPRESSED OR
NORMAL BALB/C SPLEEN CELLS

| Expt. No. | No. Spleen Cells* Transferred | TNP-BA‡ Chal-lenge | PFC/Spleen (Geom. Mean $\overset{\times}{\div}$ SE) after Transfer of Cells from | | | |
| | | | Control Donors† | | Anti-IgD-Treated Donors† | |
			19S	7S	19S	7S
1	10^7	+	14,147 $\overset{\times}{\div}$ 1.5	32,475 $\overset{\times}{\div}$ 1.3	27,454 $\overset{\times}{\div}$ 1.4	29,839 $\overset{\times}{\div}$ 1.2
	3×10^6	+	6,120 $\overset{\times}{\div}$ 1.5	30,141 $\overset{\times}{\div}$ 1.3	8,765 $\overset{\times}{\div}$ 1.2	5,627 $\overset{\times}{\div}$ 1.2
	1×10^6	+	920 $\overset{\times}{\div}$ 1.3	1,052 $\overset{\times}{\div}$ 1.6	841 $\overset{\times}{\div}$ 1.5	1,059 $\overset{\times}{\div}$ 1.5
	10^7	−	2,204 $\overset{\times}{\div}$ 1.1	1,133 $\overset{\times}{\div}$ 1.2	1,931 $\overset{\times}{\div}$ 1.2	729 $\overset{\times}{\div}$ 1.0
2	6×10^6	+	—	—	13,083 $\overset{\times}{\div}$ 1.1	13,101 $\overset{\times}{\div}$ 1.1
	4×10^6	+	—	—	7,439 $\overset{\times}{\div}$ 1.1	7,396 $\overset{\times}{\div}$ 1.1
	3×10^6	+	14,766 $\overset{\times}{\div}$ 1.1	25,895 $\overset{\times}{\div}$ 1.1	1,222 $\overset{\times}{\div}$ 1.3	1,054 $\overset{\times}{\div}$ 1.2
	2×10^6	+	8,222 $\overset{\times}{\div}$ 1.1	16,750 $\overset{\times}{\div}$ 1.0	—	—
	1×10^6	+	1,865 $\overset{\times}{\div}$ 1.1	3,775 $\overset{\times}{\div}$ 1.1	—	—
	$1 - 2 \times 10^6$	−	1,006 $\overset{\times}{\div}$ 1.1	976 $\overset{\times}{\div}$ 1.2	747 $\overset{\times}{\div}$ 1.3	903 $\overset{\times}{\div}$ 1.3

*% Ig$^+$ cells in control donor cells 36.7% (Expt. 1) and 45.5% (Expt. 2), in anti-IgD treated 9.0% (Expt. 1) and 8.2% (Expt. 2), n = 5 mice per recipient group.

†Donor mice were primed once at the age of 4 weeks (Expt. 1) or twice at ages 3 and 5 weeks by intravenous injection of 800 μg TNP-BA. Recipients received 250 mg/kg cyclophosphamide the day before transfer.

‡800 μg TNP-BA injected intravenously with the spleen cells. PFC/spleen determined seven days after transfer.

footpad, resulted in the accumulation of memory cells in the lymph node draining the site of antigen injection.[9,10] Additional experiments were performed using this type of pretreated recipient (not shown). The results indicated a markedly reduced ability of the memory cells from anti-IgD suppressed mice to enter lymph nodes. As many as 4.5×10^7 splenic cells from anti-IgD suppressed mice gave low responses in lymph nodes of recipients. The responses were roughly comparable to those of recipients of $\frac{1}{6}$ the number of spleen cells from control donors. These results have been described in more detail elsewhere.[11]

DISCUSSION

The results presented here indicate a clear difference between the spleen and lymph nodes of anti-IgD treated mice both with respect to B-cell content and functional capacity. The incidence of IgM$^+$ IgD$^-$ cells in the spleen of anti-IgD treated mice is double the incidence of such cells in the spleen of control mice. In contrast, the incidences of IgM$^+$ IgD$^-$ cells in lymph nodes of control and anti-IgD treated mice are the same. The compensatory ability of the spleen population allows for a normal response in that organ after iv immunization although in adoptive transfer studies the ability of primed spleen cells from anti-IgD treated mice to transfer a 7S response to TNP is reduced more or less in parallel with the B-cell content. The ability to transfer a 19S response is less reduced than would be expected from the number of B-cells detectable. It should be noted that the difference between splenic responses of anti-IgD treated and control mice was greater in adoptive memory studies than in intact mice. This suggests that there may be regulating effects in the normal control mice which impose a type of "ceiling" on the immune response and obscure the effects of anti-IgD treatment.

The response in lymph nodes of anti-IgD treated mice, on the other hand, is reduced to the extent that would be expected from the number of B-cells present. Even i.v. priming, which leads to the appearance of many primed cells in the spleen, does not overcome the reduced response in the lymph node. Intravenously transferred memory cells from anti-IgD suppressed donors fail to localize in lymph nodes, and recipients of such cells do not manifest memory responses in their lymph nodes after antigen challenge. This peculiar tendency of the IgM$^+$ IgD$^-$ memory cells to remain in the spleen may reflect the fact that they are a relatively immature B-cell subpopulation which localizes, according to MacLennan et al.,[12] in marginal zones rather than in follicular corona areas where IgD$^+$ cells localize. Histological observations have revealed that anti-IgD treatment primarily depletes the mantle zone area of lymphoid follicles.[3,4,13] This area is known to be the site of localization of recirculating B-cells.[14,15] In studies on the rat, chronic thoracic duct drainage leads to a depletion of the IgD$^+$, but not the IgD$^-$, spleen cell population,[12,16] suggesting that the former makes up the recirculating B-cell pool. It may be, therefore, that, upon anti-IgD treatment, the pool of B-cells that typically migrates from spleen to lymph node is principally affected. If indeed the IgD$^-$ B-cell subpopulation does not recirculate through lymph nodes, then the fact that the compensatory effects in anti-IgD treated mice are limited to the spleen would be understandable. It should be noted that the 19S/7S ratio of responding splenic PFC in anti-IgD suppressed mice was approximately twofold that of controls, suggesting a slightly reduced ability to switch to 7s antibody production. This inability was much more marked in other studies in which anti-IgD suppressed mice were immunized by the i.p. injection of a low dose of antigen.[17]

REFERENCES

1. LAYTON, J. E., G. R. JOHNSON, D. W. SCOTT & G. J. V. NOSSAL. 1978. Eur. J. Immunol. **8:** 325–330.
2. BAZIN, H., B. PLATTEAU, A. BECKERS & R. PAUWELS. 1978. J. Immunol. **121:** 2083–2087.
3. JACOBSON, E. B., Y. BAINE, Y.-W. CHEN, T. FLOTTE, M. J. O'NEIL, P. TONDA, B. PERNIS, G. W. SISKIND & G. J. THORBECKE. 1981. J. Exp. Med. **154:** 318–332.
4. METCALF, E. S., I. SCHER, J. J. MOND, S. WILBURN, K. CHAPMAN & F. FINKELMAN. 1981. Developments in Immunology **15:** 201–210.
5. ABNEY, E. R., M. D. COOPER, J. F. KEARNEY, A. R. LAWTON & R. M. E. PARKHOUSE. 1978. J. Immunol. **120:** 2041–2049.
6. MISHELL, R. & R. W. DUTTON. 1967. J. Exp. Med. **26:** 423–442.
7. JERNE N. K., A. A. NORDIN, & C. HENRY. 1963. The agar plaque technique for recognizing the antibody producing cells. *In* Cell Bound Antibody. B. Amos & H. Koprowski, Eds.: 109–117, Wistar Institute Press. Phila, Pa.
8. RITTENBERG, M. B. & K. L. PRATT. 1969. Proc. Soc. Exp. Biol. Med. **132:** 575–581.
9. PONZIO, N. M., J. M. CHAPMAN-ALEXANDER & G. J. THORBECKE. 1977. Cell. Immunol. **34:** 79–92.
10. BAINE, Y., N. M. PONZIO & G. J. THORBECKE. 1981 Eur. J. Immunol. **12:** 990–996.
11. BAINE, Y., Y.-W. CHEN, E. B. JACOBSON, B. PERNIS, G. W. SISKIND & G. J. THORBECKE. 1982. Eur. J. Immunol. In press.
12. MACLENNAN, I. C. M., D. S. KUMARARATNE, D. GRAY & H. BAZIN. 1982. Marginal zones: the major B cell compartment of the rat spleen. *In In Vivo* Immunology: Histophysiology of the Lymphoid System. P. Nieuwenhuis, A. A. van der Broek, & M. G. Hanna, Eds. Plenum Publishing Corp. In press.
13. THORBECKE, G. J., T. FLOTTE & Y. BAINE. 1982. Maturity of Precursor Cells for Germinal Centers. *In In Vivo* Immunology: Histophysiology of the Lymphoid System. P. Nieuwenhuis, A. A. van der Broek, & M. G. Hanna, Eds. Plenum Publishing Corp. In press.
14. HOWARD, J. C., J. V. HUNT & J. L. GOWANS. 1972. J. Exp. Med. **135:** 200–219.
15. KUMARARATNE, D. S. & I. C. M. MACLENNAN. 1981. Eur. J. Immunol. **11:** 865–869.
16. BAZIN, H., & I. C. M. MACLENNAN. This volume.
17. OVARY, Z., Y. BAINE, T. HIRANO, B. XUE, B. PERNIS & G. J. THORBECKE. This volume.

DISCUSSION OF THE TWO PRECEDING PAPERS

R. M. E. PARKHOUSE: The anti-δ suppressed B-cells that are activated by anti-μ don't show the increment in surface Ia expression seen on a normal B-cell. What is the normal baseline of an anti-δ suppressed mouse that you look at? Is it higher or lower or the same as in unsuppressed control mice?

E. S. METCALF: It has normal amounts of Ia on its B-cell surfaces. If anything, it's a little bit increased, but it's within normal limits. So whatever the mechanism is, it's either an absence of a sub-population for a different developmental state of these B-cells.

E. S. VITETTA: Dr. Metcalf, if one goes back to the discussion that there might be a valence difference between M and D, it seems to me that if you lack IgD, which you would postulate might be divalent, you could compensate by having an increased density of IgM on those cells. This would give you the same amount of cross linking as not having the M and having the D in its place. I was wondering if you've looked in these mice for the density of IgM on their cells?

METCALF: The answer is yes; there is an increase in the density of surface IgM and I agree that could compensate for the lack of IgD on the surface.

VITETTA: If the cells are not showing an increase in Ia following anti-μ stimulation, and you want to relate an increase in Ia to being able to receive T-cell signals and interact with T-cells, how do you explain the fact that TD responses are normal?

METCALF: Other people in our group have suggested that the increase in Ia is related to the susceptibility to T-cell help. I think there must also be other ways for the cells to accept T help. Besides, we don't know whether or not this is a specific subset of cells which doesn't require TRF receptors in order to respond to T-dependent antigens.

J. J. MOND: When our group says the expression of Ia increases on the B-cell, we mean to imply that this helps that B-cell not only in its subsequent interactions with T-cells, but also will increase the ability of that cell to present antigen. That's not to say, of course, that that cell in the absence of increased expression won't perform any of those very same functions. Neonatal cells, for example, don't appear to show the increase in Ia and we know that CBA/N-cells show this increased expression of Ia, but not to a very great extent. Still, they have very adequate responses to sheep cells and some of the other TD antigens. So it's certainly not a prerequisite for these events to happen. What we're saying is that it facilitates events to happen, but there certainly are other pathways.

D. W. SCOTT: As many people have reported today and earlier in the meeting, you see a reduction in total number of B-cells in all anti-δ suppressed animals, as Judy Layton originally reported a number of years ago. I wonder whether some of the effects, where you do find effects in such mice, need to be carefully and quantitatively correlated with the number of B-cells that are actually in the animal. I'd like to address a general question as to whether or not any of you have taken spleen or lymph node cells from these animals and done a purification of hapten-specific B-cells and then done limiting dilution analysis with equal numbers of cells from anti-δ suppressed and normal animals to see if there really is that much of a difference.

METCALF: We're in the process of doing some of those experiments and the only thing that we have right now that I can respond to it is that we increase the number of spleen cells that we put in culture to compensate for the number of B-cells, we still don't increase the LPS response up to control level which suggests that we may be looking at a subpopulation of cells.

I. SCHER: I just want to emphasize the unusual nature of the cells that are left in these animals. They really don't fit into the subsets that many of us have defined in adult normal mice. These B-cells which have no δ but have μ on their surface are not stimulated by anti-μ antibodies and yet respond very nicely to TNP Ficoll. I think that a lot of data in the literature suggest that those two functions seem to go together very nicely in normal adult mice. So these B-cells may really represent a subpopulation which is very unusual and may not even be present or only present in very low numbers in normal mice. I think it's very important in that regard to study other functions of these B-cells; for example, tolerance and MLC stimulation.

METCALF: We have been looking at *in vitro* tolerance but the evidence is still preliminary. This evidence suggests that these cells are not susceptible to tolerance induction, which would be consistent with the findings of Skelly, Baine *et al.* that they are Lyb 5 positive.

R. SKELLY: We have also found, using log amplification on the FACS, that the IgM bearing cells of anti-δ suppressed mice were very bright for IgM, while there was an absence of the dull IgM positive cells in the spleen. That would be suggestive of a very bright μ positive, δ negative cell like Dr. Metcalf just mentioned.

H. BAZIN: In the rat, a good percentage of B-cells can't recirculate and these cells are in the marginal zones of the spleen and not in the lymph nodes. It would be interesting to know, when you intravenously inject these cells, whether they can go to the lymph nodes, but we have never tried.

G. J. THORBECKE: Yes, when we injected them intravenously they did not seem to go to the lymph node that well, at least functionally, so they seem to have some difficulty in getting around which may be of very great interest as you say. That cell population may have separate properties and these observations may lead us to a tool to understand what makes cells go into lymph nodes.

H. BAZIN: John MacLennan of Birmingham has clearly demonstrated that the marginal zone cells appeared in the spleen after about three weeks of circulating. So they certainly are more mature cells. If you take immature B-cells from a fetal liver, for example, they need three weeks of circulating before you can detect them in the marginal zones.

P. W. KINCADE: It's been suggested that isotype switching is an event which might add to diversification of variable regions through somatic processes, and I wonder about the diversity of the residual B-cells in these mice. Are they like newborn type B-cells in terms of the clonal types that are there?

Y. BAINE: We briefly looked at the distribution of affinity in the secondary response to TNP in intravenously immunized mice and we found no difference between the control and suppressed mice.

METCALF: We haven't looked at the clonal types. We know that these mice respond to phosphorylcholine, a response which according to some earlier data comes up later in ontogeny, and they do make T15 idiotype responses.

G. J. THORBECKE: I think that all of us agree that, even if we don't know what δ does, anti-δ *in vivo* is a nice tool.

Part VIII. Evaluation of IgD Function

EPITOPE-SPECIFIC REGULATION OF MEMORY B-CELL EXPRESSION*

Leonore A. Herzenberg

Genetics Department
Stanford University School of Medicine
Stanford, California 94305

SUMMARY

IgG antibody responses to individual epitopes on complex antigens can fail despite the presence of fully competent populations of memory B-cells, ample carrier-specific help and the normal production of IgG antibody responses to other epitopes on the same antigen. These response failures reveal the existence of an "epitope-specific" regulatory system that selectively controls the expression of memory B-cells in antibody responses to hapten-carrier conjugates and other complex antigens.

Our earlier B-cell studies describe successive stages in memory B-cell development and consider the potential role(s) that IgD receptors on "early" memory B-cells play in determining *in situ* primary and anamnestic response characteristics.[1-5] Our more recent work, however, shows that an Igh-restricted regulatory system also plays a major role in defining such response characteristics.[6-12] This previously unrecognized system, which controls memory B-cell expression (rather than development), selectively regulates IgG antibody production to each of the individual epitopes on T-dependent antigens such as DNP-KLH and DNP-CGG (the DNP hapten on keyhole limpet hemocyanin and chicken gamma globulin, respectively)

We have shown that this system can be induced to specifically suppress IgG2a anti-DNP responses to DNP-KLH without interfering with primary or secondary antibody responses to the KLH epitopes on the same molecule. Furthermore, it can be induced to specifically suppress IgH-1b allotype responses to all DNP-KLH epitopes without interfering either with other allotype and isotype responses to DNP-KLH or with Igh-1b responses to other antigens in the same animal. Thus, under conditions where memory development is optimal, this highly versatile regulatory mechanism is key to determining the amount, specificity, affinity and Igh isotype/allotype representation of IgG antibody responses.

Since we have recently published a full description of this Igh-restricted "epitope-specific" system, we have chosen to briefly outline its properties here using a somewhat extended version of the "summary slides" prepared for the meeting. Many of the findings summarized in this outline are illustrated by evidence and presented at the meeting (and included here); however, this evidence was presented to underscore the importance of epitope-specific regulation for studies of *in situ* and adoptive memory responses and consequently does not fully document the findings discussed. (For such documentation, we refer the reader to our published work.[6-12]

*This work supported in part by grants from the National Institutes of Health (CA-04681, HD-01287).

368

1. B-cell events leading to IgG antibody production:

$$\text{Virgin B} \xrightarrow{\text{(Ag)}} \text{Early Memory} \xrightarrow{\text{(Ag)}} \text{Mature Memory} \xrightarrow{\text{(Ag)}} \text{IgG AFC}$$

Virgin B $\xrightarrow{\text{(Ag)}}$ Early Memory $\xrightarrow{\text{(Ag)}}$ Mature Memory $\xrightarrow{\text{(Ag)}}$ IgG AFC
IgD$^+$ ———————— IgD$^+$ ———————— IgD$^-$

Development   Expression

- Mechanisms that regulate memory B-cell development control the potential for IgG antibody production.

- Mechanisms that regulate memory B-cell expression control which and how many of the memory B-cells present in a given animal actually give rise to AFC.

2. Optimal development of memory B-cells requires:

- Antigen reactive precursors (virgin B-cells)

- Carrier-primed T-cells or presentation of antigens in a form that stimulates the development of carrier-primed T-cells, e.g., on alum or in complete Freunds adjuvant (CFA)

- Support for the IgD$^+$ to IgD$^-$ memory shift

3. Optimal expression of memory B-cells (maximal IgG antibody production) for a given epitope requires:

- Helper T-cells specific for the carrier on which the epitope is presented (or presentation of the antigen in a form that stimulates CTh development, e.g., on alum or in CFA)

- Active prevention of the induction of epitope-specific suppression for the response

4. Epitope-specific suppression is induced by carrier-specific suppressor T-cells that mature shortly after priming and induce suppression for antibody production to individual epitopes on the carrier protein (unless antibody production to the epitopes is already in progress).

5. Rapid initiation of primary IgG responses (before CTs mature) tends to prevent the induction of suppression for antibody responses to individual epitopes. Thus:

- Priming with a hapten-carrier conjugate enables primary and subsequent (anamnestic) IgG antibody responses to some but usually not all epitopes on the priming antigen.

- Suppression-induction protocols that induce strong suppression in animals that have not initiated an anti-epitope response are far less effective in animals already producing anti-epitope antibodies.

● Regulatory conditions that prevent initiation of selected IgG responses to epitopes on priming antigens (e.g., transient allotype suppression) result in the induction of a persistent suppression specific for those anti-epitope responses.

● The introduction of an epitope on a carrier to which the animal has previously been primed (carrier/hapten-carrier immunization) induces the epitope-specific system to selectively suppress IgG antibody responses to the "new" epitope (hapten).

6. *Induction of epitope-specific suppression by carrier/hapten-carrier immunization:*

● PROTOCOL. Immunize sequentially with a carrier protein and the "homologous" hapten-carrier conjugate, e.g., KLH/DNP-KLH; next, immunize with the hapten on an unrelated carrier molecule, e.g., DNP-CGG. (100 μg each antigen on alum).

● RESULT. Persistent and specific suppression of IgG anti-DNP antibody responses

7. *Response characteristics in KLH/DNP-KLH immunized animals:*

● Memory B-cells for all epitopes (including DNP) develop normally and are fully functional in adoptive assays.

● IgG antibody responses to the "new" epitope (DNP) on the priming carrier are specifically suppressed.

● Suppression persists after restimulation with DNP on an unrelated carrier (DNP-CGG) or on the priming carrier (DNP-KLH).

● Antibody responses to both carrier proteins proceed normally.

8. *Epitope-specific regulation is Igh-restricted. Thus selective suppression can be induced for:*

● The expression of memory B-cells committed to producing a given IgG isotype response to DNP, e.g., IgG2b or IgG3, (when carrier/hapten-carrier suppression-induction is suboptimal)

● The expression of memory B-cells committed to producing Igh-1b allotype responses to any of the epitopes on DNP-KLH (when young allotype heterozygotes are primed with DNP-KLH while allotype suppression is active)

9. *The epitope-specific system is a general regulatory mechanism (variable examined and result):*

● Epitope
   DNP, TNP   Suppression induced for both epitopes by carrier/hapten-carrier; suppression inducible for KLH epitopes by other protocols

- Carrier
  KLH, CGG, OVA, TGAL

  All prime for suppression induction; some genetic restrictions (see below); 100 μg on alum sufficient

- Adjuvant
  KLH aqueous (2X)
  KLH aqueous
  KLH on alum
  KLH CFA
  KLH on alum plus B. pertussis

  + + + + + suppression induction
  + + + + suppression induction
  + + + suppression induction
  + + + suppression induction
  No suppression induction

- Age
  KLH at 8 weeks to >6 months

  Suppression equally strong at all ages

- Timing
  1 to 13 weeks between KLH and DNP-KLH

  Suppression equally strong

- Persistance
  KLH/DNP-KLH then DNP-KLH or DNP-CGG up to 1 yr later

  Suppression equally strong

- Carrier function genes (not in MHC)
  KLH with A/J or C57BL/10

  Suppression induction by KLH/DNP-KLH impaired; (CGG/DNP-CGG OK)

- IR genes (MHC)
  TGAL/TNP-TGAL in C3H (H-2k) and C3H.SW (H-2b)

  No interference with suppression induction; stronger suppression in "nonresponder" than in responder

- Mouse Strains
  BALB/c, BAB/14, SJL, SJA, C3H, C3H.SW, A/J, (SJL × BALB/c), C57BL/10, C57BL/6

  Suppression inducible in all strains

- Chronic allotype suppression
  DNP-KLH prior to mid-life remission from Igh-1b allotype suppression

  Igh-1b responses to DNP and KLH suppressed during remission; Igh-1b responses to new antigens OK; all other IgG responses OK

- Carrier-specific suppression
  KLH Ts or KLH-TsF plus DNP-KLH to nonirradiated recipients

  Specific suppression induced for IgG anti-DNP

KLH-TsF (from thymus); DNP-KLH to irradiated recipients	Specific suppression induced for IgG anti-DNP
KLH-primed T-cells cells transferred; DNP-KLH at time of transfer	Suppression-induction favored for IgG anti-DNP in nonirradiated recipients; help for IgG anti-DNP favored in irradiated recipients

10. *In situ antibody response failures can reflect interference either with the development or the expression of memory B-cells*

		IgG2a anti-DNP Antibody in Serum	
Immunization(s)*		In situ primary	Adoptive secondary† (donor B-cells + CTh)
KLH	DNP-KLH		
		μg/ml (affinity)	μg/ml (affinity)
—	aqueous	3 (<1)	18 (<1)
alum	aqueous	5 (<1)	50 (8)
—	alum	35 (5)	73 (10)
alum	alum	< 1 (<1)	75 (8)

   * 100 μg indicated antigen at 9 and 3 (or 3) weeks prior to transfer.
   †T-depleted spleen (B-cells), supplemented with KLH primed (nylon-passed) T-cell; 1 μg aqueous DNP-KLH to recipients; *in situ* anti-DNP measured 2 weeks after DNP-KLH immunization; adoptive anti-DNP 2 weeks after transfer; RIA assay (1); affinity = Ka $\times$ M^{-1} $\times$ 10^6 by RIA

11. *T-cells in suppressed donors impair memory B-cell expression in adoptive assays*

B-cell donor immunization(s)		Cells transferred to recipients	IgG2a anti-DNP μg/ml recipient serum
KLH	DNP-KLH	spleen (T + B)	32
KLH	DNP-KLH	T-depleted spleen + CTh*	104
—	DNP-KLH	spleen (T + B)	120
—	DNP-KLH	T-depleted spleen + CTh*	90

   *KLH-primed T-cell supplement
   100 μg each antigen i.p. on alum to donors; 1 μg aqueous DNP to (irradiated) recipients; IgG2a anti-DNP (μg/ml) in recipient serum 7 days after transfer (RIA).

REFERENCES

1. HERZENBERG, L. A., L. A. HERZENBERG, S. J. BLACK, M. LOKEN, K. OKUMURA, W. VAN DER LOO, B. OSBORNE, D. HEWGILL, J. GODING, G. GUTMAN & N. WARNER. 1976. Cold Spring Harbor Symp. Quant. Biol. **41:** 33–45.
2. BLACK, S. J. & L. A. HERZENBERG. 1979. J. Exp. Med. **150:** 174–183.

3. BLACK, S. J., T. TOKUHISA, L. A. HERZENBERG & L. A. HERZENBERG. 1980. Eur. J. Immunol. **10:** 846–851.
4. HERZENBERG, L. A., S. J. BLACK, T. TOKUHISA & L. A. HERZENBERG. 1980. J. Exp. Med. **151:** 1071–1087.
5. TOKUHISA, T., F. T. GADUS, L. A. HERZENBERG & L. A. HERZENBERG. J. Exp. Med. **154:** 921–934.
6. HERZENBERG, L. A., T. TOKUHISA. 1982. J. Exp. Med. **155:** 1730–1740.
7. HERZENBERG, L. A., T. TOKUHISA, D. R. PARKS & L. A. HERZENBERG. 1982. J. Exp. Med. **155:** 1741–1753.
8. HERZENBERG, L. A., T. TOKUHISA & L. A. HERZENBERG. 1982. Eur. J. Immunol. In press.
9. HERZENBERG, L. A., T. TOKUHISA & K. HAYAKAWA. 1981. Nature **295:** 329–331.
10. HERZENBERG L. A., T. TOKUHISA & L. A. HERZENBERG. 1980. Nature **285:** 664–666.
11. HERZENBERG, L. A. 1981. Immunol. Today. In press.
12. HERZENBERG, L. A., T. TOKUHISA & L. A. HERZENBERG. 1981. Immunol. Today **2:** 40–46.

DISCUSSION OF THE PAPER

H. BAZIN: It's very amusing to see that your conclusion is very similar to the one people working with IgE in rodents have come to a long time ago. I think it was published about ten years ago that a very small dose of antigen can induce an IgE response in mice and I have published myself that the best immunization for IgE in rats or mice is to incorporate B. pertussis vaccine in the immunizing injection.

M. COOPER: It seems to me that it's pretty clear that if you stimulate an IgD bearing cell, whether with antigen or mitogens or anti-immunoglobulin, it ceases to express or it doesn't express as much IgD anymore. On that basis, since memory cells arise from stimulation of their immunoglobulin receptors, they wouldn't have IgD on them unless they have a capacity to stop making it and then expressing it later. Now that seems to me a fairly important question: Can a cell stop making IgD and then begin at another time later on?

F. R. BLATTNER: If you can sort of imagine the math that I put up on the first day where we have μ and δ close to one another and then γ way on down, and a transcript that begins at the D region and potentially can go all the way down to the most extremely distantly coded end of that transcript. There's a series of four or five transcription termination points, AATAAG sequences. The first level at which you can control the ratio of IgM to IgD is where the message is stopped. Thus, you could go from an IgM IgD positive cell to an IgM only cell just by elevating the number of enzyme molecules in the cell that clip near the AATAAG and cause a message to stop. The logical thing would be that the more you secrete of IgM, the more you express on the surface of the cell the IgM and the less IgD. I think that fits very beautifully with the type of data that we've got. But when a cell starts to secrete IgM, it stops secreting or expressing IgD on the surface. I'm not sure that has anything to do with memory. I think that has to do with just the virgin B-cell.

The next step is how you get into a γ on the surface. My prejudice is that the idea of making a messenger of 100 kilobases or more, which you would have to do to get down to γ 3, is unlikely. Honjo has published the only other way to go about it which is to delete the DNA between δ and γ. The rational way to express three classes at once, if that's really possible, would be by deleting from a point to the right of δ to a point to the left of γ 3, or some other gamma. I think the thing you'd have to look at to be sure that was happening is to rule out the possibility of a transitory stage in which some messages hang around for an immunoglobulin that was expressed early. In such a transitory cell the DNA really isn't supporting all three of the Ig classes at once. That was the big problem we thought we had to answer in the case of the double-producing cells of μ and δ, that one needed a cell line that could be kept in culture long enough for any transitory message to be eliminated. I think what you are going to see happening is a deletion of the DNA from the switch side between μ and δ up to one of the γ. At that point, you really have a memory cell and it's going to be IgD negative.

LEE HERZENBERG: When we transfer δ-negative cells and then reseparate them after they had spent some time in a host, the δ-negative cells did not generate δ-positive memory. It doesn't totally answer the question because, of course, it could have come and gone. In any event, it seems to us as though once the cell is δ-negative, it remains δ-negative. When it's δ-positive, it's very likely to go to δ-negative on the next antigenic stimulation, but it can hang up in the δ-positive state under a suboptimal condition.

G. J. THORBECKE: We should distinguish between not being able to make something and preferring not to put it on the surface, or not to make it at all. It is very peculiar that germinal center cells, where, after all, some of this is going on, don't express anything. Not only no δ, but as Dr. Bazin pointed out, in germinal centers all surface immunoglobulin is extremely low, so it might not just be a matter of δ. It might be a matter of just not expressing very much immunoglobulin at all, temporarily, and perhaps going back to whatever they were doing before. Or maybe in the process they have switched and now they produce something else. Anyway, we should perhaps not say going to a δ⁻ stage and coming back to δ⁺ is so impossible from that standpoint.

LEE HERZENBERG: I agree with your first statement absolutely. However, Eugene Butcher (and we) find that the germinal center cells early on have μ. They're bright, μ-bearing peanut agglutinin (PNA) positive cells.

THORBECKE: What I am referring to is described by Rose et al. and others. In sections, germinal centers aren't very strongly positive. But the problem is that there are some other PNA⁺ cells also. So you can't just say that because you find some very strongly μ-positive PNA⁺ cells that they were germinal center cells.

BLATTNER: The most likely sequence of events is that the first step deletes from the site between μ and δ down to γ. That makes the memory cell. And then the next step deletes from the classical Honjo-switch site, which is between J and μ, down to some point again in front of γ and that goes into an antibody secreting cell. I don't know whether you want this, but it's the simplest model at the molecular level. Now we have to see whether it fits the biological data.

ROLE OF IgD IN IMMUNOLOGICAL MEMORY

D. Lafrenz,* J. M. Teale,† and S. Strober*

*Division of Immunology
Department of Medicine
Stanford University School of Medicine
Stanford, California 94305

†Department of Cellular and Developmental Immunology
Scripps Clinic and Research Foundation
La Jolla, California 92037

INTRODUCTION

Studies involved in defining the relationship between surface immunoglobulin isotype and immune function of memory B-lymphocytes have established that memory B-cells which give rise to the secondary IgG response can express surface IgG and/or IgM.[1-8] Of concern in this communication and other studies was the immune function of memory B-cells which express surface IgD. Experiments using the fluorescence-activated cell sorter (FACS) have shown that both δ^+ and δ^- subpopulations of memory B-cells carry immunologic memory after adoptive transfer to irradiated hosts.[7,8] Other experiments indicate that a portion of memory B-cells can be protected from the lethal effects of highly radiolabeled antigen *in vitro* by preincubating the cells with anti-IgD antiserum.[6] With regard to secreted isotype after antigenic stimulation, memory cells which express surface IgM and IgD first generate an IgM response followed by an IgG response.[7,8] On the other hand, memory cells which express only surface IgD produce only an IgG response upon antigenic stimulation.

In other studies of the role of IgD-bearing memory cells, Black et al.[9] and Herzenberg et al.[10] reported that early after priming δ^+ and δ^- memory cells are present in approximately equal proportions in the spleen, but the δ^- memory cell subpopulation reconstituted the majority of the adoptive secondary response late after priming.[10] In additon to the transition from δ^+ to δ^- memory cells, it has been reported that the δ^+ memory cell subpopulation restores an appreciably lower avidity response (10–100-fold) than does the δ^- memory cell subpopulation. However, results of adoptive transfer experiments from our laboratory demonstrated the persistence of δ^+ memory cells for long periods after priming, and little or no difference in the affinity of antibody responses by the δ^+ and δ^- memory cell subpopulations.[11]

In this report, we have examined several parameters which might affect the affinity and magnitude of antibody responses restored by δ^+ and δ^- memory B-cells. We have also examined the precursor frequency and isotypes secreted by δ^+ and δ^- memory cells using the splenic focus assay system.

MATERIALS AND METHODS

Animals

(BALB/c × C57BL/Ka) F$_1$ mice bred in our own colony were derived from the colony of Dr. R. Kallman, Department of Radiology, Stanford University School

375

0077-8923/82/0399-0375 $01.75/0 © 1982, NYAS

of Medicine. All mice were maintained on acid water (pH 2.5, adjusted with HCl). One week prior to and two weeks after irradiation, adoptive recipients were maintained on antibiotic water containing 500mg neomycin sulfate (Upjohn, Los Angeles, Ca.) and 100mg polymyxin B sulfate (Sigma, St. Louis, Mo.) per liter.

Reagents

Dinitrophenylated bovine serum albumin (DNP-BSA) and dinitrophenylated keyhole limpet hemocyanin (DNP-KLH) were prepared according to the method of Little and Eisen.[12] (^{3}H)-DNP-lysine was obtained commercially (New England Nuclear Corporation, Boston, Mass.) and checked for purity by measuring the amount of known hapten bound by an excess of high-affinity antibody.

Immunization Procedures

Mice were primed with DNP-BSA (500µg protein) by i.p. injection (0.2ml) of an emulsion of equal volumes of DNP-BSA in saline and complete Freund's adjuvant (CFA; Difco Laboratories, Detroit, Mich.). In some experiments, mice were immunized by i.p. injection (0.25ml) of alum-precipitated DNP-BSA (500µg protein) with 2×10^9 killed *Bordetella pertussis* (B.p.) organisms (Department of Public Health, Boston, Mass.). Carrier primed mice were immunized by an i.p. injection (0.2ml) of BSA (500µg), as described above. DNP-KLH primed mice received an i.p. injection of (0.2ml) DNP-KLH (500µg protein) in CFA, or 0.25ml i.p. injection of alum-precipitated DNP-KLH (100µg) plus B.p. as above. KLH (Pacific Biomarine, Venice, Ca.) primed mice received an i.p. injection of KLH (500µg) in CFA as above.

Preparation of Carrier Primed T-Cells

T-lymphocytes from spleens and lymph nodes of carrier primed mice were purified by passage over a nylon wool column, as described by Julius et al.[13] or by panning, as described by Mage et al.[14] using an affinity purified rabbit anti-mouse immunoglobulin antiserum.

Irradiation

Mice were placed in Lucite containers and given 550 rads whole body X-irradiation from a 250kV, 15mA source filtered through 0.35mm Cu.

Antibody and Relative Affinity Determinations

Antibody to DNP-lysine was determined by the Farr assay, as previously described.[11] The hapten input in this assay was at a concentration of 2×10^{-7} M. The relative affinity of the anti-DNP antibodies was measured using a modification of the Farr technique, as previously described.[11] Briefly, a constant amount of antibody was mixed with 15 different concentrations of ^{3}H-DNP lysine covering a 2-$\log_{10}$ range. After overnight incubation (4°C), the equilibrium reaction was stopped by antibody precipitation using ammonium sulfate. Determination of bound and free hapten was made based upon ^{3}H-DNP-lysine present in supernatants of reaction mixtures. The average association constant was calculated from a plot of bound hapten/free hapten versus bound hapten. Relative affinity values must differ by more than twofold to be significantly different.

Antisera

Four different anti-IgD antisera were used in these experiments; 1) an antiserum to the purified fraction of spleen cell surface IgD, 2) a hybridoma antibody against the 5a allotype of IgD, 3) a hybridoma antibody against the 5b allotype, and 4) an affinity purified anti-IgD myeloma antiserum.[11] The hybridoma reagents were conjugated with NIP (4-hydroxy-3-iode-5-nitrophenylacetyl) for use in a two-stage staining procedure.

Immunofluorescent Staining and Cell Sorting

All staining utilized a two-stage procedure. All antibodies were titered over a 100-fold range of concentrations and a plateau of percentage of positively stained cells was determined for each reagent. The dilution of reagent used for staining was chosen such that the concentation was always on the plateau of the titration curve. Cell suspensions were made in minimal essential medium (MEM) containing 10% fetal calf serum (Grand Island Biological Company, Grand Island, N.Y.) (MEM-FCS). Cells were suspended in MEM-FCS and antiserum at a final concentration of 25 × 10^6 cells/ml for 30 minutes at 4°C and then spun through FCS. Cells were resuspended in fluorescein-conjugated goat anti-rabbit IgG antiserum (Meloy Laboratories, Springfield, Va.) and treated as above. The hybridoma reagents utilized fluorescein conjugated, affinity purified rabbit anti-NIP antiserum as a second-stage reagent.

Stained cells were sorted using a FACS III (Becton-Dickinson, Mountain View, Ca.). Scatter gates were set so that only small, live cells were sorted. Gates for fluorescence were set so that cells more than 10 channels to the left of the inflection point were sorted into the dull cell fraction, and cells more than 10 channels to the right of the inflection point were sorted into the bright cell fraction.

Splenic Focus Assay and Isotype Analysis

Spleen cells separated using the FACS as well as unfractionated controls (0.1 × 10^6 cells) were injected i.v. into lethally irradiated, carrier primed mice. Fragment cultures[15,16] were incubated with antigen, and culture supernatants were collected on days 9, 12, and 16. For analysis of anti-DNP antibody, a solid-phase radioimmunoassay using labeled rabbit anti-mouse class and anti-light chain specific antibodies were performed, as previously described.[17]

Experimental Design

Spleens from hapten primed donors were stained and sorted, as described above. The cell fractions were injected i.v. into syngeneic irradiated hosts at doses that corresponded to that number contained within 2×10^6 unfractionated cells or at a dose of 2×10^6 fractionated cells. Adoptive hosts also received 5×10^6 carrier primed cells. The experimental groups consisted of adoptive hosts which received bright, dull, or unfractionated cells. Control groups received T-cells alone or no cells. All experimental groups were challenged with antigen in saline i.p. within 24 hours after reconstitution at doses indicated in tables or the text.

RESULTS

Magnitude and Affinity of the Adoptive Secondary Responses to DNP-BSA with Respect to Time After Priming, Staining Reagents, and Adjuvant Used for Priming

Spleen cells from DNP-BSA (CFA) primed donors were separated into δ^+ (bright) and δ^- (dull) cell fractions at various times after priming up to 29 weeks. Cell fractions were adoptively transferred to irradiated syngeneic hosts along with carrier primed T-cells. Adoptive recipients were challenged with DNP-BSA in saline, and antibody responses were determined using the Farr assay. Representative results of antibody titers are shown in FIGURE 1, panels A and C. It can be seen that the δ^+ and δ^- cell fractions each restored approximately 50% of the response restored by unfractionated cells. This pattern of responsiveness was seen consistently regardless of the reagent used for staining or whether animals were primed with alum-precipitated DNP-BSA plus 2×10^9 B.p. organisms as adjuvant or CFA.

The affinity of the antibodies as determined by the modified Farr technique, is shown in TABLE 1. In animals primed with DNP-BSA (CFA) and with cells stained with the rabbit anti-purified spleen cell surface IgD, the affinity of the response restored by the δ^+ fraction was slightly higher than the affinity of the response restored by the δ^- fraction. However, this situation was reversed when the responses from animals primed 29 weeks earlier were examined. In both cases it must be noted that the differences in affinity, although different, are small (<tenfold) even when statistically significant.

In order to examine various anti-δ antisera, the above experiments were repeated using a hybridoma anti-δ allotype and a heterologous anti-δ myeloma reagent. As can be seen in TABLE 1, the δ^+ cell fraction restored slightly higher affinity responses with both anti-δ reagents, but again these differences were less than tenfold.

It may have been possible that the adjuvant used for priming alters the characteristics of the response on the proportion of the response restored by the δ^+ and δ^- cell fractions. To examine this point, animals were primed with DNP-BSA using alum-pertussis instead of CFA. The magnitude of the response was not altered using this priming procedure nor was the affinity of the responses restored by the δ^+ and δ^- cell fractions (TABLE 1). Even waiting up to a year after priming, no large difference in the affinity of the responses was observed.

Magnitude and Affinity of the Adoptive Secondary Response to DNP-KLH with Respect to Carrier Primed Cells, and Level of Antigen Challenge

Cells from animals primed to DNP-BSA showed no difference in affinity of the responses restored by δ^+ and δ^- cell fractions. The previous reports[9,16] wherein a difference in affinity was demonstrated, utilized the antigen DNP-KLH. We, therefore, examined the characteristics of the response to DNP-KLH using our experimental protocol. Animals were primed with DNP-KLH (100μg) using alum-pertussis. Cells from primed spleens were sorted and transferred with KLH primed T-cells as for the DNP-BSA experiments described above. As can be seen

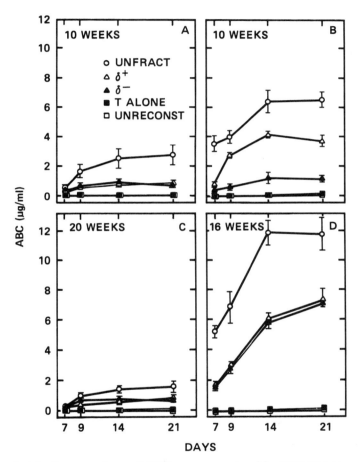

FIGURE 1. Adoptive secondary anti-DNP response restored by DNP-BSA (**A** and **C**) or DNP-KLH (**B** and **D**) primed cells sorted for surface IgD. Mice were injected with BSA primed (**A** and **C**) or KLH primed (**B** and **D**) T-cells and with a dose of bright or dull cells contained within 2×10^6 unfractionated primed spleen cells. Each point represents the mean response of 3–4 animals expressed as antigen binding capacity (ABC) ± the standard error as determined using the Farr assay.

from FIGURE 1, panels B and D, DNP-KLH elicits a greater response than does DNP-BSA. Early after priming, the response restored by the δ^+ cell fraction was greater than that restored by the δ^- cell fraction. This pattern of responsiveness was also seen in DNP-BSA animals at nine weeks after priming. At a later time

TABLE 1

RELATIVE AVERAGE AFFINITY OF ADOPTIVE SECONDARY
RESPONSE OF DNP-BSA PRIMED CELLS*

Time after priming of donor (wk)	Adjuvant used for priming	Antisera used for staining	Cell source used for reconstitution	Relative average affinity† (L/M)
9	CFA	purified spleen cell surface IgD	delta pos. delta neg. unfract.	4.76×10^8 1.55×10^8 2.5×10^8
29	CFA	purified spleen cell surface IgD	delta pos. delta neg. unfract.	1.63×10^8 2.72×10^8 8.2×10^7
20	CFA	hybridoma anti-IgD allotype	delta pos. delta neg. unfract.	6.75×10^8 3.22×10^8 2.0×10^8
20	CFA	anti-IgD myeloma	delta pos. delta neg. unfract.	1.51×10^9 4.8×10^8 7.4×10^8
20	B.p.	purified spleen cell surface IgD	delta pos. delta neg. unfract.	2.6×10^8 3.7×10^8 2.72×10^8
52	B.p.	purified spleen cell surface IgD	delta pos. delta neg. unfract.	1.13×10^9 6.2×10^8 4.17×10^8

*Donor spleen cells were stained with anti-δ antiserum and sorted. The number of cells contained with 2×10^6 unfractionated cells were injected into adoptive recipients given carrier primed T-cells and challenged with DNP-BSA (200 μg) in saline.

†Relative average affinity (κ_{50}) of anti-DNP antibodies in the serum 14 days after challenge.

TABLE 2

RELATIVE AVERAGE AFFINITY OF ADOPTIVE SECONDARY
RESPONSE OF DNP-KLH PRIMED CELLS

Time after priming of donor (wk)	Antigen used for priming	Source of carrier primed T-cells	Antigen challenge	Cell source used for reconstituion	Relative average affinity (L/m)*
15	500 μg DNP-KLH (CFA)	BSA primed	200 μg DNP-BSA	delta pos. delta neg. unfract.	1.89×10^9 2.71×10^9 3.13×10^9
10	100 μg DNP-KLH (B.p.)	KLH primed	50 μg DNP-KLH	delta pos. delta neg. unfract.	1.53×10^9 1.37×10^9 1.02×10^9
16	100 μg DNP-KLH (B.p.)	KLH primed	10 μg DNP-KLH	delta pos. delta neg. unfract.	5.57×10^9 4.9×10^9 3.95×10^9

*Relative average affinity (κ_{50}) of anti-DNP antibodies in the serum 14 days after challenge.

point (16 weeks) the responses restored by the δ^+ and δ^- cell fractions were approximately equal.

The affinity of the responses restored by these cell fractions is presented in TABLE 2. In animals primed with DNP-KHL, sorted and transferred, and challenged with two different doses of DNP-KLH (50μg and 10μg) no appreciable differences in affinity could be observed.

To assess the possibility of differential T-cell help in memory cell expression, DNP-KLH primed cells were transferred with BSA primed T-cells and animals challenged with DNP-BSA. However, even under these circumstances, no significant difference in affinities were observed.

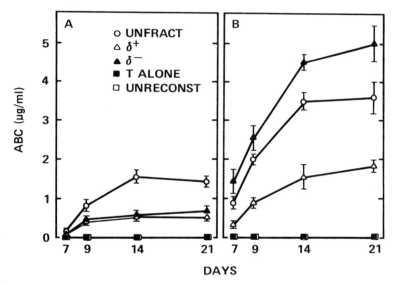

FIGURE 2. Adoptive secondary responses restored by DNP-BSA primed cells sorted for surface IgD. Mice were injected with BSA primed T-cells and with a dose of bright or dull cells contained within 2×10^6 unfractionated cells (A) or 2×10^6 cells of each cell fraction (B). Each point represents the mean response of 3–4 animals expressed as the antigen binding capacity (ABC) ± the standard error as determined using the Farr assay.

Magnitude and Affinity of the Adoptive Secondary Response to DNP-BSA with Respect to Dose of Fractionated Cells Transferred

In all of the above experiments, the number of δ^+ and δ^- cells transferred was equal to the number of cells contained in the unfractionated population. In the previous investigations[9,10] reporting a difference in affinity of the δ^+ and δ^- cell fractions, equal numbers of fractionated and unfractionated cells were transferred. Also higher numbers of cells were transferred (5×10^6 cells versus that number contained within 2×10^6 unfractionated cells). We therefore repeated the above experiments, transferring higher but equal numbers of fractionated cells (2×10^6 cells each) from DNP-BSA (CFA) primed spleen cells. As can be seen in FIGURE 2b, the magnitude of the response restored by the δ^- cell fraction exceeded both the unfractionated and δ^+ cell fraction response, as compared to the equal responses restored using the previous protocol (FIGURE 2a). The affinity of the responses restored by these higher cell numbers is presented in TABLE 3. Even though the δ^- population restored a much larger response, the affinity was not appreciably different from that restored by the δ^+ cell fraction at any of the three time periods after priming tested.

Precursor Frequency and Isotype Secretion of δ^+ and δ^- Memory Cells

The majority of the experiments presented here have utilized the adoptive transfer of δ^+ and δ^- cell fractions at cell numbers contained within 2×10^6 unfractionated cells. Under these conditions, late after priming (>12 weeks), the

TABLE 3

RELATIVE AVERAGE AFFINITY OF ADOPTIVE SECONDARY RESPONSE OF DNP-BSA PRIMED CELLS IN RELATION TO CELL NUMBER TRANSFERRED

Time after priming of donor (wk)*	Cell source used for reconstitution	Relative average affinity† (L/M)
12	delta pos.	1.48×10^9
	delta neg.	1.81×10^9
	unfract.	3.5×10^9
14	delta pos.	1.33×10^9
	delta neg.	1.2×10^9
	unfract.	1.18×10^9
52	delta pos.	2.14×10^9
	delta neg.	3.71×10^9
	unfract.	1.82×10^9

*Donor spleens were stained with rabbit anti-IgD myeloma serum and sorted. Two $\times 10^6$ cells of each fraction were injected into adoptive recipients given carrier primed T-cells and challenged with DNP-BSA (200 μg) in saline.

†Relative average affinity (κ_{50}) of anti-DNP antibodies in the serum 14 days after challenge.

δ^+ and δ^- cell fractions restored approximately equal responses. When cell fractions were transferred at a constant cell number (2×10^6 cells), the δ^- cell fraction restores a much greater response than does the δ^+ cell fraction. There are two possibilities to explain this difference of results related to number of cells transferred. One, there is a difference in precursor frequency between the δ^+ and δ^- memory cells, or there is a difference in the burst size and/or rate of immunoglobulin synthesis between the δ^+ and δ^- cell fractions. To examine these points, we examined the precursor frequency using the splenic focus assay system.

Equal numbers of DNP-KLH (CFA) sorted primed spleen cells (0.1×10^6) were transferred to heavily irradiated KLH primed mice. Fragment cultures from recipient spleens were challenged with antigen in vitro. The results of these experiments are presented in TABLE 4. It can be seen that when cells were transferred proportionally to that number contained within 2×10^6 unfraction-ated cells, approximately equal numbers of precursors are transferred to the

TABLE 4

FREQUENCY OF DNP-SPECIFIC IgD$^+$ AND IgD$^-$ PRIMED B-CELL SUBSETS

Cell Fraction Transferred*	% of Unfractionated Cells Transferred	Average Frequency of DNP Specific Clones/10^6 Cells Transferred	Approximate % of Total Response
Unfract.		33.7	100
IgD$^+$	50–55	26.6	35–40
IgD$^-$	25–30	58.3	40–45

*Spleen cells from DNP-KLH alum-pertussis primed mice were stained for IgD and sorted. Fractionated cells were injected into irradiated, carrier primed recipients for analysis of DNP responsive cells using the splenic focus assay.

adoptive recipients. Thus, when 2×10^6 of each fraction were transferred, the δ^- population received a larger number of precursors. Thus, it is improbable that the δ^+ and δ^- cells differ in their burst size and/or rate of immunoglobulin synthesis.

We also examined the isotypes which were secreted by the individual clones to examine if there were major differences in the isotype production of the δ^+ and δ^- cells. From TABLE 5 it can be seen that the majority ($>85\%$) of the clones in both the δ^+ and δ^- fractions produced IgG. The majority of the clones in the unfractionated group also produced IgG, but had a significant percentage which produced IgM alone. The finding was, however, uncharacteristic of memory cell clones[17] (J. Teale, personal observation). There was no appreciable difference in the isotypes which were secreted by the δ^+ and δ^- fractions (TABLE 6). The major isotypes secreted in all cell fractions were IgG$_1$ and IgG$_{2b}$ followed by significant levels of IgM, IgA, and IgG$_{2a}$. Furthermore, there were no apparent differences in the number of isotypes secreted per clone, with the majority of clones secreting from one to four isotypes.

DISCUSSION

We have examined the magnitude and affinity of the adoptive secondary responses restored by IgD$^+$ and IgD$^-$ memory cell subpopulations with respect to

TABLE 5

ISOTYPES SECRETED BY MEMORY B-CELL SUBSETS

Experimental Group*	No. of Clones Analyzed	% of Clones Not Secreting IgG vs. Those Secreting IgG			
		IgG$^-$		IgG$^+$	
		IgM	IgM and/or IgA	IgM + IgG ($\pm$ IgA)	IgG ($\pm$ IgA)
IgD$^+$	16	0	6.3	50.0	43.8
IgD$^-$	35	0	13.3	22.8	62.8
Unfract.	27	22.2	0	29.6	48.1

*Anti-DNP specific clones obtained from the splenic focus assay were analyzed for the isotypes secreted using a solid phase radioimmunoassay with rabbit anti-mouse heavy chain and light chain specific antisera.

TABLE 6

PROPORTION OF CLONES OF MEMORY B-CELL SUBSETS SECRETING PARTICULAR ISOTYPES

Experimental Group	No. of Clones Analyzed	% of Clones Secreting								
		IgM	IgG3	IgG1	IgG2b	IgG2a	IgE	IgA	κ	λ
IgD$^+$	16	50	12.5	56.2	62.5	12.5	6.25	37.5	68.7	25.0
IgD$^-$	35	25.7	2.9	54.3	51.4	31.4	8.6	54.3	68.6	31.4
Unfract.	27	51.8	3.7	51.8	44.4	25.9	7.4	33.3	65.6	33.3

several experimental parameters. These included: 1) time after priming of cell donors, 2) source of anti-IgD antibodies used for immunofluorescent staining, 3) adjuvant used for priming, 4) carrier protein used for priming, 5) level of antigen challenge of adoptive hosts, and 6) effect of number of cells transferred to adoptive recipients. Cells were prepared from spleens of primed donors, stained for IgD, and separated into bright (positive) and dull (negative) cell fractions using the FACS. After sorting, cells were adoptively transferred to irradiated, syngeneic mice along with an excess number of carrier primed T-cells. One day after transfer, animals were challenged with antigen in saline, and serum antibody was assayed for both the quantity and quality of anti-DNP antibody.

These studies have shown that earlier after priming (10–12 weeks) the majority of the memory response was contained within the IgD$^+$ cell fraction, whereas at later time points, it was consistently found that the IgD$^+$ and IgD$^-$ memory cell fractions each restored approximately 50% of the response restored by 2×10^6 unfractionated cells. However, when equal numbers of IgD$^+$ and IgD$^-$ cells (2×10^6) were transferred, the IgD$^-$ fraction transferred the major response. It was demonstrated using the splenic focus assay that the IgD$^-$ call fraction had a higher precursor frequency. Thus, the higher response seen from IgD$^-$ memory cells was due to larger numbers of precursors being transferred as opposed to a difference in burst size or rate of immunoglobulin secretion. Under none of the experimental parameters tested here or previously[11] was there an appreciable difference in affinity (more than tenfold) of the responses restored by the IgD$^+$ and IgD$^-$ cell fractions. This is in contrast to previous investigations wherein affinity differences of 10–100-fold have been reported. Several differences in the experimental systems could explain our contradictory findings. Black et al.[9] and Herzenberg et al.[10] used a transfer system in which donors and host differed at the H-2 and immunoglobulin allotype loci. These differences could influence the adoptive responses restored by IgD$^+$ and IgD$^-$ cells. Bosma et al.[18] reported that in congenic allotype transfer systems, Ig-Ib allotype (IgG$_{2a}$) responses were suppressed in Ig-Ia allotype hosts. The majority of the data of Herzenberg et al.[10] are based on Ig-Ib allotype responses in Ig-Ia allotype hosts. Therefore, cells bearing

TABLE 7

NUMBER OF ISOTYPES SECRETED BY CLONES OF MEMORY B-CELL SUBSETS

Experimental Group	No. of Clones Analyzed	% of Individual Clones Secreting the Following Numbers of Different Isotypes						
		1	2	3	4	5	6	7
IgD$^+$	16	25	37.5	18.7	12.5	16.3	0	0
IgD$^-$	35	34.2	34.2	11.4	14.3	2.8	0	2.8
Unfract.	27	44.4	18.5	14.8	18.5	3.7	0	0

the Ig-5b allotype may have been similarly affected. Also, the allogeneic effect may have enhanced or suppressed cell subpopulations in the allogeneic transfer system.[19-21] Finally, we have examined the affinity of the entire spectrum of antibody classes whereas the previous studies[10] have been restricted to only one allotype and class.

Several investigators have reported that memory cells producing IgG antibody can express surface IgG and/or IgM. Zan-Bar *et al.*[7,8] previously reported that IgD+ memory cells restore initially the IgM response which is followed by an IgG response. We have confirmed and extended these findings by demonstrating that both IgD+ and IgD- cells produce IgM and IgG antibodies in the splenic focus assay. These results also demonstrate that primed IgD+ and IgD- cells differ from unprimed IgD+ and IgD- cells. In unprimed populations, a percentage of IgD+ cells produce IgM alone as did an even larger percentage of IgD- cells.[22] In the primed population, we detect no clones from IgD+ or IgD- cells which produced IgM alone. However, these cells were found in the unfractionated population. The major point is that the majority of the clones produce IgG, as has been observed with other memory cell clones.[17]

In conclusion, these results have shown that although δ^- memory cells have a higher precursor frequency, they account for approximately 50% of the memory cell population *in vivo*. The results presented here also suggest that the loss of surface IgD is not a necessary intermediate stage in the maturation of memory B-cells, and that clonal selection can occur to the same extent in δ^+ and δ^- memory cells.

ACKNOWLEDGMENTS

We gratefully acknowledge the excellent technical assistance of Carol Doss, F.A. Assisi, R. Eskoz and E. Glezer, and we are indebted to Lindsay Gatenby and Claire Wolf for the preparation of this manuscript.

REFERENCES

1. ABNEY, E. R., K. O. KEELER, R. M. E. PARKHOUSE & H. N. A. WILCOX. 1976. Eur. J. Immunol. **6:** 443–450.
2. MASON, D. W. 1976. J. Exp. Med. **143:** 122–1130.
3. OKUMURA, K., M. H. JULIUS, T. TSU, L. A. HERZENBERG & L. A. HERZENBERG. 1976. Eur. J. Immunol. **6:** 467–472.
4. STROBER, S. 1976. J. Immunol. **117:** 1288–1294.
5. YUAN, D., E. S. VITETTA & J. KETTMAN. 1977. J. Exp. Med. **145:** 1421–1435.
6. COFFMAN, R. L. & M. COHN. 1977. J. Immunol. **118:** 1806–1815.
7. ZAN-BAR, I., S. STROBER & E. S. VITETTA. 1977. J. Exp. Med. **145:** 1188–1205.
8. ZAN-BAR, I., E. S. VITETTA, F. ASSISI & S. STROBER. 1978. J. Exp. Med. **147:** 1374–1394.
9. BLACK, S. J., W. VAN DU LOO, M. R. LOKEN & L. A. HERZENBERG. 1980. J. Exp. Med. **147:** 984–996.
10. HERZENBERG, L. A., S. J. BLACK, T. TOKUHISA & L. A. HERZENBERG. 1980. J. Exp. Med. **151:** 1071–1087.
11. LAFRENZ, D., S. STROBER & E. VITETTA. 1981. J. Immunol. **127:** 867–872.
12. LITTLE, J. R. & H. N. EISEN. 1967. *In* Methods in Immunology and Immunochemistry. C. A. WILLIAMS & M. W. CHASE, Eds.: 128. Academic Press. New York, N.Y.
13. JULIUS, M. H., E. SIMPSON & L. A. HERZENBERG. 1973. Eur. J. Immunol. **3:** 645–649.
14. MAGE, M. G., L. L. MCHUGH & T. L. ROTHSTEIN. 1977. J. Immunological Meth. **15:** 47–56.

15. KLINMAN, N. R. 1952. J. Exp. Med. **136:** 241–260.
16. KLINMAN, N. R. & J. L. PRESS. 1975. Transplant Rev. **24:** 41–83.
17. TEALE, J. M., D. LAFRENZ, N. R. KLINMAN & S. STROBER. 1981. J. Immunol. **126:** 1952–1957.
18. BOSMA, M. J., G. C. BOSMA & J. L. OWEN. 1978. Eur. J. Immunol. **8:** 562–568.
19. KATZ, D. H. 1972. Transplant. Rev. **12:** 141.
20. SWAIN, S. L. & R. W. DUTTON. 1977. J. Immunol. **118:** 2262–2268.
21. SWAIN, S. L. 1978. J. Immunol. **121:** 671–677.
22. LAYTON, J. E., J. M. TEALE & G. J. V. NOSSAL. 1979. J. Immunol. **123:** 709–713.

DISCUSSION OF THE PAPER

LEN HERZENBERG: It's nice to finally see some of those data. There's one question which I've been wondering about on and off for the last several years which relates to your criteria for IgD$^+$ and IgD$^-$ cells on the FACS.

D. LAFRENZ: Based upon the windows that we set in the sort, 50% of the cells are included in the δ^+ fraction and 25 to 30% in the δ^- fraction. We gate the 10 channels to either side of the inflection point. So we determine where the inflection point is and then discard cells that are ten channels to either side of the inflection point.

LEN HERZENBERG: I see, so you are eliminating those cells that might be B-cells low in δ or in fact negative for δ in favor of taking cells which don't have any apparent staining. So you might be throwing away half the δ negative cells.

PARKHOUSE: I was very interested in the data saying that memory cells were μ^+. Did I understand that correctly?

LAFRENZ: When you sort simply for μ.

PARKHOUSE: Because in fact we turned up an identical result some years ago, which we published with Keith Keeler and Erica Abney, in a system based on Williamson and Askonas' clonal limiting dilution *in vivo* technique. We had such memory cells after repeated serial challenges and transfers, some for up to 18 months. We could retrieve them and give them antigen and they would produce a Gamma-2A monoclonal, but it was quite clear in that series of experiments that these cells had membrane μ on them.

This is an area in which most people have tended to concentrate in the past on whether memory cells have the class which they produce. In fact they can have something else as well evidently and I'm interested that both you and I seem to have demonstrated that you can have IgM bearing memory cells which produce IgG.

LAFRENZ: The direct demonstration is that there is IgM on the memory cell, but that doesn't mean that they may also coexpress another isotype.

LEN HERZENBERG: We separated μ^+ cells from animals that were recently primed and showed that there was μ^+ memory in the same places where we found δ^+ memory. It looks to us as though a memory cell can at one point in its life express μ, δ and γ.

LEE HERZENBERG: Our earlier findings demonstrated that IgD$^+$ memory B-cells give rise to low-affinity antibody production in assays for adoptive secondary responses, while IgD$^-$-cells give rise to high affinity responses. Dr. Lafrenz raised doubts as to the validity of these findings.

I cannot understand why the results obtained in the laboratory of Dr. Strober and ours differ so much. If we accept that the Farr assay as he performs it can measure sub-primary level affinities of responses produced by IgD$^+$ memory cells (see FIGURE 1), then we are left with trying to ferret out the reasons for the differences in our findings from the technical details of the experiments, e.g., the amounts of antigens used for priming and boosting, and the details of the FACS

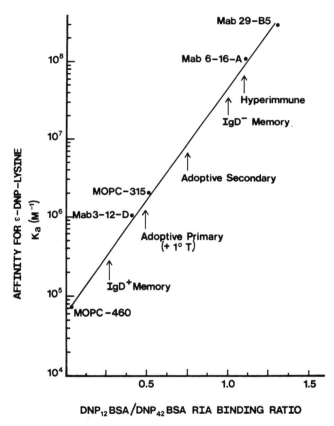

FIGURE 1. Ratio of RIA-binding to differently substituted DNP-BSA conjugates indicates anti-DNP antibody binding affinity (K_a). K_a values (points) for myeloma proteins and monoclonal antibodies were determined by fluorescence quenching. Arrows indicate $DNP_{12}BSA/DNP_{42}BAS$ ratios for various immune responses.

separations. Nothing obvious comes to mind from the data he presented although, as we shall show in our presentation, the immune system is surprisingly sensitive to immunization protocol details that one might have believed irrelevant.

In any event, I wish to make it clear that we see no reason at present to doubt our original findings. We have continued to use the affinity assay developed for the memory B-cell studies in our laboratory (see FIGURE 1) and have found it reliable. Furthermore, at least one other laboratory has confirmed its validity for measuring affinities in individual serum samples (personal communication, Dr. Fred Finkelman, Uniformed Services University of Health Science). While 2-5 fold errors in absolute affinity determinations may occur with this assay (particularly when measuring very low or very high affinity responses), it is clearly capable of measuring the large affinity differences we reported between the responses produced by long-lived IgD$^+$ memory cells and their more mature progeny that no longer carry measurable amounts of IgD.

One further point: Dr. Lafrenz suggests that the differences may derive from our having measured only IgG2a responses from transferred memory populations. We have, however, also measured IgG1 responses but presented data only for IgG2a responses because the results were similar for both isotypes. In fact, investigators who have followed our work know that we always measure at least the IgG1 and IgG2a responses and that, when working with allotype heterozygotes, we measure each allotype in these responses separately and report all significant nonconcordance.

Thus, although I sympathize with Dr. Lafrenz' attempt to explain the divergence between his results and ours, I cannot agree with the explanation he offers. I am pleased, however, that the studies he presented resolve an earlier dispute between the Strober laboratory and our own, i.e., we all now agree that both IgD$^+$ and IgD$^-$ cells are capable of transferring memory responses to adoptive recipients.

E. VITETTA: The systems which you are disagreeing about are very complex and I think it's hard for many of us to even follow the protocols. Since you are both at Stanford, I see absolutely no reason why the two groups can't get together and simply make a big pot of cells and run them through both systems. Until that's done none of us know which system we should agree with or disagree with, or why the differences exist. As a result, the whole issue is laid to rest in our minds and I think that's unreasonable because it's a very important issue.

TWO PRIMARY TRANSLATION PRODUCTS OF THE HUMAN δ CHAIN DIFFERENTIALLY N-GLYCOSYLATED TO FOUR DISCRETE FORMS *IN VIVO* AND *IN VITRO*

Joseph M. McCune, Shu Man Fu, Henry G. Kunkel, and
Gunter Blobel

Laboratories of Immunology and Cell Biology
The Rockefeller University
New York, New York, 10021

Structural differences between the heavy chain of membrane IgD (δ_m) and the heavy chain of secreted IgD (δ_s) were investigated by using a human lymphoblastoid cell line that expresses idiotypically identical IgM and IgD. In a wheat germ cell-free system, mRNA from this cell line was shown to encode two distinct δ chains that differed in molecular weight. When translated *in vitro* in the presence of dog pancreatic microsomal membranes or when synthesized *in vivo*, these two δ chains were processed to four discrete glycosylated forms, all of which shared idiotypic determinants, C-region determinants, and light chain linkage. As shown by digestion with endo-β-N-acetylglucosaminidase H, these four δ forms represent two δ polypeptide chains that are differentially N-glycosylated. Pulse-chase experiments demonstrated that, after endo-β-N-acetylglucosaminidase H treatment, δ_m has a higher molecular weight than δ_s. After integration into dog pancreatic microsomal membranes in vitro, δ_m was found not to have a large cytoplasmic domain exposed to proteolytic digestion.

The finding that δ_m and δ_s differ in primary structure is analogous to previous work showing that the corresponding heavy chains of IgM (μ_m and μ_s), synthesized by the same cell line, have identical NH$_2$-terminal amino acid sequences and idiotype, but differ in molecular weight, in topology, and in primary structure at the COOH-terminus.[1] A common feature of these membrane heavy chains, as well as the membrane heavy chain of IgA[2] appears to be inclusive of a membrane "domain" with structural characteristics underlying several functions, notably (a) information necessary for integration into the lipid bilayer of the rough endoplasmic reticulum at the time of synthesis, and (b) information relevant to the processes of B-cell activation (or inactivation), after the completed antigen receptors have been transported to the plasma membrane. The apparent dichotomy of B-cell responses mediated through either membrane IgM or membrane IgD may reflect unique COOH-terminal sequences on μ_m and δ_m, capable of initiating different intracellular cascades. The finding that the two primary translation products of the δ chain are processed *in vivo* to yield four early biosynthetic forms, a function of differential N-glycosylation, may be related to the heterogeneity of δ chains observed in earlier studies. Finally, the observation of four primary translation products (μ_m, μ_s, δ_m, and δ_s) in one cell line, each with the same V region, presents an experimental system in which to investigate the generation of the corresponding four mRNAs from the μ-δ gene complex.

REFERENCES

1. McCune, J. M., V. R. Lingappa, S. M. Fu, G. Blobel & H. G. Kunkel. 1980. J. Exp. Med. **152:** 463–468.
2. McCune, J. M., S. M. Fu, G. Blobel & H. G. Kunkel. 1981. J. Exp. Med. **153:** 1684–1689.

IN VIVO POLYCLONAL ACTIVATION OF IMMUNE DEFECTIVE B-LYMPHOCYTES BY AN ANTIBODY TO IgD*

L. Muul, I. Scher, J. J. Mond, and F. D. Finkelman

Department of Medicine
Uniformed Services University of the Health Sciences
and
Division of Immunology
Naval Medical Research Institute
Bethesda, Maryland 20814

The injection of adult BALB/c mice with 800 μg of an affinity purified isotype-specific goat antibody to mouse IgD (GaMδ) initiates a two-stage process that leads to polyclonal B-cell activation. The first stage, which is T-independent and which occurs within 24 hr of GaMδ injection, results in dramatic increases in B-cell size, DNA synthesis, and expression of B-cell surface (s) Ia antigen.[1,2] The second stage, which is T-dependent, and which occurs 5–7 days after GaMδ injection, results in further increases in B- and T-cell size and DNA synthesis, as well as the appearance of large numbers of B–lymphocytes with surface IgG and intracytoplasmic IgM and IgG.[3] Since B-lymphocytes from mice homozygous or hemizygous for the CBA/N x-linked immune defect have been reported not to proliferate *in vitro* in response to anti-Ig antibodies, or to differentiate into antibody secreting cells when stimulated *in vitro* with anti-Ig plus TRF,[4] we studied the effects of injecting (CBA/N × DBA/2)F_1 male mice (immune defective) and (CBA/N × DBA/2)F_1 female mice (phenotypically normal) with 800–1600 μg of GaMδ. B-cells from immune defective mice demonstrated definite but distinctly subnormal increases in B-cell size, ^{3}H-thymidine incorporation, and sIa one–five days after GaMδ injection (TABLE 1) but, by day 7, resembled normal B-cells in terms of increased ^{3}H-thymidine incorporation and sIa, as well as by their differentiation into cells with surface IgG and intracytoplasmic Ig (TABLE 2). These findings indicate that there are at least two separate mechanisms by which

TABLE 1

RESPONSE OF (CBA/N × DBA/2) F_1 MALE AND FEMALE SPLENIC B-CELLS THREE DAYS AFTER INJECTION OF GOAT ANTI-MOUSE δ OR NORMAL GOAT IMMUNOGLOBULIN

	% sIa⁺ Spleen Cells (Median Fluorescence Intensity)	cpm ³H Thymidine Incorporated/2 × 10⁶ sIa⁺ Cells	% sIa⁺ Cells > 429 μ^3
GaMδ male	27.9 (156)	2,390	9.1
Control male	30.8 (150)	1,360	5.4
GaMδ female	58.1 (249)	8,804	26.8
Control female	52.1 (108)	1,664	9.6

*Supported by USUHS research protocol Nos. R08308, R08315, C07305, C08310 and C08327 and Naval Medical Research and Development Command Research Task No. M0095-PN.001–1030.

TABLE 2

RESPONSE OF (CBA/N × DBA/2) F$_1$ MALE AND FEMALE SPLENIC B-CELLS SEVEN DAYS
AFTER INJECTION OF GOAT ANTI-MOUSE δ OR NORMAL GOAT IMMUNOGLOBULIN

	% sIa$^+$ Spleen Cells (Median Fluorescence Intensity)	cpm ^{3}H Thymidine Incorporated/ 2 × 10^6 sIa$^+$ Cells	% sIa$^+$ Cells >429 μ^3	% Spleen Cells with Intracyto- plasmic IgG$_1$	Serum* IgG$_1$ mg/ml
GaMδ male	25.2 (240)	10,965	11.8	5.2	1.7
Control male	27.6 (96)	2,046	4.8	0.6	0.8
GaMδ female	40.4 (242)	7,464	19.9	6.6	4.4
Control female	35.3 (37)	1,229	5.1	0.2	1.9

*Ten days after injection, GaMδ male = 7.8 mg/ml, control male 1.9 mg/ml; GaMδ female = 29.4 mg/ml, control female 3.7 mg/ml.

B-cells are activated to increase their expression of sIa and rate of DNA synthesis:
1) a direct, T-independent, ligand-sIg interaction (defective in CBA/N mice) and
2) interaction of B-cells with T-cell/macrophage generated helper substances in the presence of a ligand-sIg interaction (relatively normal in CBA/N mice). Furthermore, our data show that the differentiation of B-cells into sIgG$^+$ cells and Ig secreting cells is not directly related to the magnitude of the direct B-cell activating effects of anti-Ig antibody.

REFERENCES

1. FINKELMAN, F. D., I. SCHER, J. J. MOND, J. T. KUNG & E. S. METCALF. 1982. J. Immunol. **129:** 638.
2. MOND, J. J., E. SEHGAL, J. KUNG & F. D. FINKELMAN. 1981. J. Immunol. **127:** 881.
3. FINKELMAN, F. D., I. SCHER, J. J. MOND, S. KESSLER, J. T. KUNG & E. S. METCALF. 1982. J. Immunol. **129:** 629.
4. SCHER, E. 1981. *In* Immunological Defects in Laboratory Animals. M. E. Gershwin & B. Merchant, Eds. **1:** 163. Plenum Publishing Co.

EFFECT OF ANTI-IgD ON THE GROWTH AND DIFFERENTIATION OF HAPTEN-SPECIFIC B-CELL COLONIES

Margaret Piper, P. S. Pillai, and David W. Scott

Division of Immunology
Duke University Medical Center
Durham, North Carolina 27710

It has been previously shown that fluorescein (FL)-specific B-cells can be cloned in semisolid agar cultures and that individual colonies, placed in secondary microcultures, can be triggered by FL-antigen to differentiate to anti-FL PFC (Pillai and Scott, 1981). This system has been used to investigate the growth and subsequent differentiation of FL-specific B-cells cloned in the presence of anti-IgD antibodies. When the agar cultures include both LPS and SRBC as potentiators of cell growth, the presence of a monoclonal anti-IgD (10-4.22) causes a 50–60% maximal reduction in colony numbers. These results are in agreement with published data obtained by cloning normal spleen cells under similar conditions (Kincade, Lee, Scheid, and Blum, 1980). However, when these FL-specific B-cell colonies are placed in microculture in the presence of irradiated spleen cell fillers and FL-POL, the results show that the colonies which grow in the presence of anti-IgD respond with an equal or greater frequency when compared to normal colonies. Therefore, although anti-IgD inhibits the growth of a percentage of the colony-forming B-cells, it has no effect on the ability of the remaining colonies to differentiate and respond to FL-POL. In contrast, when FL-specific B-cells are cloned in the presence of an affinity purified goat anti-IgM, colony numbers are again reduced 40–60% but the ability of the colonies to respond upon stimulation with FL-POL is reduced nearly 100%. When both anti-IgD and anti-IgM are present in the agar cultures, colony numbers are inhibited to a significantly greater degree than when either antibody alone is present. These results show that FL-specific B-cells which form colonies in semisolid agar cultures are differentially sensitive to anti-IgD and anti-IgM antibodies, and suggest that separate B-cell subpopulations are being detected.

MURINE IgD IS STRUCTURALLY HETEROGENEOUS WHEN IT FIRST APPEARS DURING ONTOGENY

Roberta R. Pollock* and Matthew F. Mescher

Department of Pathology
Harvard Medical School
Boston, Massachusetts 02115

Murine IgD, unlike membrane IgM, is structurally heterogeneous. Two membrane δ chains are seen upon sodium dodecyl sulfate (SDS) electrophoresis, δ_1 (70,000 daltons) and δ_2 (68,000 daltons).[1-4] These δ chains contain different amounts of sialic acid and probably different amounts of neutral sugars.[4,5] McCune et al.[6] have shown that the primary translation product of the human membrane δ chain is differentially N-glycosylated to yield two chains.

Two IgD structures, IgD_I and IgD_{II}, exist on the cell surface.[3,7-12] IgD_I is a four chain molecule containing two δ chains and two light chains. IgD_{II} is a "half-molecule" composed of one δ chain and one light chain. Each IgD form contains both of the two δ chains.[12]

The relative amounts of IgD_I and IgD_{II}, expressed as the IgD_I to IgD_{II} ratio, is constant within each strain but varies among strains. The value of this ratio is linked to the Igh-5 allotype.[13] Mice of the Igh-5^a or Igh-5^b allotype have a high ratio of 1.4 (determined as the ratio of net cpm in each IgD band) while mice of the Igh-5^e allotype have a low ratio of 0.4.

The appearance of IgD during ontogeny has been studied extensively.[14-17] However, these studies did not examine the expression of IgD's structural heterogeneity. If δ_1 and δ_2, or IgD_I and IgD_{II}, serve different functions, they might appear at different times during development. Therefore we have studied the expression of δ_1, δ_2, IgD_I and IgD_{II} in neonatal mice.

Both δ_1 and δ_2 appear simultaneously during development. Neonatal spleen cells from all strains examined (BALB/c, C57B1/6 and A) express equal amounts of δ_1 and δ_2, as do adult spleen cells.

IgD_I and IgD_{II} also appear simultaneously during ontogeny. The IgD_I to IgD_{II} ratio expressed on neonatal spleen cells is the same ratio expressed on adult cells. Thus, neonatal cells show the same strain variation in the IgD_I to IgD_{II} ratio seen for adults: BALB/c (Igh-5^a) and C57B1/6 (Igh-5^b) mice have high ratios while A (Igh-5^e) mice have low ratios.

These results show that when IgD first appears during ontogeny it exhibits the same structural heterogeneity observed in adult mice. Thus it seems unlikely that δ_1 and δ_2, or IgD_I and IgD_{II}, serve different functions which appear at different times. Further studies on the basis of this heterogeneity and its expression during B-cell activation may reveal any functional differences.

REFERENCES

1. MELCHER, U. & J. W. UHR. 1976. J. Immunol. **116:** 409–415.
2. PEARSON, T., G. GALFRÉ, A. ZIEGLER & C. MILSTEIN. 1977. Eur. J. Immunol. **7:** 684–690.

*Current address: Department of Cell Biology, Albert Einstein College of Medicine, 1300 Morris Park Avenue, Bronx, N.Y. 10461.

3. SITIA, R., G. CORTE, M. FERRARINI & A. BARGELLESI. 1977. Eur. J. Immunol. **7:** 503–507.
4. MESCHER, M. F. & R. R. POLLOCK. 1979. J. Immunol. **123:** 1155–1161.
5. GODING, J. W. & L. A. HERZENBERG. 1980. J. Immunol. **124:** 2540–2547.
6. McCUNE, J. M., S. M. FU, H. G. KUNKEL & G. BLOBEL. 1981. Proc. Natl. Acad. Sci. **78:** 5127–5131.
7. MELCHER: U., E. S. VITETTA, M. McWILLIAMS, M. E. LAMM, J. M. PHILIPS-QUAGLIATA & J. W. UHR. 1974. J. Exp. Med. **140:** 1427–1431.
8. ABNEY, E. R. & R. M. E. PARKHOUSE. 1974. Nature **252:** 600–602.
9. LISOWSKA-BERNSTEIN, N. & P. VASSALLI. 1975. In Membrane Receptors of Lymphocytes. M. Seligmann, J.L. Preud'hommé & F.M. Kourilsky, Eds.: 39–49. American Elsevier Publishing Co. New York, N.Y.
10. CORTE, G., G. VIALE, E. COSULICH, A. BARGELLESI & M. FERRARINI. 1979. Scand. J. Immunol. **10:** 275–280.
11. EIDELS, L. 1979. J. Immunol. **123:** 896–902.
12. POLLOCK, R. R. & M. F. MESCHER. 1980. J. Immunol. **124:** 1668–1674.
13. POLLOCK, R. R., M. E. DORF & M. F. MESCHER. 1980. Proc. Natl. Acad. Sci. **77:** 4256–4259.
14. VITETTA, E. S., U. MELCHER, M. McWILLIAMS, M. E. LAMM, J. M. PHILLIPS-QUAGLIATA & J. W. UHR. 1975. J. Exp. Med. **141:** 206–215.
15. ABNEY, E. R., I. R. HUNTER & R. M. E. PARKHOUSE. 1976. Nature **259:** 404–406.
16. KEARNEY, J. F., M. D. COOPER, J. KLEIN, E. R. ABNEY, R. M. E. PARKHOUSE & A. R. LAWTON. 1977. J. Exp. Med. **146:** 297–301.
17. ABNEY, E. R., M.D. COOPER, J. F. KEARNEY, A. R. LAWTON & R. M. E. PARKHOUSE. 1978. J. Immunol. **120:** 2041–2049.

IgD-Fc RECEPTORS (Fc$_\delta$) ON NORMAL AND NEOPLASTIC HUMAN B-LYMPHOCYTES

Richard A. Rudders and Janet Andersen

Lymphocyte Typing Laboratory
Tufts University School of Medicine
New England Medical Center Hospital
Boston, Massachusetts 02111

Cells from normal peripheral blood and human lymphoid neoplasms were studied for the presence of Fc receptors for IgD utilizing fluorescent labelled IgD aggregates (TABLE 1). In normal blood 2.0–3.7% of mononuclear cells bound IgD aggregates. Binding increased with enrichment for SmIg$^+$ B-lymphocytes and decreased with enrichment for T-lymphocytes. In double fluorescent labelling studies Agg IgD binding cells were also SmIg$^+$. IgD Fc fragments were prepared by trypsin digestion. Agg IgD binding was shown to be Fc fragment specific in blocking experiments. Fc$_\delta$ fragments inhibited IgD binding whereas IgM and IgG did not inhibit IgD binding.

When the monoclonal human B-cell neoplasms, chronic lymphocytic leukemia (CLL) and malignant lympyhoma (ML) were studied, 13/22 bound IgD

TABLE 1

FL AGG IgD BINDING BY NORMAL HUMAN
BLOOD LYMPHOCYTES

Populations	% Positive Cells*	
	SmIg$^+$	Agg IgD$^+$
Unfractionated	7	3
B-Enriched	32	11
T-Enriched	1	0

*Numbers represent mean values for experiments with several donors.

TABLE 2

BINDING OF FL AGG IgD BY HUMAN MONOCLONAL
B-NEOPLASMS

Tumor (Lineage)	Monoclonal SmIg Heavy Chains	% Cells Positive for Agg IgD*
CLL (B)	$\mu\delta$	62
	μ	0
	λ	0
	(λ only)	0
ML (B)	$\mu\delta$	12
	μ	1
	$\mu\alpha$	0
ML-CLL (T)	none	1

*Mean value for several tumors in each category.

395

aggregates (TABLE 2). T-derived neoplasms displayed no Agg IgD binding. Agg IgD binding to B-cell clones was restricted to those expressing a surface membrane Ig δ chain. Clones expressing other membrane heavy chains failed to bind Agg IgD.

We conclude that Fc receptors for Agg IgD are present on a subset of normal peripheral B-lymphocytes. The study of neoplastic cells suggests that Fc_δ receptors are present on B-derived neoplasms and the expression of Fc_δ correlates with the membrane expression of SmIgD.

ANTI-IgD TREATED STIMULATOR SPLEEN CELLS ENHANCE THE MURINE MIXED LYMPHOCYTE REACTION*

John J. Ryan, James J. Mond, Fred D. Finkelman,
and Irwin Scher

Immunology Branch
Infectious Diseases Program Center
Naval Medical Research Institute
and
Department of Medicine
Uniformed Services University of the Health Sciences
Bethesda, Maryland 20814

Previous studies have shown that splenic B-cells from mice injected intravenously with rabbit anti-mouse δ antibody (RaMδ) exhibited enhanced expression of cell surface Ia molecules.[1] These antigens are the most potent lymphocyte activating determinants (LAD) which trigger proliferation of T-responder cells in a H-2-defined mixed lymphocyte reaction (MLR).[2] They may also play a role in the recognition of the non-H-2-linked Mls determinants which trigger proliferation in an allogeneic H-2-compatible MLR.[3] Therefore to test for a functional change in MLR stimulatory capacity of H-2 and/or Mls-associated antigens that might occur with increased expression of Ia determinants, spleen cells from mice injected 24 hr beforehand with RaMδ were utilized as stimulator cells across both an entire H-2 haplotype or an Mls difference.

In a typical experiment (TABLE 1), Dl.C/Sn (H-2^d, Mls^a) (d, a) mice were injected with either 100 μg Ramδ or 100 mg RaKLH. Twenty-four hours later the spleen cells were removed and used as stimulator cells in a Mls-defined MLR with BALB/c (d, b) responder cells or in a H-2-defined MLR with Dl.LP (b, a) responder cells. At concentrations of 1×10^5 or 2×10^5 the RaMδ treated Dl.C/Sn spleen cells exhibited more than a tenfold increase in stimulatory capacity over the control group in a Mls-defined MLR and approximately a twofold increase in H-2 defined MLR stimulatory capacity. It was consistently observed that only anti-δ treated spleen cells from those strains of mice which possessed the strongly stimulatory Mls^a or Mls^d determinants exhibited this markedly enhanced capacity to trigger responder cells to proliferate across a non-H-2 barrier.

Injection of 100–200 μg of RaMδ into recipient animals 24 hr beforehand optimally enhanced the Mls and H-2 stimulatory capacity of spleen cells from these animals. The increase in Mls and H-2 stimulatory capacity induced with

*This work was supported in part by the Naval Medical Research and Development Command Research Task No. MR041.20.01.0439; the Uniformed Services University of the Health Sciences Research Nos. C08310, R08307, and R08308; and the National Naval Medical Center Clinical Investigator No. 3-06-132. The opinions and assertions contained herein are the private ones of the writers and are not to be construed as official or reflecting the views of the Navy Department or the naval service at large. The experiments reported herein were conducted according to the principles set forth in the current edition of the *Guide for the Care and Use of Laboratory Animals*, Institute of Laboratory Animal Resources, National Research Council.

TABLE 1

EFFECT OF ANTI-δ TREATMENT ON THE ABILITY OF SPLEEN CELLS TO INDUCE PROLIFERATION IN A MLs OR A H-2 DEFINED MLR

Responder Cells	Locus at which Stimulator Differs from Responder	Strain	Treatment	Mean uptake of ^{3}H-TdR (cpm ± S.E.M.) Stimulator Cells		
				1×10^5	2×10^5	4×10^5
BALB/c		BALB/c	anti-KLH	2,442 ± 386	3,489 ± 583	3,330 ± 614
			anti-δ	3,364 ± 258	3,844 ± 592	5,026 ± 593
	Mls	Dl.C/Sn	anti-KLH	5,422 ± 1,019	16,539 ± 1,609	34,175 ± 2,216
			anti-δ	76,946 ± 4,637	193,884 ± 9,567	259,386 ± 7,703
D1.LP/Sn		D1.LP/Sn	anti-KLH	7,633 ± 706	7,441 ± 798	8,047 ± 847
			anti-δ	11,181 ± 1,211	11,161 ± 1,025	13,672 ± 1,129
	H-2	Dl.C/Sn	anti-KLH	24,914 ± 2,531	39,102 ± 2,292	69,694 ± 2,627
			anti-δ	48,083 ± 3,723	71,000 ± 2,396	102,158 ± 5,008

different doses of RaMδ was paralleled by an increase in median fluorescence intensity of cell surface Ia antigen expression on splenic B-cells contained in the stimulator cell populations.

Hybridoma as well as heterologous anti-δ antibody was also shown to enhance the MLR stimulatory capacity of spleen cells from mice injected 24 hr beforehand.

Anti-IgD treatment of spleen cells from B-cell-defective (CBA/N × DBA/2)F$_1$ male mice, that lack the mature Lyb5$^+$ population of B-cells that expresses Mls determinants, were unaffected by treatment with RaMδ antibody in terms of their capacity to stimulate in a Mls defined MLR. In contrast, spleen cells from phenotypically normal (DBA/2 × CBA/N)F$_1$ male mice showed a dramatically enhanced capacity to stimulate responder cell proliferation across a Mls-defined MLR after being exposed to anti-δ *in vivo*.

Since the injected anti-δ antibodies presumably have their major initial effect on surface IgD bearing B-cells, and not on T-cells or accessory cells, it seems most reasonable that B-cells from the anti-IgD-treated stimulator population may have a role in the presentation of alloantigens such as Ia or Mls to unprimed responder T-cells.

REFERENCES

1. MOND, J. J., E. S. SEGHAL, J. KUNG & F. D. FINKELMAN. 1981. J. Immunol. **127:** 881–888.
2. MEO, T., J. VIVES, V. MIGGIANO & D. C. SHEFFLER. 1973. Transplant. Proc. **5:** 377–381.
3. JANEWAY, C. A., E. A. LERNER, J. M. JASON & B. JONES. 1980. Immunogenetics **10:** 481–497.

NONSPECIFIC FACTORS INDUCE sIgD ON A CLASS
OF INTERMEDIATE "PRE-PROGENITOR" B-CELLS

Ken Shortman, Judy Layton, and James W. Goding

The Walter and Eliza Hall Institute
Royal Melbourne Hospital
Melbourne, Australia 3050

Adoptive immune responses derive from a distinct, minor subset of B-cells we have termed "pre-progenitors." Such responses appear to proceed in two stages, the first being a nonspecific (macrophage dependent) activation of pre-progenitors into cell cycle and further differentiation into "direct progenitors," the second being a specific antigenic response of the resultant "direct progenitors" to produce antibody secreting cells (AFC).[1] In previous work using spleen cells from specific pathogen free mice we found these B-cells initiating hapten-specific primary adoptive responses (pre-progenitors) to be predominantly s-IgM[+]IgD[-].[2] However, this result was in conflict with the work of others,[3,4] who found the progenitors of primary adoptive responses to be mainly sIgD[+]. Did the adoptive assay systems used register a different B-cell subset than in our assay? Or could the surface IgD status of the pre-progenitor subset vary with the state of the donor mice? The following experiments suggest the latter was the correct explanation.

Specific pathogen free (SPF) C57BL/6 mice were used, either unprimed, or primed intraperitoneally (i.p.) with horse erythrocytes (HRC) or low doses of lipopolysaccharide (LPS), or both, for 24 hr. A fixed number of spleen cells were treated with a monoclonal, allotype-specific anti-IgD and rabbit complement, to destroy all sIgD[+] cells, or with complement alone as a control. The cells remaining in the two samples were transferred to irradiated recipients, which then received a sequential nonspecific (HRC at day 0) then specific (the hapten NIP on bacterial flagellin at day 3) priming schedule.[1,2] NIP-specific IgM secreting AFC in the recipient spleens were then assayed 8 days post cell transfer. Results are shown in TABLE 1.

Spleen cells from unprimed mice gave the same response regardless of whether sIgD[+] cells were present or not, as we have found before.[2] Thus all the activity was in the minor, sIgD[-] subset. Priming with HRC alone, or with LPS alone, caused only a minor shift to sIgD[+] activity. However if both stimuli had been applied, much of the activity was lost when sIgD[+] cells were removed. Adoptive activity had shifted from the sIgD[-] to the sIgD[+] B-cell compartment. In some experiments (about one in five) LPS alone caused such a shift; we assume that the mice in these experiments had received some natural stimulus resembling that given by HRC. In some early experiments HRC alone appeared to give such a shift; this effect was traced to endotoxin or LPS-like material in the saline used for suspending the HRC. With care to ensure endotoxin-free reagents, injection of HRC alone does not cause the massive shift to sIgD[+] adoptive activity.

This requirement for two distinct stimuli to change the responding population from sIgD[-] to sIgD[+] appears to differ from the requirement for non-specific activation of the same subset into cell cycle, since the latter can be accomplished

400

TABLE 1

THE EFFECT OF PRIMING WITH HRC AND LPS ON THE sIgD STATUS OF
"PRE-PROGENITORS"*

Donor Priming Stimulus	Treatment of Cells	NIP-specific IgM AFC per recipient spleen per 5×10^6 pretreatment cells	% Activity IgD†
Unprimed	Complement alone	$6,430 \pm 1,010$	0
	and anti-IgD	$7,800 \pm 2,320$	
HRC	Complement alone	$8,640 \pm 1,400$	17
	and anti-IgD	$7,180 \pm 1,240$	
LPS	Complement alone	$6,960 \pm 1,280$	5
	and anti-IgD	$6,620 \pm 980$	
LPS and HRC	Complement alone	$17,100 \pm 2,180$	57
	and anti-IgD	$7,300 \pm 1,360$	

*The basic conditions are given in text. The stimuli were injected i.p. in saline, HRC at a level of 5×10^6, LPS at a level of 2 μg. The spleen cells from pools of 6 SPF C57BL/6 donor mice were treated with a monoclonal anti-IgD (5b) and rabbit complement, as described elsewhere,[2] which killed an average of 39% of all spleen cells. The cell numbers transferred were based on a pretreatment count. Twenty recipients were used in each group in each experiment. Results are the means ±S.E.M. of the pooled data from two experiments. The effect of anti-IgD treatment was significant at the p = 0.001 level in the LPS and HRC group, but was not statistically significant in the other groups.

by HRC injection alone.[1] We have confirmed this difference in side-by-side tests using priming with HRC suspended in endoxin-free saline.

We conclude that the reported differences in the sIgD status of B-cells initiating primary adoptive responses reflect differences in the status of the donor animals. Natural infections in a mouse colony might be expected to cause the shifts we have produced experimentally, as would adjuvant prepriming schedules used to activate helper T-cells. Lack of IgD can only serve as a marker for the pre-progenitor subset if the animals are maintained in an infection-free and unstimulated state. An additional conclusion is that the pre-progenitor subset does not lose its basic capacity for nonspecific expansion merely because of the acquisition of sIgD. The transition from intermediate pre-progenitor to mature direct progenitor, although usually associated with an increase in sIgD, must be determined by other factors.

REFERENCES

1. SHORTMAN, K. & M. HOWARD. 1979. *In* B-Lymphocytes in the Immune Response. M. Cooper, D. E. Mosier, I. Scher & E.S. Vitetta: 97–106. Elsevier North-Holland.
2. COFFMAN, R. L. & M. COHN. 1977. J. Immunol. **118:** 1806–1815.
3. ZAN-BAR, I., E. S. VITETTA & S. STROBER. 1977. J. Exp. Med. **145:** 1206–1215.
4. LAYTON, J. E., J. BAKER, P. BARTLETT & K. SHORTMAN. 1980. J. Immunol. **126:** 1227–1233.

POSSIBLE INDUCTION OF A TRF RECEPTOR BY
ANTI-IgD ANTIBODY*

L. J. Yaffe and Fred D. Finkelman

Naval Medical Research Institute
Bethesda, Maryland 20817
and
Uniformed Services University of the Health Sciences
Bethesda, Maryland 20814

T-cell replacing factor (TRF) prepared by concanavalin A (Con A) stimulation of normal mouse spleen cells has the capacity to replace T-cells in a primary *in vitro* T-dependent antibody response.[1] We have found that spleen cells from mice immunized seven days earlier with sheep red blood cells (SRBC) were more potent absorbers of TRF activity than were spleen cells from nonimmune mice. To examine whether an interaction between antigen and cell surface immunoglobulin (sIg) might be involved in this enhancement, mice were injected with goat anti-mouse IgD (GaMδ) and their spleen cells tested subsequently for the ability to absorb TRF.

Con A supernatants containing TRF activity were prepared similarly to previously described procedures.[2] For TRF absorption, mice were immunized one to seven days prior to sacrifice with 1×10^8 SRBC, 800 μg affinity-purified GaMδ, or 800 μg normal goat IgG (NGIg). One ml of TRF supernatant was absorbed twice for 30 min at 37°C with 1×10^5 to 1×10^8 spleen cells from the immunized animals. Absorbed TRF supernatants were tested for residual activity by their ability to reconstitute an *in vitro* T-cell-depleted B-cell response to SRBC. Results in TABLE 1 demonstrate that spleen cells from DBA/2J mice immunized with SRBC were able to absorb TRF activity from supernatants, whereas spleen cells from unimmunized animals showed significantly less absorptive capacity. Interestingly, CBA/N and DBA/2Ha mice, TRF unresponsive strains,[3] failed to absorb TRF activity even when immunized earlier with SRBC.

DBA/2J mice treated with GaMδ showed an increased ability to absorb TRF activity compared to animals given NIgG (TABLE 2). Most significantly, spleen cells from GaMδ treated mice absorbed TRF activity earlier with fewer spleen cells than following SRBC immunization. Additionally, TABLE 2 indicates that at one or three days following immunization, GaMδ treated mice had 100 to 1000 times the TRF absorptive capacity of spleen cells from NGIg treated mice. Spleen cell from nude mice similarly immunized were able to absorb TRF activity (TABLE 3). These results suggest that the cross-linking of surface IgD by GaMδ and possibly the cross-linking of sIg by antigen, may induce the expression of B-cell receptors for one or more components of TRF. It appears that the initial interaction of B-cells with antigen, or as we have shown early cross-linking with GaMδ, may induce the appearance of helper factor receptors, in particular a TRF receptor, which subsequently can interact with this late-acting helper factor. Spleen cells from CBA/N and DBA/2Ha mice may fail to completely absorb TRF activity because of a defect in receptor induction. Possibly B-cell activation and

* This work supported by the Naval Medical Research and Development Command Task No. MR041.20.01.0440.

TABLE 1

ABSORPTION OF TRF ACTIVITY WITH SPLEEN CELLS FROM SRBC IMMUNIZED MICE*

| TRF Absorption before Assay | | Anti-SRBC PFC/10^6 Cultured | |
Spleen Cells From	Treated With	T-cell-depleted DBA/2J Spleen Cells	[% Reduction]
No TRF Added		1 (1.00)	—
Unabsorbed TRF		109 (1.09)	—
DBA/2J	Untreated	77 (1.16)	[94]
DBA/2J	SRBC	5 (2.30)	
DBA/2Ha	Untreated	177 (1.07)	[35]
DBA/2Ha	SRBC	115 (1.09)	
(CBA/N × DBA/2)$F_1\delta$	Untreated	150 (1.13)	[38]
(CBA/N × DBA/2)$F_1\delta$	SRBC	93 (1.16)	

*TRF was prepared using Balb/c spleen cells cultured at 1×10^6 cells/ml in RPMI 1640 supplemented with 1 μg/ml Con A. Cultures were maintained at 37°C for 48 hr, then supernatants were passed over Sephadex G100. The fraction eluted at 40,000 ± 7,500 daltons was used as a Con A-depleted, TRF-enriched fraction. Spleen cells used for TRF absorption were from mice treated seven days earlier with 1×10^8 SRBC. 1×10^8 spleen cells from treated and control mice were used to absorb 1 ml of TRF supernatant. Residual TRF activity was assayed by reconstitution of in vitro anti-SRBC B-cell responses using Mishell-Dutton cultures and the Cunningham plaquing technique to count plaque forming cells (PFC). T-cell-depleted spleen cells were prepared by a double treatment with monoclonal anti-Thy 1.2 plus complement. Twenty-five μl of absorbed TRF supernatant per 200 μl well volume was tested. Data represent geometric means ×/÷ standard errors.

TABLE 2

ABSORPTION OF TRF ACTIVITY WITH SPLEEN CELLS FROM MICE TREATED ONE AND THREE DAYS EARLIER WITH GaMδ*

| TRF Absorption with DBA/2J Spleen Cells | | Anti-SRBC PFC/10^6 Cultured T-cell-depleted DBA/2J Spleen Cells Number of Spleen Cells From Treated Mice Used for TRF Absorption | | | |
Days After Treatment	Treated With	1×10^5	1×10^6	1×10^7	1×10^8
	NGIg	59 (1.22)	50 (1.26)	58 (1.23)	54 (1.12)
1	GaMδ	43 (1.13)	20 (1.15)	13 (1.36)	10 (1.19)
	[% Reduction]	[27]	[60]	[78]	[82]
	NGIg	53 (1.35)	65 (1.19)	59 (1.11)	61 (1.23)
3	GaMδ	68 (1.09)	19 (1.27)	15 (1.19)	13 (1.18)
	[% Reduction]	[0]	[71]	[75]	[79]

*Spleen cells used for TRF absorption were from mice treated one or three days earlier with 800 μg GaMδ or 800 μg NGIg. One × 10^5 to 1×10^8 spleen cells from treated and control mice were used to absorb 1 ml of TRF supernatant and residual TRF activity was assayed on T-cell-depleted spleen cells as described in TABLE 1. Data represent geometric means ×/÷ standard errors with 3 PFC subtracted for background plaques in the absence of TRF supernatant.

TABLE 3

ABSORPTION OF TRF ACTIVITY WITH SPLEEN CELLS FROM NUDE MICE TREATED ONE DAY EARLIER WITH GaMδ*

TRF Absorption with NIH Swiss nu/nu Spleen Cells Treated With	Anti-SRBC PFC/10^6 Cultured T-Cell-depleted DBA/2J Spleen Cells
NGIg	79 (1.17)
GaMδ	5 (1.18)
[% Reduction]	[94]

*Spleen cells for TRF absorption were from nude mice treated one day earlier with 800 μg GaMδ or 800 μg NGIg. One × 10^8 spleen cells from these treated mice were used to absorb 1 ml of TRF supernatant, and residual TRF activity was determined, as described in TABLE 1. Data represent geometric means ×/÷ standard errors with 4 PFC subtracted for background plaques in the absence of TRF.

the generation of antibody forming cells may proceed under the influence of antigen-sIg interactions, together with factor signals, which are able to induce TRF receptor sites, thereby permitting terminal differentiation of B-cells into antibody-secreting cells in the presence of TRF.

ACKNOWLEDGMENT

The authors wish to thank Ms. Clara Shields for her excellent editorial assistance.

REFERENCES

1. SCHIMPL, A. & E. WECKER, 1975. Transplant. Rev. **23**: 176.
2. HÜNIG, T., A. SCHIMPL & E. WECKER, 1977. J. Exp. Med. **145**: 1216.
3. TOMINAGA, A., K. TAKATSU & T. HAMAOKA, 1980. J. Immunol. **124**: 2423.

EFFECT OF TREATMENT WITH ANTI-IgD FROM BIRTH ON THE PRODUCTION OF DIFFERENT CLASSES OF ANTIBODIES IN BALB/c MICE*

Z. Ovary, Y. Baine, T. Hirano, B. Xue, B. Pernis,† and
G. J. Thorbecke

Department of Pathology
New York University School of Medicine
New York, New York 10016

†Department of Microbiology
Columbia College of Physicians and Surgeons
New York, New York 10032

BALB/c mice treated with anti-IgD from birth were shown previously to produce excellent primary and secondary IgM and IgG responses to trinitrophenylated-B. abortus injected intravenously.[1] In view of the reduced B-cell content (spleen approx. 8%, lymph node 2%) in such mice, shown previously,[1,2] and because of reports in the literature showing reduced antibody production after intraperitoneal (i.p.) immunization in mice[3] and low IgE production in similarly suppressed rats,[4] it seemed of interest to study IgE antibody production in anti-IgD suppressed mice.

BALB/c mice received three weekly i.p. injections of monoclonal 10-4.22 anti-Ig-5a antibody from birth: 5 μg per injection until 10 days of age, 10 μg between 10 and 20 days, and 50 μg per injection from age of 20 days on. At eight weeks of age anti-IgD treated mice and littermate controls were immunized in such a way to produce IgE and IgG antibodies[5]: 0.2 μg dinitrophenylated ovalbumin and 1 mg $Al(OH)_3$ ip. The mice were bled weekly and they were boosted after three weeks with the same antigen in the same amount i.p. IgE antibody was titrated by passive cutaneous anaphylaxis (PCA) in Sprague-Dawley rats,[6] IgG1 by PCA in mice,[7] IgG2a by PCA in guinea pigs,[7] passive hemolysis was used to detect complement fixing antibodies (IgG and IgM). Hemagglutination without and with 0.1M Mercaptoethanol (ME) was used as an additional estimate of IgM and IgG antibody titers. The results of a typical experiment are shown for IgE (FIGURE 1), for IgG1 (FIGURE 2), and for complement fixing antibodies (FIGURE 3). The sera of three mice in the experimental and five in the control groups were pooled and the mean antibody titers are shown in the figures. It is evident that in mice injected with the monoclonal anti-Ig-5a, no IgE (FIGURE 1) or IgG1 (FIGURE 2) was detectable, whereas in the controls good primary and very good secondary antibody formation of these classes was seen. The titers of complement fixing antibodies were the same in treated and control animals.

In another experiment, the secondary response serum titers of individual mice were determined one week after boosting (TABLE 1). The experimental animals produced little, if any, anti-DNP IgE, IgG1 or IgG2a. Hemagglutination titers for 19S antibody gave similar results to those obtained with passive lysis; both were slightly lower than in control mice. However, 7S hemagglutinating antibody was

*This work was supported by research grants from the National Institutes of Health, U.S.P.H.S.: AI-03075, AI-03076 and AI-14398.

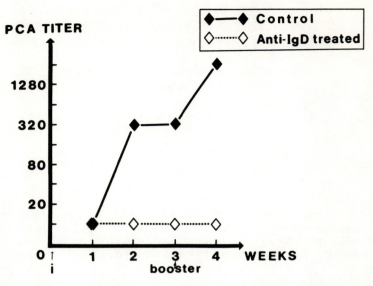

FIGURE 1. Serum IgE anti-DNP titers of anti-IgD treated and control mice. Titers determined on rats challenged with 1 mg DNP-BSA i.v. two hours after intracutaneous injections of serum dilutions.

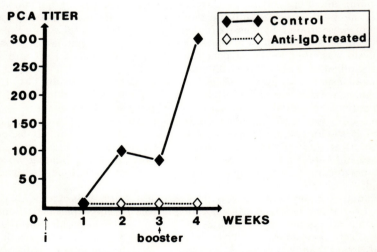

FIGURE 2. Serum IgG1 anti-DNP titers determined on mice challenged with 0.5 mg DNP-mouse albumin 1.5 hours after intracutaneous injection of serum dilutions.

TABLE 1

SECONDARY RESPONSE ONE WEEK AFTER BOOSTER*

Mouse No.	IgE	IgG1	IgG2a	Passive Lysis	Hemagglutination		PCF/Spleen‡	
					Without Me†	With Me	19S	7S
Anti-Ig-5a								
1	10	<10	<10	320	640	<20	$11,482 \times\div 1.23$	$1,479 \times\div 1.45$
2	<10	<10	<10	80	320	<20		
3	80	10	<10	1280	1280	<20		
Control								
4	2560	320	800	2560	2560	1280	$4,365 \times\div 1.29$	$30,902 \times\div 1.10$
5	1280	320	800	1280	2560	2560		
6	2560	320	800	1280	2560	2560		

*Reciprocals of highest serum dilutions of individual mice giving positive test results

†ME = 0.1M mercaptoethanol

‡PFC (geom. mean $\times\div$ SE; n = 3) determined seven days after booster injection. 7S PFC were assayed in the presence of anti-μ in agar and developed by anti-Ig and C.

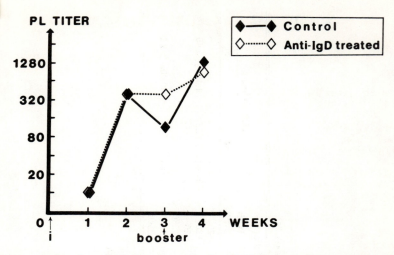

FIGURE 3. Passive hemolysis titers determined on DNP-sheep erythrocytes using guinea pig C.

not detected in the sera of experimental animals, whereas the sera of the control mice contained primarily ME resistant antibody (TABLE 1). It was therefore concluded that the complement fixing antibodies in the sera of suppressed mice were probably also of the IgM and not of the IgG2b class.

The numbers of 19S and 7S (in presence of anti-μ in the agar) plaque forming cells (PFC) was also examined four days after boosting and are shown in the last column of TABLE 1. The 19S PFC response of treated animals was equal to or higher than that in control mice. However, 7S PFC were greatly reduced in the suppressed mice. It was concluded that, with this immunization schedule, IgE and all classes of IgG were suppressed in animals treated from birth with anti-Ig-5a, whereas IgM anti-DNP antibody production was not suppressed.

REFERENCES

1. JACOBSON, E. B., Y. BAINE, Y.-W., CHEN, T. FLOTTE, M. J. O'NEIL, B. PERNIS, G. W. SISKIND, G. J. THORBECKE & P. TONDA. 1981. J. Exp. Med. **154:** 318–332.
2. BAINE, Y., Y.-W., CHEN, E. B. JACOBSON, B. PERNIS, G. W. SISKIND & G. J. THORBECKE. Submitted, J. Immunol.
3. LAYTON, J. E., G. R. JOHNSON, D. W., SCOTT & G. J. V. NOSSAL. 1978. Eur. J. Immunol. **8:** 325–330.
4. BAZIN, H., B. PLATTEAU, A. BECKERS & R. PAUWELS. 1978. J. Immunol. **121:** 2083–2087.
5. ITAYA, T. & Z. OVARY. 1979. J. Exp. Med. **150:** 507–516.
6. OVARY, Z., S. S. CAIAZZA & S. KOJIMA. 1975. Int. Arch. Allergy Appl. Immunol. **48:** 16–21.
7. HIRAYAMA, N., T. HIRANO, G. KOHLER, A. KURATA, O. KO & Z. OVARY. 1982. Proc. Natl. Acad. Sci. **79:** 613–615.

Index of Contributors

(Italicized page numbers refer to comments made during DISCUSSION)